Gasping for Air and Grasping Air in Medicine

Equity, Diversity, and Inclusion on the Medical Frontlines

Edited by

Mariam Abdurrahman, Ana Hategan and Caroline Giroux

Gasping for Air and Grasping Air in Medicine: Equity, Diversity, and Inclusion on the Medical Frontlines

Edited by Mariam Abdurrahman, Ana Hategan and Caroline Giroux

This book first published 2023

Ethics International Press Ltd, UK

British Library Cataloguing in Publication Data

A catalogue record for this book is available from the British Library

Print Book ISBN: 978-1-80441-034-9

eBook ISBN: 978-1-80441-035-6

Dedication

There are still chapters that cannot be read aloud for fear, for shame, for keeping the peace. Yet they sit heavy like an albatross. So heavy, it stifles the breath. This book is dedicated to those unable to tell that story but who know it well, and will someday read it out loud. And for those listening, learning, unlearning and quietly applauding- speak up! And for those hearing and deliberating- please ask. And for those talking loudly from the first space- yield the floor.

Table of Contents

Part 3. Opening Eyes and Opening Minds: Leading with Equity, Diversity and Inclusion

Foreword

Achieving equity, diversity and inclusion is critical in achieving optimal health – both for us as medical professionals as well as for our patients. In recent years, with growing awareness of social justice, this issue has received increasing attention. The more we address this, the more we recognize there remains progress to be made.

We are increasingly recognizing the need to diversify our medical workforce, reduce healthcare disparity and improve patient outcomes. Our patients experience barriers to inclusion, leading to disparities in access and outcome. Providing patient-centered care includes ensuring that care providers understand the unique needs of the patient, which is enhanced when the healthcare professional looks, prays, speaks or loves like them. Research shows that such commonality between the healthcare providers and their patients leads to improved communication, decision-making, adherence with care plans, patient satisfaction and patient outcomes.

The value of diversity in healthcare is also noted by learners, educators, researchers and clinicians. Diverse training environments have been shown to improve learning outcomes, such as empathy, critical thinking, motivation, and comfort and effectiveness in working in diverse communities. Increasing the diversity of researchers in medicine may enhance clinical trial enrollment within underrepresented communities. Healthcare providers could also enjoy a greater quality of life as part of a more diverse workforce. Thus, diversity offers a richness of experience and an opportunity to learn from each other, and can foster a greater sense of identity, appreciation and belonging.

This book is a much-needed resource. *Gasping for Air and Grasping Air in Medicine: Equity, Diversity, and Inclusion on the Medical Frontlines* offers us an opportunity to understand the importance of enhancing equity, diversity and inclusion in medicine. The editors have collaborated with a team of co-authors to share knowledge and expertise collectively in order to comprehensively address the issue. They have added much-needed context to help us fully understand the crucial aspects of medical history that have led to discrimination, trauma and medical mistrust, and to the current gaps in equity, diversity and inclusion in medicine.

Exploring our past will be important in assisting us in dismantling the structural barriers that persist. Each chapter focuses on a specific aspect of structural discrimination, including minorities of race, gender, disability, sexual orientation and gender identity. Expert knowledge about the issues is balanced with practical guidance for reflection, with rich clinical vignettes, opportunities to pause and reflect, glossaries of terms, and summaries of key takeaways.

While this book courageously tackles overt discrimination that must be addressed, it also identifies and discusses more insidious forms of bias that occur. The chapter, Smokescreens: Sanitized Racism through Race Correction, Tolerance and Privilege, hit particularly close to home. Compared to many of my colleagues from a minority background, I had always felt grateful that, as an immigrant, I grew up in a supportive community with no discrimination. While there was no overt racism, I now realize that the racism was sanitized. As the only racialized family in this small community, there were rules and norms that we had to satisfy in order to participate. Being bright and highly capable, we were tolerated, and felt indebted to the community. We strove to fit in and be liked. We gave up our linguistic culture, holidays, dress and food to be more like our new neighbors.

I recall being a young, brown woman in my first year of medical school. The message was very clear: "Be grateful to be here and fit in". As a bright person, I learned this lesson well. I learned to hide my identity so as not to offend anyone. I now recognize that what I thought was generosity was actually tolerance that perpetuates a feeling of being less than, not measuring up, and being othered. Not surprisingly, I have devoted my career in medicine to supporting and uplifting those with less privilege – treating colleagues with burnout and mental illness, advocating for racial and ethnic minorities, and developing women leaders in medicine.

I am truly grateful to the editors for their insights and wisdom. This book serves to inspire us all to be leaders and change-makers, working together towards a future healthcare system that is inclusive of all people.

Mamta Gautam, MD, MBA, FRCPC

Psychiatrist, Expert in Physician Wellbeing and Physician Leadership, University of Ottawa, Canada. CEO, PEAKMD Inc.

Prologue

❖

Sure, there is a problem, but I'm not the problem,
society is the problem, society needs to fix the problem.

❖

The authors and editors of this volume are delighted to share this work on equity, diversity, and inclusion (EDI), issues that are much discussed yet paradoxically also a source of silence, discomfort and sensitivity - the proverbial elephant in the room. The COVID-19 Pandemic has cast a spotlight on long-standing issues of structural discrimination and systematized brands of propagating othering as evident in the highly publicized deaths of unarmed racialized men, the repeat incidents of civilian casualty during police response to mental health calls and the repeat incidents of shocking fatal healthcare outcomes for minorities. These events have triggered mass reckoning, with effects ricocheting through the clinical microcosm, including calls for critical examination of equity, diversity and inclusion in healthcare delivery, and more internally in terms of applying the same core principles amongst our own peers.

In the creed to save lives, clinicians euphemistically aim to deliver a lifesaving breath, yet some of us charged with the very task cannot ourselves "breathe." The issue is magnified given our role in the care of the most vulnerable and the long-standing history of the othering of minority groups in medicine, both staff and patients alike. This book is designed to elicit reflection, facilitate conversation and promote critical dialogue on what remains an uncomfortable issue for many.

Although the formal publication of this book occurs now, its genesis started years before for each contributor. The seeds were likely sown quietly as we each progressed through our journey in medicine, recognized instances of being othered or oppressed, questioned the fact of our legitimacy as physicians when questioned by peers and patients alike whilst also paradoxically inhabiting the cloak of the impostor syndrome, likely in response to the body checking that still occurs too often in the culture of medicine.

Once we decided to commit to this book, the editor team began workshopping proposals with publishers and the experience proved to be both instrumental and reaffirming of the need to increase the dialogue on EDI in medicine. The proposal to publishers was largely met with excitement and interest. Our desire was to create something with a narrative lens that not only drew from contributing authors' experiences as physicians but was also shaped by current events such as those that pushed this book from the ideas stage to the tangible stage. We wished to avoid replicating the contemporary EDI "problem" in medicine, namely, that of sanitizing the discourse and making it palatable by presenting it in the familiar academic language and format. Given that much has been written about EDI with the patient lens and EDI within the realm of academic medicine, our goal was to avoid a purely academic treatise and engage readers in an accessible dialogue with an experiential lens. Presenting it in a different format would essentially stifle the conversation and thus engage us in an inauthentic dialogue about the issue.

Why now and why in this format? Contemporary events have been instrumental in directing attention to seminal EDI issues and health equity. In choosing to utilize pivotal events as a backdrop in examining each EDI topic, we wish to utilize the captive moment to engage readers in further reflection, interprofessional discussion and ultimately a more EDI-informed practice. The rationale for this book also stems in part from our observation of the role of EDI matters in discussions about burnout amongst physicians and more broadly in the healthcare profession.

Many of the authors and editors of this volume had done some work on physician burnout and through some of our discussions recognized a quiet but important theme around equity, bias and burnout. Not surprisingly, burnout and EDI both came up as concurrent issues when potential chapter topics were canvassed, and we discussed the experiential lens to this book. Some of the imagery relayed included that of being stifled, suppressed and relegated to restricted roles because of inbuilt biases within the medical system. Being stifled has the twin effect of limiting our efficacy as patient advocates while also impinging on wellbeing and self-efficacy. Thus, the problem is two-fold: struggling to stay afloat whilst also trying to hold patients afloat with our limited breath.

The growing prevalence of burnout concurrent with increasing recognition of deeply rooted structural bias in the medical field signaled a loud and clear message to us: time is of the essence, act now. The COVID-19 Pandemic has emphasized this message and we are now in crisis as the systematized inequity in clinical care is also mirrored on the physician workforce side. Our motivation in formulating this book is to provide a venue for examining an essential topic that shapes both the process and the outcome of care delivery.

The editors are psychiatrists working in different clinical academic settings in North America. This is perhaps fitting given that historically, psychiatry has had to battle for its legitimacy as a medical specialty. From this origin and the continued experience of being professionally othered, comes a genuine interest in fostering a dialogue about the ways in which diversity, equity and inclusivity constitute determinants of health, resilience and wellness for both healthcare providers and their patients alike.

As female physicians of varying backgrounds, united in a specialty that leans heavily on narrative, the editors have often occupied the voyeur and advocacy seat interchangeably with respect to the impact of systemic bias in shaping opportunity and health outcomes. We have had many a conversation about our roles as agents, silent witnesses and casualties of the status quo in medicine. Nonetheless we recognize our various levels of privilege including the privilege to gather a community of peers on this project. Over the past few years we reflected on the societal biases replicated in medicine, particularly within our ranks as physicians and not just in regard to patient care. We discussed the influence of ethnoracial and socioeconomic bias on the dynamics amongst our healthcare teams and recognized that it was not productive to expect change to start from the top and percolate through the ranks.

While the power structures in medical leadership can orchestrate institutional and cultural changes, the momentum at the frontline level can be even more potent. As we became increasingly uncomfortable with the

EDI "elephant in the room", we contemplated various ways of contributing to the dialogue. The book materialized out of these discussions. We were jolted beyond musings with the occurrence of parallel seminal events in medicine and society, including a series of fatal police encounters with persons in psychiatric crisis, adverse medical outcomes for racialized patients, recurring questions about our debt as colonial settlers, and the indelible impacts of personal events in our journey as physicians charting the COVID-19 Pandemic.

As we continue to liaise with contributing authors, all from various medical specialties, we recognize that the conversation is even more critical and our very survival as an ecosystem depends on taking action on inequity. If the life jackets for the medical workforce are battered, how can we extend intact life jackets to patients and peers?

Mariam Abdurrahman

Toronto ON, Canada

Preface

In this book, we explore the issues associated with equity, diversity and inclusion (EDI), examine the gaps and opportunities for growth, and then we explore the exciting possibilities for inclusion strategies that can help propel forward momentum, including those that are already unfolding.

The book is organized into three parts, with the first section dedicated to introducing the topic and exploring how we got here. The second part is devoted to exploring the issues as they stand today. The third part focuses on exploring the opportunities to lead with an EDI-informed practice and practical considerations of the way forward. The recommendations and reflections may not be practical for every setting, but certainly the intent and the principles remain true as guideposts to gaining momentum towards a more inclusive professional practice. An EDI Lexicon is included to facilitate a mutual understanding starting with a common language. The lexicon is not exhaustive, nor is it static as the EDI conversation is rich with new ideas, new insights and nuances.

Along with each EDI topic explored is a combination of reflective exercises and vignettes. Through the exercises, vignettes, and a closing creative corner, we hope to increase attention to the less salubrious messaging in the silent curriculum of medicine, whilst concurrently improving the recognition of bias, inequity, microaggressions and options to intervene with microaffirmations and allyship.

The "Pause and Reflect" exercises are designed to engage readers in a reflection of their experiences with the issue and facilitate consideration of equity-bridging possibilities. Ideally, the reflective exercises stimulate dialogue with colleagues, peers and learners as many of these topics remain unaddressed or continue to masquerade in plain sight. Continued silence on these palpable issues promotes a form of violence that moderates further oppression in the culture of medicine, particularly the silent curriculum which has powerful reach in the development of physicians' professional identity.

The professional vignettes are vignettes about physician experiences of inequity in the trenches, so to speak. The professional vignette presents an experiential perspective with a view towards stimulating more explicit discussion of the salient points, particularly as they affect our interactions in the medical microcosm and in effect, sort our medical community into echelons that mirror the societal fabric of bias. Although there is growing discussion, there is still a wealth of silence, with many harboring a quiet belief that "other people are biased, not me", "I'm not the problem, it's others who are". The issue of silence is one of structural violence, and violence need not be overt or physical to diminish the soul or obstruct the breath. We use the analogy of breathing as identity differences are as fundamental to life as a vital sign that results in a metaphorical death when oppressed or suppressed.

The clinical (i.e., patient level) vignettes are designed to enhance increased attendance to the fifth Quintuple Aim of healthcare improvement- health equity. In contrast, the professional vignettes and personal reflections are designed to capture the physician experience of EDI issues. The vignettes are designed as patient and professional level vignettes as the two are closely intertwined. For full disclosure, the clinical vignettes contained in this book have been specifically composed for the publication and are not based on real cases. Any similarity to actual clinical cases in the clinical vignettes presented in this volume is purely coincidental. The professional vignettes represent a combination of both personal experiences and composites of professional encounters, current events and historical events that shape the profession.

In summary, without recognition of the EDI issues that chart a patient's course, we cannot truly be effective care providers, nor will we be able to recognize the same equity issues as they affect our colleagues from equity-deprived groups. These colleagues will continue to grasp for air in a profession that prides itself on administering the lifesaving breath. We hope this book remains on bookshelves during medical training, professional medical practice, and beyond.

Mariam Abdurrahman, MD, MSc., University of Toronto

Ana Hategan, MD, McMaster University

Caroline Giroux, MD, University of California, Davis

Contributors

Mariam Abdurrahman, MD, MSc, FRCPC, Assistant Clinical Professor, Department of Psychiatry, University of Toronto Temerty Faculty of Medicine, UHT- St. Joseph's Health Centre, Toronto, ON, Canada

Muri Abdurrahman, MD, FRCPC, Toronto, ON, Canada

Zainab Abdurrahman, MMath, MD, FRCPC, Assistant Clinical Professor (Adjunct), Pediatrics, Faculty of Health Sciences, Michael G. DeGroote School of Medicine, McMaster University, Hamilton, ON, Canada

Sabrina Agnihotri, MD, PhD, Department of Psychiatry, Postgraduate Medical Education, University of Toronto Temerty Faculty of Medicine, Toronto ON, Canada

Olubimpe Ayeni, MD, MPH, FRCSC, FACS, Department of Surgery, Southlake Regional Health Centre, Newmarket, ON, Canada

Shania Bhopa, Ph.D Candidate, Global Health, School of Health Research Methods, Evidence & Impact, Faculty of Health Sciences, McMaster University, Hamilton, ON, Canada

Tara Burra, MD, MSc, FRCPC, Assistant Clinical Professor, Department of Psychiatry, University of Toronto Temerty Faculty of Medicine, Mount Sinai Hospital, Toronto, ON Canada

Mamta Gautam, MD, MBA, FRCPC, Assistant Clinical Professor, Department of Psychiatry, Faculty of Medicine, University of Ottawa, ON, Canada

Caroline Giroux, MD, FRCPC, Clinical Professor, Department of Psychiatry and Behavioral Sciences, UC Davis Health System, Sacramento, CA, USA

Emma Gregory, MD, FRCPC, Clinical Fellow, Geriatric Psychiatry, Department of Psychiatry, University of Toronto Temerty Faculty of Medicine, Toronto ON, Canada

Smrita Grewal, MD, FRCPC, Lecturer, Department of Psychiatry, University of Toronto Temerty Faculty of Medicine, Mount Sinai Hospital. Toronto, ON, Canada

Richard Hae, MD, FRCPC, Clinical Scholar, Division of Nephrology, Department of Medicine, Faculty of Health Sciences, Michael G. DeGroote School of Medicine, McMaster University, St. Joseph's Healthcare Hamilton, Hamilton, ON, Canada

Ana Hategan, MD, FRCPC, Clinical Professor, Department of Psychiatry & Behavioural Neurosciences, Faculty of Health Sciences, Michael G. DeGroote School of Medicine, McMaster University, Hamilton, ON, Canada

Marissa Joseph, MD, MScCH, FRCPC , Department of Medicine, University of Toronto Temerty Faculty of Medicine, Division of Dermatology, Women's College Hospital, Toronto, ON, Canada

Meera Joseph, MD, FRCPC, Assistant Clinical Professor, Division of Nephrology, Department of Medicine, Faculty of Health Sciences, Michael G. DeGroote School of Medicine, McMaster University, Hamilton, ON, Canada

Tara La Rose, MSW, RSW, Ph.D, Associate Professor, School of Social Work, Faculty of Social Sciences, McMaster University, Hamilton, ON, Canada

Chase Everett McMurren, MD, CCFP, Assistant Clinical Professor, Department of Family & Community Medicine, Theme Lead, Indigenous Health, MD Program, Office of Indigenous Health, University of Toronto Temerty Faculty of Medicine, Toronto, ON, Canada

Irina Mihaescu, MD, FRCPC , Clinical Lecturer, Department of Psychiatry, Faculty of Medicine & Dentistry, University of Alberta, Edmonton, AB, Canada

Umberin Najeeb, MD, FCPS (Pak), FRCPC, Associate Clinical Professor of Medicine, Department of Medicine, University of Toronto Temerty

Faculty of Medicine, Toronto ON, Canada. Division of General Internal Medicine, Sunnybrook Health Sciences Centre, Toronto, ON, Canada

Crystal Pinto, MD, FRCPC, Lecturer, Department of Psychiatry, University of Toronto Temerty Faculty of Medicine, UHT- St. Joseph's Health Centre, Toronto, ON, Canada

Noam Raiter, MD, CCFP, Department of Family and Community Medicine, University of Toronto Temerty Faculty of Medicine, Toronto, ON, Canada

Heather Sylvester, MD, CCFP, Stratford Family Health Team, Stratford, ON, Canada

Albina Veltman, MD, FRCPC, Associate Chair, Equity Diversity Inclusion & Indigenous Reconciliation and Associate Clinical Professor, Department of Psychiatry & Behavioural Neurosciences, Faculty of Health Sciences, Michael G. DeGroote School of Medicine, McMaster University, Hamilton, ON, Canada

Part 1.
How Did We Get Here?

Chapter 1
Medicine: Yesterday, Today and the Lingering Shadow of Yesterday

Mariam Abdurrahman, MD, Ana Hategan, MD, Muri Abdurrahman, MD

❖

Hark, who goes there?
Tis I the physic come to balance ye humours.
I bring the leech and the trepan.
What manner of quackery is that?
Away with your chicanery, lest you purloin my soul!
For there is nary a physic to be trusted
—Mariam Abdurrahman, 2023

❖

Abstract: This chapter examines key aspects of medical history that have shaped the practice of medicine today and concurrently explores the historical residue that manifests as contemporaneous equity, diversity and inclusion gaps. Diversity-related demographic changes in the field are examined against their historic origins, with a focus on the presence of women and ethnoracial minorities in medicine. The chapter considers the ways in which history has shaped our view of various populations and the paradoxical persistence of primacy in medicine despite the vow to do no harm and treat all patients equally. The origins of enduring patient distrust of the establishment are examined in order to better understand the relevance in today's social justice discourse.

Keywords: *equity, diversity, history of medicine, inclusion, medical history, medical mistrust*

Introduction

Indeed today's physician has journeyed far from the ancient ways of medicine offered in the days of balancing humours, bloodletting, trepanation and mechano-stimulatory treatments of hysteria. Medicine began its historical journey as an apprenticeship, with practicing physicians teaching the art and science to acolytes. Training was not restricted to the corporeal tract of knowledge as the process also inculcated apprentices in the ways of seeing the world. In the modern era, the formal organization of medical education and training has significantly altered the training process. Nonetheless, despite the modernization of medical education and clinical practice, the ways of past remain a palpable influence to varying degrees today.

It is often said that one cannot move forward without understanding the past and this certainly rings true in medicine. In this context, history is instructive in demonstrating the ways in which culture, institutions, knowledge, society and power intersect to perpetuate primacy and inequity in medicine. Without knowledge of the origins of historical medical artifacts and their influences on today's medical establishment, attempts to gauge current purpose and level of relevance are unlikely to be fruitful. How do we gauge historical cultural residues and sort the good from the bad if we do not even recognize the origins of current perceptions and practices in medicine?

The practice of medicine has been present in various forms since the dawn of time. As the practice of medicine became more formalized as a profession, so too did a uniting creed focused on the principle to do no harm, and in contemporary times, a commitment to provide all patients with the same quality and standard of care. However, the reality is that the clinical climate is not neutral and the culture of science has never been apolitical or color blind. In fact the very concept of medicine and science being color blind and noble is itself a troublesome fallacy that casts a curtain over key accountabilities in social justice. Continued amaurosis detracts from meaningful and sustained action on creating equity-responsive environments in Western medical settings where colonialism and racism constitute systemic issues. The concept of color-blindness and other identity-blindness is also dangerous as it disregards the contextual factors that shape health, thus allowing equity gaps to continue and potentially deepen further.

Science served colonialism primarily by codifying race, with the sequelae continuing to reverberate in academic and clinical spaces (Amster, 2022). The specter of colonialism in medicine is receiving increased attention. However, attempts to decolonize medicine may have paradoxically driven racism "underground, to continue invisibly in medical structures and cause misdiagnosis, poor patient care, dysfunction, abuse and public backlash" (Amster, 2022).

Society and the prevailing culture have always exerted a strong influence on the practice of medicine and healthcare delivery, with seismic contributions from colonialism, genderism and slavery (Amster, 2022; Daffe et al., 2021; Fraser et al., 2021; Jensen and Carmen-Lopez, 2022; Tilley, 2016). The residual effects of imperialism and the history of medical racism are instructive in attempts to dually understand the underrepresentation of physicians from minority groups and the experiences of minoritized physicians in medicine. The literature shows improved access, care experiences and outcomes for minoritized patients who receive care from physicians of similar backgrounds, added to which minority physicians provide a disproportionate share of care to underserved populations (Greenwood et al., 2020; Marrast et al., 2014; Shen et al., 2018). This speaks to the power of diversity in the physician workforce.

The science and practice of medicine are strongly influenced by historical artifacts that shape the role of physicians, the diversity of the medical establishment and the differential treatment that patients of varying backgrounds receive. As such, cultural imperialism is not restricted to society and continues to shape the agenda in clinical practice (Amster, 2022; Tilley, 2016). These influences have shaped medicine today in a variety of key areas, of which the following will be examined: (i) perspectives on diseases and populations, (ii) minority groups in medicine, (iii) the acquisition and dissemination of knowledge, (iv) gender and medicine, and (v) generational shifts and the future of medicine.

Perspectives on Diseases and Populations

Medical evaluation, diagnosis and treatment are strongly affected by the surrounding culture, society and norms of the time. This closely intertwined relationship is exemplified by the evolution of clinical approaches and diagnostic entities over time, with societal biases conspicuously reflected in the classification of gender, sexuality and race, including the practice of race-based correction. Whilst this close dance with society can be positive when society exerts pressure on medicine to adapt to the changing face of society, the converse is also true in that medicine also shapes society to adapt and shift viewpoints about diseases, populations and treatments. However, medicine has not always been successful in attempts to exert pressure on society to reduce the denigration and ostracism of patients and populations that bear the burden of certain conditions.

The history of leprosy, syphilis and HIV/AIDS provide classic examples of medical complicity in devising and perpetuating discrimination. For example, HIV/AIDS was initially classified as a gay-related immunodeficiency (GRID) syndrome by the medical establishment during the early days of the disease (Singer, 1994). In spite of very early indications that HIV/AIDS appeared to be evolving amongst multiple socially disadvantaged groups rather than being a "GRID condition" as it had been characterized, there was reluctance to shed the notion of HIV/AIDS as a "gay disease" (Singer, 1994), largely driven by the subtext of sexuality-based discrimination. In labelling HIV/AIDS a "GRID condition", the wages of sin rhetoric quickly branded men who have sex with men as being an inferior patient group with no expectation of equitable or inclusive access to care. While there has been much growth in the care of people living with HIV/AIDS in Western settings, the specter of stigma and discrimination persist for the non-heteronormative non-cis gender White male as explored in Chapters 5-12.

Historical views on what were then described as the venereal diseases were very much affected by perceptions of excess and wages of sin in non-European races. One only needs to consider the early views of syphilis to understand the ways in which disease is used to demonize non-European races and once more, underscore prevailing beliefs of racial superiority.

The concept of "exotic syphilis" was coined by Bertherand, a French colonial era physician in North Africa in the mid to late 1800s. He devised a theory of Arab hypersexuality causing a form of hereditary syphilis and constitutional differences including underdeveloped brains and primitive nervous systems (Amster, 2016; Amster, 2022). The observations were also seen with the lens of Islam-as-pathology, a medico-social framework that continued to influence scientific inquiry even after Pasteur's contributions to germ theory (Amster, 2016). This spawned a view of syphilitic endemicity and racial inferiority that was widely disseminated globally about non-White races. In fact, the egregious Tuskegee Study was intended to test the theory of "exotic syphilis" and observe the natural course of disease amongst African Americans who were seen as being promiscuous, lacking in moral fibre and inferior to White Americans (Cartwright, 1851; Park, 2017); we explore the Tuskegee Trial in greater detail with the discussion on medical mistrust. The Tuskegee Trial is of particular relevance given its juxtaposition against the Hippocratic oath and its continuation to 1972, well beyond the development of the Nuremberg Code in 1947.

The originating observations that resulted in the theory of "exotic syphilis" were based on a physician's incidental observations of syphilis amongst prostitutes and soldiers while he was in North Africa. There was no systematic examination of disease prevalence before drawing a conclusion of endemicity at "80%" prevalence (Colombani, 1924 as cited in Amster 2016 p. 322). Nonetheless, these flawed observations were retained and perpetuated throughout the medical field globally in an all-too-common pattern that has been replicated throughout the history of medicine. The same sequence of events unfolded within nephrology and respirology, with unsubstantiated observations being used to devise and perpetuate algorithm-based bias through the use of race correction factors.

Algorithm bias is prevalent across the medical field, with varying degrees of recognition and examination of the provenance of the bias. Structural competence applies an understanding of structural inequities and social determinants including race to clinical care (Hansen and Metzl, 2017; Metzl and Hansen, 2014) rather than inaccurate conflations of race with biology as occurs in algorithm bias which inevitably perpetuates medical racism. The Human Genome Project (1990-2003) illustrated that human beings are 99.9% identical genetically, thus reiterating that race has no genetic basis (USDE, 2019). Given that "how we think about disease pathologies affects how we design policies and deliver care to those most affected by social and economic inequities" (Mendenhall, 2017), the role of socio-pathological factors like racism as a determinant of health cannot be underscored enough. Racism shapes health, race does not; so, why does medicine continue to tie race to biology?

The continued conflation of race and biology is highly problematic as the effects of noxious social conditions are reported as racial differences which in effect redirect the focus from investment in structural solutions. Thus, race insidiously became the reason for disease rather than racism, and the perception of a noble apolitical profession has remained uncontested for much of the history of medicine. It is now recognized that upstream social, political, and structural determinants contribute more to health inequities than factors such as biology, race, and personal choices (Willen et al., 2017). The recent discourse on race correction has forced a moment of reckoning upon the profession, raising questions about the relevance of the process and the moral implications of overlooking the role of racism on health equity (Opara et al., 2021). Is race correction just another form of maintaining health inequity?

Although it is recognized that lower forced vital capacity is associated with social conditions, notably poverty, historic observations of reduced respiratory capacity in Black slaves were reported as a *deficit of the pulmonary apparatus* (Cartwright, 1851; Jefferson, 1832) which was then modified into a correction factor that was embedded in the standard spirometry equipment that is in continued use today (Braun et al., 2013; Braun, 2014; Lujan and DiCarlo, 2018). In nephrology, this is seen in the race correction factor applied to estimates of glomerular filtration rates for Blacks. The origin of race correction factors is covered later in this chapter and the concept of race correction is explored in detail in Chapter 11.

Although many advances have been made in germ theory, ethics and the understanding of diseases, the damage done by historical "experiments" and views such as "exotic syphilis" and "the deficit of the pulmonary apparatus" illustrate how medicine can perpetuate racist ideas in pathology, research, conferences, journals, institutions, grants and medical careers (Amster, 2022). Fast forward to modern day, and the residues of racialized medicine and healthcare persist, although "driven underground" into the fabric of medical institutions and the silent medical curriculum, manifesting in misdiagnosis, poor patient care, and disproportionate rates of diseases and deaths amongst various groups (Amster, 2022), as evident with the COVID-19 Pandemic.

The Pandemic had initially been thought to be the great equalizer, but this notion was quickly dispelled as it became evident that older adults and ethnoracial minorities had a significantly increased risk of infection and mortality (Bowleg, 2020; Marmot and Allen, 2020; Sandset, 2021). In fact, the Pandemic precipitated further racial reckoning alongside the publicized deaths of Joyce Eshaquan and George Floyd. Their deaths highlighted systemic racism that was deeply entrenched in medicine, policing and other key infrastructures. The Pandemic revealed health infrastructure predilections for what they are: healthcare for all, modified by the underpinnings of racialized and class-based health disparities and vulnerabilities (Parker and Ferraz, 2021; Sandset, 2021).

The *necropolitics* (Mbembe, 2003) of COVID-19 are such that certain minoritized groups disproportionately bear the brunt of morbidity and mortality (Sandset, 2021). However, the racialized morbidity and mortality rates of the COVID-19 Pandemic are not unique to this disease or the patient realm. While infected patients are gasping for breath, so too are some of their providers. In particular, minoritized healthcare professionals are similarly fighting for breath in the inequitable infrastructure of the Western healthcare system.

The physician workforce does not resemble the diversity seen in the general populations served, particularly in cosmopolitan settings (Boynton-Jarrett et al., 2021; Rodriguez et al., 2015a/2015b). Historically, many were explicitly excluded from medical careers, for example women and racialized minorities. These groups were relegated to the role of patients and unwitting or unwilling research subjects exposed to much structural violence, through which arises a long memory of medical mistrust as subsequently discussed (Alsan et al., 2020; Amster, 2022; Jaiswal and Halkitis, 2019; Shen et al., 2018).

Minority Groups: Immortality, Elephant-like Memories, and Medical Mistrust

The history of medical mistrust is deeply rooted for certain minority groups and serves as an intergenerational memory, underpinning continued racial trauma and medical mistrust (Alsan et al., 2020; Boynton-Jarrett et al., 2021; Breault et al., 2021; Freimuth et al., 2001; Shen et al., 2018; Wasserman et al., 2007). The gaze cast on minorities is shaped by historical valuation of their very humanity, their entitlements as patients and societally imposed limitations on their level of self-actualization. In addition, knowledge of the health differences across ethnoracial groups is still influenced by flawed historic information, liberally laced with the conflation of race and biology which perpetuate continued structural violence (see Chapter 10 and 11).

The dangers of conflating race and biology are profound and wide ranging; in fact, the conflation has historically allowed the pathologization of attempts to fight oppression on the gender and racial front. Samuel Cartwright's work serves as a case in point, as attempts to flee slavery were pathologized as a diagnosis of *drapetomania* while "lazy" slaves were diagnosed with an ailment "peculiar to negroes" termed *dyaesthenia aethiopica*.

Cartwright (1793-1863) was an American physician and a slave owner who observed a 20% difference in spirometry results between Whites and enslaved Blacks; he concluded that this was a racial deficit of Blacks which gave credence to the idea that forced labor was a form of exercise that improved the pulmonary function of slaves (Cartwright, 1851). Prior to this, an American president (Jefferson) had reported similar observations (Jefferson, 1832; Lujan and DiCarlo, 2018). Together, this slavery era work, which was entirely without any scientific rigour, spawned the widespread practice of race-correction in pulmonary function tests (Braun et al., 2013; Braun, 2014; Lujan and DiCarlo, 2018). The prototype for the modern-day spirometer arose from this slavery era work.

Many pulmonary function studies followed Jefferson and Cartwright's work, reporting the same findings in journals and reiterating an observed difference as a racial deficit or dysfunction. These findings were used to promulgate the idea of racial inferiority through medical establishments, medical symposia and journal publications. Thus, racist publications that were accepted as fact gained uptake into normative practices, constituting one of the most egregious ways in which the history of medicine persists in today's practice of medicine. Are budding respirologists taught the origins of the spirometer? Do they understand the racial connotations of the correction factor? Or are they like most, who trust their medical education and would be in disbelief about the 1700's slavery era origins of a correction that persists to current day scientific practice?

The historical spirometry findings form the basis of modern-day spirometry, yet the level of scientific rigour exercised in the index studies would almost certainly fail the mark today. The index studies on which today's spirometers are built do not appear to recognize context, in that there is no acknowledgment that social factors such as poverty and environmental exposures likely play a greater role in pulmonary capacity despite clear evidence that the social determinants of health and biosocial context exert a far greater influence on health status than do race, culture, ethnicity and behavioural factors (Braun et al., 2013; Braun, 2014; Lujan and DiCarlo, 2018; Singer and Clair, 2003; Singer et al., 2017). In the 226 articles included in Braun, Wolfgang and Dickersin's systematic review (2013) of publications comparing lung function between races, 94% of articles published between 1922 and 2008 did not examine race in the context of socioeconomic status.

In addition to the spirometry contributions described above, Cartwright made other contributions that cast a long shadow to present day. He proposed the term, drapetomania, as a diagnostic entity to describe the "disease of the mind" which "induces the negro to run away" (Cartwright, 1851; AMS Press, 1851; Pilgrim, 2005). He believed that escape attempts were a clear manifestation of mental illness as autonomy and freedom were contrary to God's will for slaves. He declared that "the Creator's will in regards to the negro [declares] him to be a submissive knee-bender" and proposed the diagnostic entity, drapetomania, to capture this mental defect of slaves who attempted to escape (Cartwright, 1851). Cartwright expressed concern about a failure of medical attention to mental diseases of slaves, stating "that it should have escaped the attention of the medical profession, can only be accounted for because its attention has not been sufficiently directed to the maladies of the negro race" (Cartwright, 1851). As with any medical condition, signs, symptoms, prevention and treatment were examined, with Cartwright recommending to "whip the devil out" of slaves who displayed warning signs of drapetomania, while other medical authorities endorsed the removal of both big toes to prevent escape (Cartwright, 1851; Pilgrim, 2005).

The disorder of "rascality" (*dysaesthesia aethiopica*) was also proposed with drapetomania and although debunked, its residue persists to present in the form of the rhetoric about the work ethic of Blacks. This likely shaped the societal framework of withheld opportunities on a supposition of a lack of internal drive. The drapetomania paper was published in a reputable medical journal, *The New Orleans Medical and Surgical Journal*, demonstrating yet again how academic publications have historically provided a powerful conduit for the dissemination of racist propaganda under the guise of medicine and science.

Drapetomania has long since been debunked as junk science, however its connotations certainly linger. Although no longer enslaved by shackles, members of the Black, Indigenous and people of color (BIPOC) community are still attempting to flee the modern-day shackles imposed on them by society and exercised on them in institutions such as medicine. The impact of oppression is not restricted to a social experience, but rather permeates through the skin and into biology as explicated in the Minority Stress Model (Flentje, 2020; Meyer, 2003). Social adversity is transmitted biologically and becomes embodied within individuals and populations, which in turn perpetuates further vulnerability to poor health and disease (Singer, 1994). Thus, structural conditions come to be embodied at the biological level and foster further synergistic interactions that drive poor health status and an increased burden of disease (Singer, 1994).

Disease clusters and differences in health status arise from the complex interplay of structural and systemic factors with biology (Abdurrahman et al., 2022; Bulled et al., 2022; Singer et al., 2017). In turning a blind eye to vectors such as systemic bias, we disregard the clear impacts of inequity on health status and thus allow privilege to supersede patient outcomes. In choosing to overlook the structural drapetomania that oppresses our minoritized peers in medicine, we accept the status quo that limits their wellbeing, professional inclusion and self-actualization, which in turn limits the collective strength of our medical establishments.

The health of members of the BIPOC community consistently reflects the impact of structural myopia and inequity. This is further exacerbated by inequitable access to health and social services, misdiagnosis, poorer outcomes, and appropriation of the racialized body for medical use (Amster, 2022; Browne et al., 2016; Fraser et al., 2021; Jensen and Carmen-Lopez, 2022; Nuriddin et al., 2020; Rouse, 2021; Tilley, 2016; USPHS, 2023). There have been recurring instances of bodily appropriation of minorities over the course of the history of medicine to present. These include medical experimentation, the deliberate infliction of disease to cull populations, forced or withheld treatment and the appropriation of biological material without knowledge and/or consent (Alsan and Wanamaker, 2018; Alsan et al., 2020; Park, 2017; Skloot, 2010; Leason, 2021; Nuriddin et al., 2020; Zingel, 2019).

The medical establishment has been complicit in these unethical actions, at times leading the charge, in parallel with the broader racist structures of society that permitted and justified these actions (Wasserman et al., 2007). For example, James Marion Sims, a renowned gynecologist, made most of his discoveries through vicious experimentation on enslaved women in the 19th century (Amster, 2022; Nuriddin et al., 2020). Sims' ethics reflected the prevailing racist social structure of his time, and the fact that he experimented without anaesthesia was unremarkable of his era (Wasserman et al., 2007). Although abhorrent, it is important to note the context in which many of these events occur, rather than judging them solely on present day outlooks as this precludes the learnings gained over time, particularly in medical and research ethics (Wasserman et al., 2007).

One of the most egregious instances of forced treatment occurred with the implementation of early 20th century eugenics laws which overwhelmingly targeted Native American, African American, and Puerto Rican women for involuntary, coercive, and compulsory sterilisation

(Nuriddin et al., 2020). In Canada, the forced sterilization of Indigenous women continued until very recently, with the last of the provincial Sexual Sterilization Acts being repealed in the 1970s (Leason, 2021) although the sterilizations continued beyond the repeal of laws (Zingel, 2019).

In terms of illicit appropriation of biological material, the extraction of Henrietta Lacks' cervical tumour cells stands out in scope. **H**enrietta **La**cks' (HeLa) cells constitute one of the most noteworthy examples of the appropriation of BIPOC bodies given the worldwide scope or *viral spread* of Lacks' cells. Billions of the global population have been touched directly by these cells or indirectly by biotechnology stemming from these cells. The origin of this long-lived lineage of cervical cancer cells originated from a horrific disease that allowed the appropriation of tumour samples from Henrietta Lacks (1920-1951), a Black American woman, without her knowledge or permission. Where other tumour cells died rapidly in the lab at that time, Lacks' cells doubled every 20 to 24 hours (Johns Hopkins Medicine, 2023). Lacks died from cervical cancer within months of diagnosis, at the age of 31.

Although HeLa cells constitute the first immortalized human cell line and one of the most important cell lines in medical research, Henrietta Lacks was never compensated for the use of her cells. In terms of acknowledgment, Johns Hopkins proposed to break ground on a research building to be named after Lacks in 2022 (Johns Hopkins Medicine, 2023). However, HeLa cells have generated immeasurable profit to pharmaceutical corporations, unparalleled research opportunities for many institutions and scientists globally, whilst also advancing innumerable benefits in kind to medicine and society. Research that helped create the polio and COVID-19 vaccines, gene mapping and IVF treatment all relied on HeLa cells (Johns Hopkins, 2023). In addition, HeLa cells are used to study the effects of toxins, drugs, hormones and viruses on the growth of cancer cells without experimenting on humans, to name a few medical and scientific milestones that were made possible by Henrietta Lacks' after life.

Henrietta Lacks legacy lives on full force today, however it is debatable that patients and physicians who derived benefit from HeLa cell research and technology are aware of the origins of these cells. The teaching of medical education and clinical ethics without an exploration of events such as this one is unconscionable and reinforces the view of a salubrious medical and scientific establishment. Similarly, the attempts to decolonize research and shift towards reconciliation are yet to gain traction for Indigenous peoples and racialized groups who have been subject to scientific inquiry that has been of greater benefit to the medical establishment than the subjects.

Without knowledge of historical events and their everlasting residue, one cannot appreciate the scope of potential reasons for medical mistrust by minoritized groups. Without this frame of reference, it is difficult to provide structurally competent care. Furthermore, medical research on minoritized populations will continue to meet cynicism and suspicion about who ultimately benefits and whether the research is in fact a recreation of imperialism: another route of confirming health differences and the "positional superiority ingrained in the psyche of western researchers" (Prior, 2007).

The 1932 to 1972 Tuskegee Study of Untreated Syphilis in the Negro Male (USPHS, 2020) constitutes another milestone of medical distrust that lingers in the present. The Study was conducted by the United States government and constitutes the longest running non-therapeutic study in medicine. Black men were enrolled in the observational study but the cohort who had syphilis were not made aware of their disease nor were they given treatment even after the advent of penicillin, thus facilitating disease progression as well as transmission to the subjects' family members (Alsan and Wanamaker, 2018; Alsan et al., 2020; Park, 2017). The Study was founded on imperial racial ideology about the poor hygiene, increased susceptibility and promiscuity of the Black race (Park, 2017).

Alsan and colleagues (2020) posit mistrust as the peripheral trauma from a specific historical injustice such as those described in this chapter and elsewhere in the book. Although the seeds of medical mistrust were sown before Tuskegee and draw from other events post-Tuskegee, following the Study, a decline was observed in health-seeking behavior concurrent with a rise in mortality and medical mistrust among African-American men who were not enrolled in the Tuskegee Study (Alsan et al., 2020). Recently, it has raised much debate about how much the Study contributes to Black vaccine hesitancy given the low uptake of COVID-19 vaccines.

While the COVID-19 vaccine offers comparatively short-term humoral immunity, the memory of the egregious syphilis trial is ever living. This single but colossal historical failure of a key public health authority will need to be considered by public health authorities attempting to understand and address ongoing vaccine hesitancy by communities already experiencing a disproportionately high incidence of COVID-19 cases. In the absence of this, history becomes the sentry that deters preventive measures such as vaccination, thus exacerbating preexisting health disparities.

The peripheral trauma of the Tuskegee Study is one example of the importance historical knowledge can impart in increasing physicians' structural and cultural competence (Alsan et al., 2020). It is important to also consider other contributory factors in medical mistrust, including vicarious mistrust associated with medical miscarriages, structural trauma and violence against minoritized groups, as well as the misreporting and media sensationalization of distal events (Wasserman et al., 2007).

To overlook history in the present day bodes poorly for advancing the discourse on race and minority relations whether within the medical establishment or beyond. Medical learners entrust their education to the medical establishment and should reasonably expect to receive an honest, well-rounded education if they are to engage in inclusive interactions with their peers and patients alike. Learners who are minorities may face a "minority tax" as they progress into practice. This tax is comprised of an array of additional duties, expectations and challenges that accompany being an exception; it takes the form of expectations to contribute to diversity initiatives by the institution, mentor new minority trainees and recruits, and generally act as diversity champions (Rodriguez et al., 2015b).

In combination with the minority tax, the daily experiences of oppression and discrimination create a burden that drives further inequity and inevitably results in health systems impacts (Esparza et al., 2022; Johnson, 2017; Rodriguez et al., 2015; Xierali et al., 2021). To practice medicine as explicitly taught and implicitly modelled through the silent curriculum is to be complicit in perpetuating the inbuilt inequity in the system. Thus, shifting away from historically embedded biases and moving towards an equity-responsive environment is imperative for health system integrity and sustainability.

Alsan and colleagues (2020) recommend that educating the medical profession on the history of peripheral trauma is an important first step to addressing persistent health disparities whilst further work is concurrently done to increase diversity in medicine and "debias" physicians in practice. Furthermore, re-educating the medical profession is a key responsibility in unlearning biased messages, seeing anew and questioning structural gaps, and in turn inculcating new learners with an equity-responsive mindset. Re-education and unlearning require an examination of the ways of seeing and knowing, thus the next section explores information and knowledge in medicine.

Medical Misinformation: Acquisition and Dissemination of Knowledge in Medicine

Information, whether in its creation, dissemination, scholarship or acclamation, constitutes a key area of inequity in medicine as evidenced by the relative absence or skewed presence of minorities in the academic literature, whether as authors, study participants or gatekeepers (Abdalla et al., 2023; Jensen and Lopez-Carmen, 2022; Ogedegbe, 2020; Rakhra et al., 2021). The historical methods of sharing information in medicine and science include society meetings, symposia, publications and current events media used to varying degrees over the course of time. While there are many avenues to the creation and diffusion of information, publication in leading medical journals has remained critical to knowledge dissemination and career advancement alike (Abdalla et al., 2023).

Abdalla and colleagues (2023) examined two major medical journals (JAMA and NEJM), with JAMA having the highest global circulation and NEJM having the highest impact factor amongst medical journals. They noted some striking trends: it will take more than a century for both journals to reach gender parity at the current rate of increase of female authorship. They also observed that despite attention to structural inequalities in medical academia, authorship by ethnoracial minorities has remained stagnant for the past three decades.

Rakhra et al. (2021) examined medical journal leadership and reported near absence of minorities as editors-in-chief and very low minority representation on journal editorial boards. The stark underrepresentation of minoritized groups in high-impact medical journal authorship and leadership is not unique and has raised robust discussion, with many journals acknowledging and decrying the inequities, whilst endorsing a commitment to redress the balance. Medical journals can play an important role in achieving health equity by diversifying their content, authorship, and leadership (Abdalla et al., 2023; Ogedegbe, 2020; Rakhra et al., 2021).

The issue of visibility is a broadly ranging one, with some under-represented groups describing the issue as one of erasure both in their voices as scholars and as patients. Jensen and Lopez-Carmen (2022) note that Indigenous health professionals must perpetually advocate for visibility in healthcare, with medical students learning little about Indigenous health and cultural practices. Furthermore, they note the relatively tiny Indigenous footprint in the academic literature as studies often exclude Indigenous persons, thus creating a cycle of data inequity and continuing to perpetuate structural racism (Gee et al., 2022; Jensen and Lopez-Carmen, 2022; Morey et al., 2022).

Data inequity is replicated to varying degrees for various racialized groups who concurrently experience both erasure and hyper focus: they are not studied adequately to generate accurate or objective information but at the same time when they are studied, they are often identified by their race and minority identities in a manner that appears to racialize risks and adverse health conditions, effectively continuing to conflate race and biology (Amutah et al., 2021; Deyrup and Graves, 2022; Gee et al., 2022; Morey et al., 2022). The paradox is noteworthy when one considers that despite the extent of discussion about antiracism and decolonization in medicine and science, the voices of the colonized and racialized are relatively quiet (Abdalla et al., 2023; Amster, 2022; Jensen and Lopez-Carmen, 2022; Morey et al., 2022; Tilley, 2016). As such, medical literature constitutes another component in the widely entrenched sources of bias within the medical establishment.

The issue of who is studied, how they are studied and reported, as well as the ethics of the process including participant acknowledgment, are noteworthy sources of enduring medical racism. The HeLa cell line reflects a tale of immortality and paradoxical erasure of the source but for recent outcry. While the scope of Henrietta Lacks' story is unique in its unparalleled global reach, the associated issues of non-consent, exploitation and experimentation on racialized and colonized persons within the medical establishment are not unique.

Rebecca Skloot (2010) publicized Henrietta Lacks' story in her book, The Immortal Life of Henrietta Lacks, with much outcry thereafter about issues of non-consent and exploitation. In its rebuttal statement to Skloot's book and the vigorous publicity that followed its release, Johns Hopkins (2010) issued a statement noting that *"at the time the cells were taken from Mrs. Lacks' tissue, the practice of obtaining informed consent from cell or tissue donors was essentially unknown among academic medical centers. Sixty years ago, there was no established practice of seeking permission to take tissue for scientific research purposes......Johns Hopkins never patented HeLa cells, nor did it sell them commercially or benefit in a direct financial way"*. Although Johns Hopkins did not have direct financial benefit from HeLa cells, certainly many pharmaceutical, research, developmental enterprises have done so with no acknowledgment of the generative source of cells.

The use of the racialized body in research dates back to the early history of medicine and colonialism, with Tilley (2016) noting that "establishing medical services tended to go hand-in-glove with launching research programs on a range of subjects, turning the African continent writ large into a vast arena for experimentation". Smith (1955), a prominent British physician at Oxford University enthusiastically described that "clinical material is unlimited" and the scope of inquiry unfettered in Africa. Smith's view is not unique, with low-income countries being appealing to Western medical researchers seeking more permissive settings. The power inequalities within colonial empires are embedded in the Western medical establishment and continue to nurture primacy in medicine.

While the ownership of racialized bodies may no longer be in overt practice in Western medicine and clinical research, the social factors and systemic conditions that create vulnerability to medical exploitation and experimentation remain prevalent and continue to influence the quality of care received by those who are Black, Indigenous and People of Color

(Amster, 2022; Jensen and Carmen-Lopez, 2022). As Amster (2022) notes, the residue of colonial empires warps healthcare systems in consistent and structural ways as race is the historic basis for resource allocation. Thus, the profession faces the challenge to disentangle race from biology, privilege, power and advancement.

Gender and Medicine: The Evolving Role of Women in Medicine

Gender and medicine yesterday

The history of women in medicine perhaps represents the greatest story of minority advancement, despite the persisting gender equity gap. The history of women and medicine is a complex one for female patients and physicians alike. Historically, women were chattel, overseen by fathers, brothers, husbands and sons. Men were largely in charge of the *fairer sex*, from what they occupied their mind with to what they did with their bodies and how their health needs were addressed (Lippi et al., 2020). Furthermore, the patient space was the chief space women occupied in medicine.

In those early times, the presence of women as healthcare professionals was exclusively in the context of nursing and midwifery. In fact, throughout the 14th to 17th century witch-hunting period, midwifery was the only clinical profession that women were allowed to practice although that field also came to be dominated by men (Achterberg, 1991; Lippi et al., 2020; Wynn, 2000). Women's practice of midwifery is thought to have been permitted because male medical practitioners did not find the lower status of midwifery appealing, particularly as they had the option of the more prestigious obstetrician role (Achterberg, 1991; Jefferson et al., 2015). At the same time women were dying of childbed fever because the gendered establishment could not accept Semmelweiss' findings with respect to hand hygiene (Hellman, 2001).

Whilst male physicians were attending to women in parturition, so too were midwives, however midwives faced an occupational battle to practice in such a way that they were not branded as witches (Lippi et al., 2020). The introduction of the magic instrument, the obstetric forceps, was a game changer in that men took even greater control of the birthing environment-only members of the all-male Barber Surgeon Guild were allowed to use these surgical instruments (Jefferson et al., 2015). It would take some time for the forceps to be utilized by women physicians. Similarly, other instruments were developed and applied in a gendered fashion, with male physicians utilizing electromechanical stimulators to treat women with "hysteria".

As women gained a voice and the vote, attempts to fight gender oppression inevitably resulted in pathologization, as outspoken women received asylum committals and forcible medical treatment, suffragettes were force-fed or incarcerated, and generally the troubled and troublesome were institutionally hidden (Coleborne, 2012; Lippi et al., 2020; National Archives, 2011; Williams, 2008; Wynn, 2000).

Fast forward to modern day medicine and we continue to see the residue of a gendered experience of care for females, including the under-recognition and delayed diagnosis of acute coronary syndromes, under-diagnosis of ischemic heart disease, the differential recognition of attention deficit hyperactivity disorder, and the relative differences both in the care experiences and treatment outcomes for female patients treated by female physicians versus those treated by male physicians (Baumhäkel et al., 2009; Berthold et al., 2008; Healy, 1991; Jefferson et al., 2013; Tsugawa et al., 2017; Vaina et al., 2015;Wallis et al., 2022).

The residue of the history of medicine is very much alive and present in the treatment of female patients and the professional experience of women physicians, both as clinicians and as clinician scientists. The DNA helix controversy perhaps presents the most extreme case of the gendered gaze in medicine and science. Few are aware that Watson, Crick and Wilkins' final discovery of the helical structure of DNA was made on the basis of Rosalind Franklin's work (Hellman, 2001 pp.144-164) and the 1962 Nobel Prize should have in fact been awarded to Franklin (posthumously), Watson, Crick and Wilkins.

❖

"Higher education in women produces monstrous brains and puny bodies, abnormally active cerebration and abnormally weak digestion, flowing thought and constipated bowels."
—Edward H. Clark, 1873 (in Jefferson et al., 2015)

❖

From the gurney to the bedside: women and medicine today

Women have taken the great leap from the gurney to the bedside. However, the bedside experience is yet to be on par with men physicians, with the gendered gap evident across all specialties and tied to an increased risk of burnout for women physicians (Adesoye, 2017; McMurray et al., 2000; Shanafelt, 2022; West et al., 2018).

Over the past number of decades, women have increasingly chosen medicine as their profession in growing numbers. Some have described this trend as a "feminization" of medicine (Steiner-Hofbauer et al., 2022). But what does this mean? For centuries previously, almost all physicians were men and interestingly, there was never discourse about the masculinization or "masculinity" of medicine (Steiner-Hofbauer et al., 2022). In a society with roughly equated gender distribution, it should not be necessary to orchestrate equal participation of women and men in medicine. Rather, it would be expected that the representation from the gender spectrum roughly approximates population proportions and that there is gender representation across the medical specialties (Steiner-Hofbauer et al., 2022).

Women only participate in medicine to the same extent as they are part of the public (Steiner-Hofbauer et al., 2022). In the North American context, women comprise 40 to 60% of medical students in Canada and the U.S.A. today. In 2020, women represented 44% of the Canadian physicians (Canadian Institute for Health Information, 2020). Yet, in Canada women make up only about a third (32%) of surgical specialists, while it is already near even (48%) in family medicine (Canadian Institute for Health Information, 2020).

In medical specialties, 41% of physicians are female (Canadian Institute for Health Information, 2020). The biggest representation of female physicians is found in child and adolescent medical specialties (Steiner-Hofbauer et al., 2022). Psychiatry is also a specialty with a growing representation of women. One recent study showed that the growth in the U.S. workforce representation of women psychiatrists between 2009 and 2019 was slightly slower (37.1% to 42.9%) when compared with the increasing representation of female speakers at their annual national meetings (37% to 45%), and this was believed to be due to promoting female representation and career development (Sebbane et al., 2022). Interestingly, this study also showed that female speakers in 2019 were more interested in diversity and health disparity matters as they may have felt more directly concerned.

Women appear to be overrepresented in less lucrative specialties. However, even within specialties, women earn less than men (Steffler et al., 2021). There remains a sizeable pay gap in lower-paying specialties, which are dominated by women, as well as in higher-paying specialties, which are dominated by men. Dossa et al. (2022) showed that female surgeons earn 24% less in hourly wages than male surgeons. They showed that male surgeons made more per hour than women in almost every surgical specialty, including gynecology (Dossa et al., 2022).

Despite the fact that women may work less outside the home for various reasons (e.g., women are still undertaking the majority of unpaid domestic labour), the differences in hours and pay do not line up. In a recent study, female primary care physicians in British Columbia, Canada, earned 36% less than their male counterparts, but worked just about three hours less a week (Cohen and Kiran, 2020). It is disappointing to see that this trend holds true even when both spouses are physicians (Ly et al., 2017).

The evidence that women are not given as many opportunities as men does not appear to have triggered sufficient progress on addressing the gender pay gap problem. Although the number of female physicians is increasing, their salaries are paradoxically decreasing. Many theories have been proposed to explain this phenomenon including the observation that fields that are less prestigious and attractive to men become "opportunities" for women (Steiner-Hofbauer et al., 2022). When a medical field becomes less prestigious and attractive to men, women enter but only close the physician shortage gap (Steiner-Hofbauer et al., 2022); their earnings do not match that earned by men who left the field, nor are they commensurate to the earnings of men who remain in the specialty.

Addressing gender bias and equity in medicine is just and necessary if we are to foster safer work environment characterized by a greater sense of solidarity and inclusion among physicians. Furthermore, examining the history of women in medicine, both as patients and physicians, is essential to understanding gender relations in medicine today. Looking backwards is critical to moving forward and managing the effects of gender bias on patient care experiences, patient outcomes, professional quality of life for women and gender diverse physicians, and ultimately the sustainability of the physician workforce.

Generational Shifts and the Future of Medicine

Physician shortage is a palpable problem in most settings, with the etiology of the shortage being multifactorial. One factor in the shortage is the socio-cultural phenomenon that unpaid care work is still seen as "women's business". A recent U.S. study showed that during the COVID-19 Pandemic, 24.6% of female physicians were responsible for child care and schooling compared to only 0.8% of male physicians (Frank et al., 2021). In some Scandinavian nations, parental leave is shared equally between parents (Lidbeck et al., 2021). The engagement of both parents in raising young children needs to be recognized as changes in gender norms evolve in modern family life (Lidbeck et al., 2021). Discriminatory gender stereotypes are still a predicament and will need to shift in order to better balance the gendered differences in personal and professional workload. An improved balance between professional and personal obligations could facilitate a reduction in burnout risk whilst also improving the opportunity for physicians to achieve fulfillment in their roles as parents and/or caregivers regardless of gender.

The issue of physician shortage is one that is of particular concern in the context of the ageing population, which is mirrored by an ageing physician population, and exacerbated by the COVID-19 Pandemic. The generation of "baby boomer" physicians (born between 1946 and 1964) will retire in the foreseeable future. People of generation X (born between 1965 and 1979) and generation Y (born between 1980 and 1996), followed by generation Z (born between 1997 and 2010) will take over in medicine (Elenga and Krishnaswamy, 2023; Steiner-Hofbauer et al., 2022). Work-life balance and leisure-time is assigned higher value by generation Y and Z (Steiner-Hofbauer et al., 2022). In contrast, the "baby boomers" ethos is one of strong professional identification, granted many were male physicians acting in the assigned gender role of breadwinner.

These shifting demographic trends and personal values of the younger generations entering medicine will gradually force a shift in traditional gender role ascriptions and stereotypes, but the profession cannot afford to passively absorb the shifting trends. With the majority of physicians soon to belong to generations Y and Z, the healthcare employer will need to pivot to meet the generational differences in work identity in order to fill their job vacancies (Steiner-Hofbauer et al., 2022). The structure and operation of the medical workforce will look very different. It will be important to combine quality of care, professional satisfaction, and quality of life in a variety of ways including: (1) use of telemedicine, (2) delegating certain medical tasks to other healthcare professionals such as physician assistants or advanced practice nurses in hospitals and private practices in order to reduce the workload, and (3) allowing time for relaxation and recreation with loved ones, among other changes (Elenga and Krishnaswamy, 2023).

Building an inclusive and diverse medical profession requires that the diverse physician workforce be recognized as valuable contributing members. As such, the focus of the gendered discussion needs to shift from that of the "feminization" of a formerly "masculine" medicine towards "individualization" (Steiner-Hofbauer et al., 2022). The shift to individualization would better capture the underrepresentation of the gender diverse spectrum of physicians and other minority physician identities.

There have been seismic shifts in the historical role of women in medicine, most notably the shift from the gurney to the bedside as attending physicians. Despite the growing representation of women within the medical profession, discrimination and bias, including the "feminization" rhetoric, continues to create barriers to the advancement and livelihood of women physicians. The gendered history of medicine continues to exert its effects today. Thus, the task of gender equity is one that requires careful examination of lingering historical residues on gender valuation and continued concerted effort to shift away from the shadow of yesterday.

Key Takeaways

- The seeds to contemporary equity, diversity and inclusion problems were planted early in the history of medicine.
- Historically, fighting oppression has been pathologized in the guise of medical diagnoses such as drapetomania; medicine has also been a carceral system of sorts used to suppress voices of dissension as exemplified by the suffragette movement.
- The medical profession is strongly influenced by historical artifacts that shape the role of physicians, the diversity of the medical establishment and the differential treatment that patients of varying backgrounds receive.
- Medical mistrust continues to shape health seeking behaviour by racialized groups.
- Medical mistrust can only be understood by examining key historical influences and attempting to account for its intergenerational presence in the exam room.
- Understanding and addressing equity, diversity and inclusion issues in medicine today requires recognition of the shadows cast by yesterday.
- The complex interplay of historical, structural and systemic factors must be taken into account in attempts to shift towards an equity-responsive environment.
- History is instructive in elucidating the intersection of culture, society, institutions, knowledge, and power, and how their intersection perpetuates primacy and inequity.
- Exploring the residues of the past on the present constitutes an enduring responsibility that must be discharged in order to dismantle structural barriers and approach structural competence.

Conclusion

Although this book focuses on equity, diversity and inclusion (EDI) issues in medicine today, the seeds to contemporary problems were planted long ago, in the nascent origins of medicine. In Western societies, the seeds have been watered by intolerance of diversity as societies expanded and reduced in homogeneity. The reaction to diversity has been problematic from a medical standpoint as the ways of knowing are influenced by society and its valuation of who should study and who should be studied, why they are studied and how they are studied. Furthermore, societal valuation has historically shaped access to care and the quality of care provided. This valuation has resulted in some appalling historical events in medicine. However, these same events serve as invaluable fodder for analyzing and learning how such miscarriages were facilitated, what the medical establishment's role was and how that role has since evolved, as this knowledge is critical to navigating how to carry out the four important tasks we face today: accountability, health equity, structural competence and systems sustainability.

Exploring the residues of the past on the present constitutes an enduring responsibility so that we can dismantle structural barriers that chart an inequitable course of patient care and hold back minoritized physicians. To make a concerted shift towards structural competence and structural integrity will thereby shift the medical establishment towards a system that resembles and celebrates the diverse population it serves.

Personal Reflection: On Time and Turbulence in Medicine
by Muri Abdurrahman, MD, FRCPC

My journey in medicine started over 50 years ago. I completed residency training as a pediatrician in Toronto, Canada, in 1973. Thereafter, I taught in various medical schools in Nigeria and the Middle East before returning to Canada where I remained in practice for almost thirty years. Over the course of my career, I held administrative positions, such as chief of pediatrics in different institutions and assistant dean in a medical school. Thus, I had the opportunity of seeing and being in medicine in various capacities and settings.

During this time I saw and experienced instances of the issues raised in Chapter 1. The topic of the chapter says it all: Medicine: Yesterday, Today and the *Lingering Shadows of Yesterday* (italics mine). Recently, advances in medical technology have been so exponential that what was science fiction a decade ago is now a reality. Personalized medicine, for example molecularly targeted treatment, is becoming the norm. In contrast, progress on the psychosocial front has been glacially slow in the context of social justice. The concept of the need for Equity, Diversity, and Inclusion (EDI) in medicine is receiving increasing attention. Unfortunately, there are still physicians and clinical systems that stubbornly cling to the lingering shadow of yesterday: they opine that race underlies ill health, rather than racism, despite strong evidence to the contrary. This stand is still championed by some "experts" and "opinion makers," aided and abetted by some respectable medical journals. Chapter 1 contains evidence that shatters the lingering shadow of yesterday. How else does one justify the continued existence of gendered career advancement, unsubstantiated race correction and under-representative teaching materials that overlook the diversity of the population?

An illustrious African singer, Miriam Makeba, aptly sums up the situation: "The conqueror writes history. They came, they conquered, and they write. You don't expect the people who came to invade us to tell the truth about us."

The EDI revolution has started. We must recognize and acknowledge the existence of the many -isms that plague the profession. We must not be complicit in perpetuating the myths that reinforce oppression in its various guises. The medical school curriculum should be revised to include a balanced history of medicine: the good, the bad, the ugly. At the same time critical thinking must be emphasized at all levels of medical training and practice. We should not tolerate lip service to EDI, and we must avoid tokenism.

Miriam Makeba Quotes [online]. Available from:
https://afrolegends.com/2017/06/16/great-quote-by-miriam-makeba/

References

Abdalla, M., Abdalla, M., Abdalla, S., Saad, M., Jones, D. S., & Podolsky, S. H. (2023). The Under-representation and Stagnation of Female, Black, and Hispanic Authorship in the Journal of the American Medical Association and the New England Journal of Medicine. *Journal of racial and ethnic health disparities*, 10(2), 920–929. https://doi.org/10.1007/s40615-022-01280-z

Abdurrahman, M., Pereira, L.F., Bradley, M.V. (2022). HIV Syndemics. In: Bourgeois, J.A., Cohen, M.A.A., Makurumidze, G. (eds) *HIV Psychiatry*. Springer, Cham. https://doi.org/10.1007/978-3-030-80665-1_14.

Achterberg, J. (1991). *Woman as Healer: A Comprehensive Survey From Prehistoric Times to the Present day*. London: Rider.

Adesoye, T., Mangurian C., Choo E.K. et al. (2017). Perceived discrimination experienced by physician mothers and desired workplace changes: a cross-sectional survey, JAMA Intern Med, 177(7), p1033-6. https://doi.org/10.1001/jamainternmed.2017.1394.

Alsan M, Wanamaker M. (2018). Tuskegee and the Health of Black Men. *Qtrly J of Econ*, 133(1), pp.407–55.

Alsan, M., Wanamaker, M., Hardeman, R.R. (2020). The Tuskegee study of untreated syphilis: a case study in peripheral trauma with implications for health professionals. *J Gen Intern Med*, 35(1), pp.322-325. https://doi: 10.1007/s11606-019-05309-8. Epub 2019 Oct 23.

AMS Press. (1851). Diseases and peculiarities of the negro race by Dr. Cartwright. *De Bow's review* [online]. New Orleans: AMS Press. Available from: https://www.pbs.org/wgbh/aia/part4/4h3106t.html

Amster E. (2016). The syphilitic Arab? A search for civilization in disease etiology, native prostitution, and French colonial medicine. In: Lorcin P, Shepherd T, editors. *French Mediterraneans*. Lincoln, Nebraska: University of Nebraska Press; 320-46.

Amster E. J. (2022). The past, present and future of race and colonialism in medicine. *Canadian Medical Association Journal*, 194(20): E708–E710. https://doi.org/10.1503/cmaj.212103.

Amutah, C., Greenidge, K., Mante, A., Munyikwa, M., Surya, S.L., Higginbotham, E., Jones, D.S., Lavizzo-Mourey, R., Roberts, D., Tsai, J., Aysola, J. (2021). Misrepresenting race - the role of medical schools in propagating physician bias.

N Engl J Med., 384(9), pp.872-878. https://doi: 10.1056/NEJMms2025768. Epub 2021 Jan 6.

Baumhäkel, M., Müller, U., and Böhm, M. (2009). Influence of gender of physicians and patients on guideline-recommended treatment of chronic heart failure in a cross-sectional study. *Eur J Heart Fail,* 11(3), pp. 299–303. https://doi.org/ 10.1093/eurjhf/hfn041.

Berthold, H.K., Gouni-Berthold, I., Bestehorn, K.P. et al. (2008). Physician gender is associated with the quality of type 2 diabetes care. *J Intern Med,* 264(4), pp. 340-50. https://doi.org/10.1111/j.1365-2796.2008.01967.x.

Boynton-Jarrett, R., Raj, A., & Inwards-Breland, D. J. (2021). Structural integrity: Recognizing, measuring, and addressing systemic racism and its health impacts. *EClinicalMedicine, 36,* 100921. https://doi.org/10.1016/j.eclinm.2021.100921.

Bowleg, L. (2020). We're not all in this together: On COVID-19, intersectionality, and structural inequality. *American Journal of Public Health, 110*(7), p. 917. https://doi.org/10.2105/AJPH.2020.305766

Braun L, Wolfgang M, Dickersin K. (2013). Defining race/ethnicity and explaining difference in research studies on lung function. *Eur Respir J,* 41(6), pp. 1362-70. https://doi:10.1183/09031936.00091612. Epub 2012 Aug 9.

Braun L. Breathing Race into the Machine: The Surprising Career of the Spirometer from Plantation to Genetics. (2014). Minneapolis, MN: University of Minnesota Press. https://doi:10.5749/minnesota/9780816683574.001.0001.

Breault, P., Nault, J., Audette, M., Échaquan, S., & Ottawa, J. (2021). Reflections on Indigenous health care: building trust. *Canadian family physician Medecin de famille canadien, 67*(8), pp. 567–568. https://doi.org/10.46747/cfp.6708567.

British Medical Association. (1992). Medicine betrayed: the participation of doctors in human rights abuses. London: Zed Books. p. 65.

Browne, A. J., Varcoe, C., Lavoie, J., Smye, V., Wong, S. T., Krause, M., Tu, D., Godwin, O., Khan, K., & Fridkin, A. (2016). Enhancing health care equity with Indigenous populations: evidence-based strategies from an ethnographic study. *BMC health services research, 16*(1), p. 544. https://doi.org/10.1186/s12913-016-1707-9.

Bulled, N., Singer, M., and Ostrach, B. (2022). Syndemics and intersectionality: A response commentary. *Social science & medicine (1982), 295,* 114743. https://doi.org/10.1016/j.socscimed.2022.114743.

Cartwright S. (1851). Report on the diseases and physical peculiarities of the Negro race. *N Orleans Med Surgical J,* (7), pp. 691-715.

Cartwright, S. A. (1851). "Diseases and Peculiarities of the Negro Race" [online]. DeBow's Review. XI. Available from: https://www.pbs.org/wgbh/aia/part4/4h3106t.html

Cohen, M., & Kiran, T. (2020). Closing the gender pay gap in Canadian medicine. *CMAJ, 192*(35), pp. E1011-E1017. https://doi.org/10.1503/cmaj.200375.

Coleborne C. (2012). Insanity, gender and empire: women living a 'loose kind of life' on the colonial institutional margins, 1870-1910. *Health and history, 14*(1), pp. 77–99. https://doi.org/10.5401/healthhist.14.1.0077.

Daffé, Z. N., Guillaume, Y., & Ivers, L. C. (2021). Anti-racism and anti-colonialism praxis in global health-reflection and action for practitioners in US academic medical centers. *The American journal of tropical medicine and hygiene, 105*(3), pp. 557–560. https://doi.org/10.4269/ajtmh.21-0187.

Deyrup, A., & Graves, J. L., Jr (2022). Racial Biology and Medical Misconceptions. *The New England journal of medicine, 386*(6), 501–503. https://doi.org/10.1056/NEJMp2116224.

Delgado, C., Baweja, M., Crews, D.C., Eneanya, N.D., Gadegbeku, C.A., Inker, L.A., Mendu, M.L., Miller, W.G., Moxey-Mims, MM., Roberts, GV.., St. Peter, W.L., Warfield, C., Powe, N.R. (2021). A unifying approach for GFR estimation: recommendations of the NKF-ASN task force on reassessing the inclusion of race in diagnosing kidney disease. *Journal of the American Society of Nephrology, 32*, pp. 2994–3015.

Dossa, F., Zeltzer, D., Sutradhar, R., Simpson, A.N., & Baxter, N.N. (2022). Sex differences in the pattern of patient referrals to male and female surgeons. *JAMA Surg, 157*(2), pp. 95-103. https://doi:10.1001/jamasurg.2021.5784.

Elenga, N., & Krishnaswamy, G. (2023). A new generation of physicians-The Generation Z. Are you ready to deal with it?. *Frontiers in Public Health, 10*, p. 1015584. https://doi.org/10.3389/fpubh.2022.1015584.

Esparza, C. J., Simon, M., Bath, E., & Ko, M. (2022). Doing the Work-or Not: The Promise and Limitations of Diversity, Equity, and Inclusion in US Medical Schools and Academic Medical Centers. *Frontiers in public health, 10*, 900283. https://doi.org/10.3389/fpubh.2022.900283.

Frank, E., Zhao, Z., Fang, Y., Rotenstein, L. S., Sen, S., & Guille, C. (2021). Experiences of work-family conflict and mental health symptoms by gender among physician parents during the COVID-19 Pandemic. *JAMA network open, 4*(11), e2134315. https://doi.org/10.1001/jamanetworkopen.2021.34315.

Gee, G. C., Morey, B. N., Bacong, A. M., Doan, T. T., & Penaia, C. S. (2022). Considerations of Racism and Data Equity Among Asian Americans, Native Hawaiians, And Pacific Islanders in the Context of COVID-19. *Current epidemiology reports, 9*(2), pp. 77–86. https://doi.org/10.1007/s40471-022-00283-y.

Flentje, A., Heck, N.C., Brennan, J.M. and Meyer, I.H. (2020). The relationship between minority stress and biological outcomes: A systematic review. *Journal of Behavioral Medicine*, [online] 43(5), pp.673–694. https://doi.org/10.1007/s10865-019-00120-6.

Fraser, S. L., Gaulin, D., & Fraser, W. D. (2021). Dissecting systemic racism: policies, practices and epistemologies creating racialized systems of care for Indigenous peoples. *International journal for equity in health, 20*(1), p. 164. https://doi.org/10.1186/s12939-021-01500-8.

Freimuth, V. S., Quinn, S. C., Thomas, S. B., Cole, G., Zook, E., & Duncan, T. (2001). African Americans' views on research and the Tuskegee Syphilis Study. *Social science & medicine (1982), 52*(5), pp. 797–808. https://doi.org/10.1016/s0277-9536(00)00178-7.

Greenwood, B.N., Hardeman, R.R., Huang, L. and Sojourner, A. (2020). Physician–patient racial concordance and disparities in birthing mortality for newborns. *Proceedings of the National Academy of Sciences*, 117(35), pp. 21194-21200. https://doi.org/10.1073/pnas.1913405117.

Hansen, H., & Metzl, J. M. (2017). New medicine for the U.S. health care system: training physicians for structural interventions. *Academic medicine: journal of the Association of American Medical Colleges, 92*(3), pp. 279–281. https://doi.org/10.1097/ACM.0000000000001542.

Healy B. (1991). The Yentl syndrome. *The New England journal of medicine, 325*(4), pp. 274–276. https://doi.org/10.1056/NEJM199107253250408.

Hellman, H. (2001). Great Feuds in Medicine. New York: John Wiley & Sons, Inc.

Hunt S. B. (1855). Dr. Cartwright on "Drapetomania". *Buffalo Medical Journal*, 10(7), pp. 438–442.

Jaiswal, J., and Halkitis, P. N. (2019). Towards a More Inclusive and Dynamic Understanding of Medical Mistrust Informed by Science. *Behavioral medicine (Washington, D.C.)*, 45(2), pp. 79–85. https://doi.org/10.1080/08964289.2019.1619511.

Jefferson T. (1832). Notes on the State of Virginia [online]. Available from: https://www.loc.gov/item/03004902/

Jefferson, L., Bloor, K., Birks, Y. et al. (2013). Effect of physicians' gender on communication and consultation length: a systematic review and meta-analysis. *J Health Serv Res Policy*, 18(4), pp. 242-8. https://doi.org/10.1177/1355819 613486465.

Jefferson, L., Bloor, K., Maynard, A. (2015). Women in medicine: historical perspectives and recent trends. *British Medical Bulletin*, 114(1), pp. 5–15. https://doi.org/10.1093/bmb/ldv007.

Jensen, A., & Lopez-Carmen, V. A. (2022). The "elephants in the room" in U.S. global health: Indigenous nations and white settler colonialism. *PLOS global public health*, 2(7), e0000719. https://doi.org/10.1371/journal.pgph.0000719.

Johns Hopkins Medicine. (2010). A statement from Johns Hopkins Medicine about HeLa cells and their use, February 1, 2010 [online]. Available from: https://www.hopkinsmedicine.org/news/media/releases/a_statement_from_jo hns_hopkins_medicine_about_hela_cells_and_their_use

Johns Hopkins Medicine. (2023). The Legacy of Henrietta Lacks [online]. Available from: https://www.hopkinsmedicine.org/henriettalacks/

Johnson, T. (2017). The minority tax: an unseen plight of diversity in medical education. *IM Diversity* [online]. Available from: https://imdiversity.com/ diversity-news/the-minority-tax-an-unseen-plight-of-diversity-in-medical-education/

Leason J. (2021). Forced and coerced sterilization of Indigenous women: strengths to build upon. *Can Fam Physician*, 67(7), pp. 525-527. https://doi: 10.46747/cfp.6707525.

Lippi, D., Bianucci, R., & Donell, S. (2020). Gender medicine: its historical roots. *Postgraduate medical journal*, 96(1138), 480–486. https://doi.org/10.1136/ postgradmedj-2019-137452.

Lidbeck, M., & Boström, P. K. (2021). "I believe it's important for kids to know they have two parents": Parents' experiences of equally shared parental leave in Sweden. *Journal of Social and Personal Relationships*, 38(1), pp. 413-431. https://doi.org/10.1177/0265407520961841.

Lujan, H.L., DiCarlo, S.E. (2018). Science reflects history as society influences science: brief history of "race," "race correction," and the spirometer. *Adv Physiol Educ*, 42(2), pp. 163-165. https://doi: 10.1152/advan.00196.2017.

Ly, D.P., Seabury, S.A., & Jena, A.B. (2017). Hours worked among US dual physician couples with children, 2000 to 2015. *JAMA Intern Med*, 177(10), pp. 1524-1525. https://doi:10.1001/jamainternmed.2017.3437.

Marmot, M., & Allen, J. (2020). COVID-19: exposing and amplifying inequalities. *Journal of Epidemiology and Community Health*, 74(9), pp. 681–682. https://doi.org/10.1136/jech-2020-214720.

Marrast, L. M., Zallman, L., Woolhandler, S., Bor, D. H., & McCormick, D. (2014). Minority physicians' role in the care of underserved patients: diversifying the physician workforce may be key in addressing health disparities. *JAMA internal medicine*, 174(2), 289–291. https://doi.org/10.1001/jamainternmed.2013.12756.

Mbembe, A. (2003). Necropolitics. *Public Culture*, 15(1), pp.11–40. https://doi.org/10.1215/08992363-15-1-11

McMurray, J. E., Linzer, M., Konrad, T. R., Douglas, J., Shugerman, R., & Nelson, K. (2000). The work lives of women physicians results from the physician work life study. The SGIM Career Satisfaction Study Group. *Journal of general internal medicine*, 15(6), pp. 372–380. https://doi.org/10.1111/j.1525-1497.2000.im9908009.x.

Mendenhall E. (2017). Syndemics: a new path for global health research. *Lancet (London, England)*, 389(10072), 889–891. https://doi.org/10.1016/S0140-6736(17)30602-5.

Metzl, J. M., & Hansen, H. (2014). Structural competency: theorizing a new medical engagement with stigma and inequality. *Social science & medicine (1982)*, 103, pp. 126–133. https://doi.org/10.1016/j.socscimed.2013.06.032.

Meyer, I.H. (2003). Prejudice, social stress, and mental health in lesbian, gay, and bisexual populations: conceptual issues and research evidence. *Psychological Bulletin*, 129(5), pp. 674–697. https://doi.org/10.1037/0033-2909.129.5.674.

Morey, B. N., Chang, R. C., Thomas, K. B., Tulua, , Penaia, C., Tran, V. D., Pierson, N., Greer, J. C., Bydalek, M., & Ponce, N. (2022). No equity without data equity: data reporting gaps for Native Hawaiians and Pacific Islanders as structural racism. *Journal of health politics, policy and law*, 47(2), pp. 159–200. https://doi.org/10.1215/03616878-9517177.

National Archives. (2011). *The Suffragettes: Deeds Not Words* [online] December 8, 2011. Available from: https://cdn.nationalarchives.gov.uk/documents/education/suffragettes.pdf

New Directions. https://newdiscourses.com/tftw-minoritize/

Nuriddin, A., Mooney, G., White, A.I. (2020). Reckoning with histories of medical racism and violence in the USA. *Lancet*. 396(10256), pp. 949-951. https://doi:10.1016/S0140-6736(20)32032-8.

Ogedegbe G. (2020). Responsibility of medical journals in addressing racism in health care. *JAMA network open*, 3(8), e2016531. https://doi.org/10.1001/jamanetworkopen.2020.16531.

Opara, I.N., Riddell-Jones, L., Allen, N. (2021). Modern day drapetomania: calling out scientific racism. J *Gen Intern Med*, 37(1), pp. 225–6. https://doi:10.1007/s11606-021-07163-z.

Pilgrim, D. (2005). Drapetomania [online]. Available from: https://www.ferris.edu/HTMLS/news/jimcrow/question/2005/november.htm

Park J. (2017). Historical origins of the Tuskegee experiment: the dilemma of public health in the United States. *Uisahak*, 26(3):545-578. https://doi:10.13081/kjmh.2017.26.545. PMID: 29311536.

Parker, R., & Ferraz, D. (2021). Politics and pandemics. *Global public health, 16*(8-9), pp. 1131–1140. https://doi.org/10.1080/17441692.2021.1947601.

Prior D. (2007). Decolonising research: a shift toward reconciliation. *Nursing*, 14(2), pp. 162-8. https://doi:10.1111/j.1440-1800.2007.00361.x.

Rabatin, J., Williams, E., Baier Manwell, L., Schwartz, M. D., Brown, R. L., & Linzer, M. (2016). Predictors and outcomes of burnout in primary care physicians. *Journal of primary care & community health*, 7(1), pp. 41–43. https://doi.org/10.1177/2150131915607799.

Rakhra, A., Ogedegbe, G., Williams, O., Onakomaiya, D., & Ovbiagele, B. (2021). Representation of Racial/ Ethnic Minority Individuals in the Leadership of Major Medical Journals. *Journal of health disparities research and practice, 14*(4), pp. 69–81.

Rodriguez, J. E., Campbell, K. M., & Adelson, W. J. (2015a). Poor representation of Blacks, Latinos, and Native Americans in medicine. *Family medicine, 47*(4), 259–263.

Rodríguez, J.E., Campbell, K.M. & Pololi, L.H. (2015b). Addressing disparities in academic medicine: what of the minority tax?. *BMC Med Educ*, 15(6). https://doi.org/10.1186/s12909-015-0290-9.

Rouse C. M. (2021). Necropolitics versus biopolitics: spatialization, white privilege, and visibility during a pandemic. *Cultural anthropology : journal of the Society for Cultural Anthropology, 36*(3), pp. 360–367. https://doi.org/10.14506/ca36.3.03.

Sandset, T. (2021). The necropolitics of COVID-19: race, class and slow death in an ongoing pandemic. *Global Public Health, 16*(8–9), pp. 1411–1423. https://doi.org/10.1080/17441692.2021.1906927

Scanlon, P.D., Shriver, M.D. (2010). "Race correction" in pulmonary-function testing. *N Engl J Med*, 363(4), pp. 385-6. https://doi: 10.1056/NEJMe1005902.

Sebbane, S., Bailly, S., Lambert, W. C., Sanchez, S., Hingray, C., & El-Hage, W. (2022). Representation of women at American Psychiatric Association annual meetings over 10 years (between 2009 and 2019). *PloS one*, 17(1), e0261058. https://doi.org/10.1371/journal.pone.0261058.

Shanafelt, T.D., West, C.P., Sinsky, C. et al. (2022) Changes in burnout and satisfaction with work-life integration in physicians and the general US working population between 2011 and 2020, *Mayo Clin Proc*, 97(3): p.491-506. https://doi.org/10.1016/j.mayocp.2021.11.021.

Shen, M.J., Peterson, E.B., Costas-Muñiz, R., Hernandez, M.H., Jewell, S.T., Matsoukas, K. and Bylund, C.L. (2018). The effects of race and racial concordance on patient-physician communication: a systematic review of the literature. *Journal of Racial and Ethnic Health Disparities*, 5(1), pp.117–140. https://doi.org/10.1007/s40615-017-0350-4.

Singer M. (1994). AIDS and the health crisis of the U.S. urban poor: the perspective of critical medical anthropology. *Soc Sci Med*, 39, pp.931-48.

Singer, M., and Clair, S. (2003). Syndemics and public health: reconceptualizing disease in bio-social context. *Medical anthropology quarterly*, 17(4), pp. 423–441. https://doi.org/10.1525/maq.2003.17.4.423.

Singer, M., Bulled, N., Ostrach, B., & Mendenhall, E. (2017). Syndemics and the biosocial conception of health. *Lancet (London, England)*, 389(10072), pp. 941–950. https://doi.org/10.1016/S0140-6736(17)30003-X.

Skloot R. (2010). The Immortal Life of Henrietta Lacks. New York: Crown Publishers.

Smith H. (1955). Medicine in Africa as I have seen it. *Afr Aff*, 54(214), pp. 28-29.

Steffler, M., Chami, N., Hill, S., et al. (2021). Disparities in physician compensation by gender in Ontario, Canada. *JAMA network open*, 4(9), e2126107. https://doi.org/10.1001/jamanetworkopen.2021.26107.

Steiner-Hofbauer, V., Katz, H.W., Grundnig, J.S., & Holzinger, A. (2023). Female participation or "feminization" of medicine. *Wien Med Wochenschr*, 173, pp. 125-130. https://doi:10.1007/s10354-022-00961-y.

Tilley H. (2016). Medicine, empires, and ethics in colonial Africa. *AMA journal of ethics*, 18(7), 743–753. https://doi.org/10.1001/journalofethics.2016.18.7.mhst1-1607.

Tsugawa, Y., Jena, A.B., Figueroa, J.F. et al. (2017). Comparison of hospital mortality and readmission rates for Medicare patients treated by male vs female physicians. *JAMA Intern Med*, 177(2), pp. 206-13. https://doi.org/10.1001/jamainternmed.2016.7875.

USDE- United States Department of Energy. (2019). Human Genome Project Information [online]. https://web.ornl.gov/sci/techresources/Human_Genome/index.shtml

USPHS- United States Public Health Service. The U.S. Public Health Service Syphilis Study at Tuskegee [online]. Available from: https://www.cdc.gov/tuskegee/timeline.htm

Vaina, S., Milkas, A., Crysohoou, C., & Stefanadis, C. (2015). Coronary artery disease in women: From the yentl syndrome to contemporary treatment. *World journal of cardiology*, 7(1), pp. 10–18. https://doi.org/10.4330/wjc.v7.i1.10.

Vyas DA, Eisenstein LG, Jones DS. (2020). Hidden in plain sight - reconsidering the use of race correction in clinical algorithms. *N Engl J Med*, 383(9), pp. 874-882. https://doi:10.1056/NEJMms2004740. Epub 2020 Jun 17.

Wallis, C.J.D., Jerath, A., Coburn, N. et al. (2022). Association of surgeon-patient sex concordance with postoperative outcomes. *JAMA Surg*, 157(2), pp. 146-56. https://doi.org/10.1001/jamasurg.2021.6339.

Wasserman, J., Flannery, M. A., & Clair, J. M. (2007). Raising the ivory tower: the production of knowledge and distrust of medicine among African Americans. *Journal of medical ethics*, 33(3), pp. 177–180. https://doi.org/10.1136/jme.2006.016329.

West, C. P., Dyrbye, L. N., & Shanafelt, T. D. (2018). Physician burnout: contributors, consequences and solutions. *Journal of internal medicine*, 283(6), pp. 516–529. https://doi.org/10.1111/joim.12752.

Willen, S. S., Knipper, M., Abadía-Barrero, C. E., & Davidovitch, N. (2017). Syndemic vulnerability and the right to health. *Lancet (London, England)*, 389(10072), 964–977. https://doi.org/10.1016/S0140-6736(17)30261-1.

Williams E. A. (2008). Gags, funnels and tubes: forced feeding of the insane and of suffragettes. *Endeavour*, 32(4), pp. 134–140. https://doi.org/10.1016/j.endeavour.2008.09.001.

Wynn, R. (2000). Saints and sinners: women and the practice of medicine throughout the ages. *JAMA*, 283(5), pp. 668-669.

Xierali, I. M., Nivet, M. A., Syed, Z. A., Shakil, A., & Schneider, F. D. (2021). Recent trends in faculty promotion in U.S. medical schools: implications for recruitment, retention, and diversity and inclusion. *Academic medicine : journal of the Association of American Medical Colleges, 96*(10), pp.1441–1448. https://doi.org/10.1097/ACM.0000000000004188.

Zingel A. (2019). Indigenous women come forward with accounts of forced sterilization, says lawyer. *CBC News* Apr 18, 2019 [online]. Available from: https://www.cbc.ca/news/canada/north/forced-sterilization-lawsuit-could-expand-1.5102981

Chapter 2
The Ways of Teaching Medicine:
The Formal Curriculum

Umberin Najeeb, MD, Marissa Joseph, MD

❖

"Education consists mainly of what we have unlearned."
—Mark Twain, 1899

❖

Abstract: This chapter will examine the presence and influence of oppression in the formal medical education curriculum with a view towards the teaching of medicine with an equity, diversity, and inclusion lens. The development and incorporation of anti-racism curricula and innovative pedagogical approaches are essential to enhancing the ways of teaching medicine so that physicians recognize the spectrum of disease pathology across diverse patient groups and can distinguish a normative spectrum of presentations. The lack of diversity and representation in curricular materials and the impact on clinical dexterity are discussed. Through a critical analysis of the status quo, strategies are identified to reshape whom, how, and what we teach in learning spaces.

Keywords: anti-racism, curriculum, diversity, equity, inclusion, injustice, medical education, teaching, innovative pedagogy

Introduction: Lack of Diversity in Medical Education

Canada's first medical school was founded at McGill University in 1829, with subsequent faculties of medicine formed across Canada. The tenets of medical education have evolved greatly since. Sir William Osler (1849-

1919) has been described as the father of modern medicine in North America (National Library of Medicine, undated), credited with shifting towards patient-centred care. Osler established the first residency training program and brought medical students to the patient bedside.

Osler opined in his address, titled "Chauvinism in Medicine", four great features of the guild of medicine: (1) noble ancestry (2) remarkable solidarity (3) progressive character, and (4) singular beneficence (Bryan and Podolsky, 2019; Osler, 1979). The notion of **noble ancestry** deserves critical thought and reflection. Does noble ancestry include individuals with diverse social identities, for example individuals with ethnic, racial, or socioeconomically diverse backgrounds? Who is included in this portrait that Osler paints?

> *"A White, cisgender, apolitical, heteronormative man not living with a disability has long been upheld as the model 'professional,' in line with a system that centres on a series of characteristics that institutionalize whiteness and Westernness as both normal and superior to other ethnic, racial and regional identities and customs."* (Sharda et al., 2021, p. E101)

The Importance of Diversity in Medical Education

North America continues to see an increase in ethno-cultural diversity, with evolving needs of the communities served by healthcare systems. For example, it has been estimated that by 2041, 1 in 4 Canadians will have been born in Asia or Africa. In a similar trend, it is estimated that in 2041, 4 out of 5 Torontonians will be foreign born or born to immigrant parents (Statistics Canada, 2022).

The Indigenous population in North America has historically been underserved and reconciliation requires a paradigm shift to address health inequities. As a result, healthcare providers need to enhance their skillset and develop competencies to provide, as well as teach, how to deliver culturally safe patient-centered care to diverse patient populations. The changing demographics and social identities of learners in both undergraduate and postgraduate settings as well as within the teaching pool have also enhanced diversity in the academic and clinical learning spaces. Recognizing and supporting the diversity of patients, learners and faculty is a critical component in enhancing a sense of inclusiveness and promoting equity within the learning environments, and by extension, within the patient-care environments.

The Issues

Is the History of Medicine Relevant in Medical Education Curricula?

In order to explore this further, one must consider the impact that medicine has on societal notions of race, ethnicity, gender, sexuality and social class. Conversely, it is also imperative to recognize the impact of these factors on an individual's experience within medicine. One must also acknowledge the role of medicine in advocacy for justice, opposition to threats to humanity and harm reduction. Medicine cannot address health injustice in the present, without teaching the injustices of the past as elucidated in Chapter 1. The historical context matters, as does thoughtful analysis of the present in order to identify opportunities for change.

Jones et al. (2015) articulate that history is an essential component of medical knowledge, reasoning and practice. History offers insights about the cause of disease and efficacy of therapeutic interventions. The authors also note the importance of the interplay of medical knowledge and practice amid the social, economic and political context of medicine as this interplay shapes the lens through which patients from minority groups are seen.

A review of the inclusion of the history of medicine in undergraduate medical education in Canada in 2012 found that it was more deeply incorporated in the core curriculum when compared with surveys in 1939, 1968, and 1999, but half of Canada's medical schools did not require it (Fuller and Olszewski, 2013). The incorporation into curricula varies considerably across institutions, and even over time at the same institution. Fuller and Olszewski (2013, p. 207) examined a 70-year span of survey results for all 16 Canadian medical schools and noted that all the schools *"included history of medicine in the core curriculum at some point in their history, before removing it (and sometimes including it again later)"*. Box 2.1 lists some potential benefits of incorporating the history of medicine in the undergraduate medical education curriculum (Fuller and Olszewski, 2013).

Box 2.1 Benefits of Incorporating the History of Medicine in the Core Undergraduate Medical Curriculum (adapted from Fuller and Olszewski, 2013)

- Contextualize medical practice
- Illustrate the uncertainty associated with medical practice: medical knowledge as temporal, fallible and provisional
- Foster an approach shaped by humility and prudence in scholarship

---

It is useful to analyze the potential benefits of including the history of medicine from the postgraduate medical education perspective, utilizing the CanMEDS Framework in the Canadian system, as an example (Figure 2.1) (CanMEDS, 2022; Frank et al., 2015). This framework describes the *"abilities physicians require to effectively meet the health care needs of the people they serve"* (CanMEDS, 2022). These abilities are identified as seven CanMEDS roles and competencies. According to the framework, physicians, as professionals, must *"reflect contemporary society's expectations ... which include ... promotion of the public good ... and values such as ... humility, respect for diversity. In their role as health advocates, they are called to promote the health of the communities they serve"* (Frank et al., 2015). It has been recognized that medical humanities are relevant to the professional sphere of the framework (Jones et al., 2015). Medical students may demonstrate resistance to content they perceive as irrelevant, the proverbial "is it on the exam?" response. Currently, Canadian and U.S. licensing and certification exams do not specifically test knowledge of medical history.

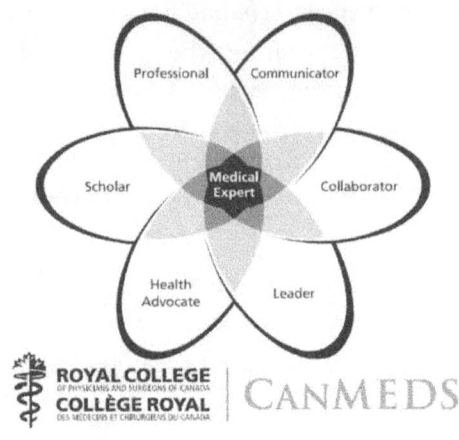

Figure 2.1 *CanMEDS roles (reproduced with permission from the Royal College of Physicians and Surgeons of Canada, Copyright 2015)*

Reviewing the historical context of medicine and engaging in critical analysis of issues beyond pathogenesis of disease and exam findings is essential to providing a well-rounded medical education. Medical expertise in the core competencies (i.e., health advocate, scholar, professional, communicator, collaborator, leader) is needed to address racism and discrimination in the healthcare systems. Enhancing the education of both learners and faculty will facilitate an understanding of the importance of such critical analysis and reflection on the origins of medical culture.

Professional Vignette

A 12-month-old boy of South Asian descent presented to an outpatient pediatric dermatology clinic for evaluation of multiple bluish/black patches over his buttocks, upper thighs and proximal arms. In reviewing the case with the medical student, the supervising faculty member discussed the diagnosis of "dermal melanocytosis". The student exclaimed "aren't these just Mongolian spots? It's easier to remember, why complicate things"? The supervising physician explained the problematic use of such terms because of their origin and the collective responsibility to avoid using them just because they are easier or have been in use for a long time. The student expressed surprise and lack of awareness around the concern in using such terms. The student was given time to explore the term and to further discuss it at the end of the clinic day.

The student presented their findings and a fulsome discussion ensued including:

- *In 1881 Erwin Bälzin coined Mongolian spots after observing blue spots on Japanese babies (Yale et al., 2021). He married a Japanese woman and had two multiracial Asian children of his own. He named these spots "Mongolenfleck", erroneously believing that the appearance was characteristic of Johann Bluembach's "Mongoloid" race (Yale et al., 2021).*

- *In the 1770s, Johann Bluembach had introduced the Western concept of race: Caucasian, Malayan, Ethiopian, Mongolian, and American. He believed that Mongolians were a "degeneration" of the original Caucasian race due to a new natural environment (Westby, 2020).*

The student was reflective and thoughtful, expressing surprise at the term's problematic origin, and regret about not appreciating the importance of its origin.

Key reflections: Teaching the history of problematic terms allows critical reflection. Terms that specifically stigmatize a culture, region, people, country, communities, and ethnic group have **no place in medicine**. They should be replaced by more descriptive terms. We should teach to unlearn and at the same time to relearn and know more. When we know better, we do better.

What is the History of Racism in Medical Culture?

Scholarly analysis of history (including the voices of those violated, not considered, or traumatized by medicine) is required to shift the knowledge, culture, and practice of medicine. A common criticism of applying an EDI lens to historical events in medicine is judging past behaviors with a present-day lens (Westby, 2020). Sir William Osler was purported to:

1) be a proponent of eugenics by his attendance at the first International Eugenics Conference in 1912 (Bryan, 2021) and

2) to have made the statement on May 28th, 1914, *"But we have to safeguard our country. Therefore, we shall be bound to say, 'We are sorry, we would if we could, but you cannot come in on equal terms with Europeans.' We are bound to make our country a White man's country"* (Bryan, 2021, p.195), expressing the pervasive anti-Asian attitudes of White Canadians at the time. Offensive commentary about Latin American, African American and Indigenous peoples have also been attributed to Osler including *"Every primitive tribe retains some vile animal habit not yet eliminated in the upward march of the race"* (Persaud et al., 2020, p. E1415)

In 2019, medical students at McGill University (Osler's alma mater) passed a motion in favour of dropping Osler eponyms due to his treatment of racialized people (Medical Students' Society of McGill University, 2019). Osler is a revered and respected figure in medicine, oft praised for his humanism, and criticisms of his legacy have been challenged, with the argument that his statements were just reflecting the societal sentiments and expectations at the time (Bryan, 2021).

Pause and Reflect

An Exercise in Self-Reflection: Sir William Osler's Legacy

1. What is your immediate reaction to the motion to drop Osler eponyms?
2. What are the critical elements to consider in reflecting on Osler's historic contributions to medical education and modern-day depictions of him?
3. Are similar historical events mitigated by a "present day lens" when applying an EDI viewpoint?

What about Present Day Medicine and Medical Education?

❖

"Wherever the art of medicine is loved, there is also a love of humanity"
— Hippocrates, nd (Stone and Gordon 2013; Wald et al., 2019)

❖

Over the past number of decades, there have been considerable advancements in the science of medicine. The teaching and practice of medicine have also evolved over the course of time. The focus of medical education has largely been on the sciences, however, the art of teaching medicine and practicing patient-centered evidence-based medicine is of utmost importance as well. Providing faculty with a fulsome understanding of concepts such as equity, diversity, and inclusiveness, allyship and advocacy with anti-oppressive practices have an important effect, on both (a) the curricula developed and formally transmitted to learners, and (b) on the medical culture (or "hidden curriculum") that faculty enact with their patients and learners (and thus role model for their learners) (see Chapter 3). Faculty development initiatives to equip teaching faculty with skills and resources to incorporate health inequities and racism into curriculum have been shown to have positive effects: the initiatives enhance faculty members' awareness, attitudes and personal commitments to incorporate anti-oppressive approaches in medical education (White-Davis et al., 2018).

Most medical schools have only recently begun to consider the historical legacy of racial injustice. Racialized students, trainees, and faculty are underrepresented in most medical schools and universities (Ahmad and Shi, 2017; Hess et al., 2020). Many of the traditional criteria for selecting medical students disproportionately disadvantage students of color (Boatright et al., 2017). As a result, there is a growing push to address bias and discriminatory practices in the selection process of medical schools and post graduate training programs. Development of specific Black and Indigenous entry pathways in various Canadian MD programs are examples of initiatives aimed at enhancing diversity and inclusion in medical schools.

Despite the growing push, there are very few residency programs providing specific entry pathways in postgraduate programs for Black and Indigenous learners in Canada. In the University of Toronto Core Internal Medicine Program, the "CaRMS equity group" was created to *embrace the Department of Medicine's strategic commitment of promoting equity and diversity"* and to ensure that the Canadian Resident Matching Service (CaRMS) selection process for under-represented students is fair and equitable (Norris et al., 2022). A specific pathway for Black and Indigenous Canadians into the Core Internal Medicine Residency Program at University of Toronto was developed and implemented in 2019-2020 CaRMS postgraduate matching year; the pathway has continued with enhancements in the subsequent years (Norris et al., 2022). Chapter 4 provides further coverage of under-representation in medical education, training and leadership.

❖

"Prejudice is a burden that confuses the past, threatens the future, and renders the present inaccessible"
—Maya Angelou, 1986

❖

Building Anti-racist and Anti-oppressive Medical Curricula

An increasing number of Canadian medical schools are actively developing and incorporating anti-racist curricula into their teaching framework. However, the medical education curriculum is still yet to adequately prepare physicians to respond to the needs of Indigenous people. There is a need to train physicians to provide quality, non-racist, culturally appropriate care to Indigenous populations (Asiniwasis et al., 2021; Fournier and Smith, 2021; Indigenous Health Writing Group, 2019; Richardson et al., 2021). The Royal College of Physicians and Surgeons of Canada is now asking all Canadian postgraduate residency training programs to include Indigenous health education content in their curricula (Indigenous Health, 2022) and to provide tools and resources to practitioners (Fournier and Smith, 2021; Richardson et al., 2021). For example, the University of Manitoba's Rady Faculty of Health Sciences, has introduced an Indigenous health curriculum with anti-racism content (Sharda et al., 2021).

The University of Toronto Temerty Faculty of Medicine's (UTTFoM) key strategic initiative is *"to make inclusion and equity essential components of how we define and foster excellence in scholarship, practice and health outcomes" and* to *"embed principles of equity and inclusion into curricula and teaching across the*

Faculty to create a safe and healthy learning environment for all" (UTTFoM, 2022). This has led to various curricular innovations, with a few of the examples shared below.

- **Cultural Safety and Anti-oppression:** In 2016, a working group was created to develop a unique curriculum on cultural safety and anti-oppressive practices. The curriculum provides an overview of important concepts like power, privilege, bias, oppression, reflexivity, intersectionality, health equity, social justice, cultural safety, allyship, and advocacy. The working group also provides strategies to learners about approaching structures and processes in healthcare settings with an anti-oppressive lens. The curriculum has continued to evolve and is delivered to date as a lecture and workshop in the University of Toronto Medical Doctorate Program. Both lecture and small group teaching in workshop settings have continued to be highly valued by both learners and teachers (Goel et al., 2018).

- **Religious Discrimination in Medical Education:** A small working group was established to design a novel curriculum and module to define religious discrimination, identify various forms of religious discrimination, and characterize the impact of religious discrimination on medical education and the learning environment. The module provided resources on how to share, disclose, and report experiences of religious discrimination in the learning environment. The inaugural session was delivered in April 2021 in the University of Toronto's MD program and is now delivered annually (Lefkowitz et al., 2021).

- **Learner Mistreatment:** A working group was established to design, implement, and evaluate a workshop to define mistreatment, identify various forms of mistreatment, communicate the impact of mistreatment on the learning environment, and make learners aware of available supports and resources. The workshop highlighted how learners can discuss, disclose, or report witnessed or experienced mistreatment in the learning environment. The inaugural session was delivered in the University of Toronto's MD program in November 2020 and is now delivered annually (Agarwal et al., 2021).

- **Dialogic Teaching:** A pilot working group on person-centered and dialogic teaching initiative was established in the University of Toronto's Department of Medicine in 2018. The group co-created and delivered faculty development sessions on *"ways to prepare for and implement dialogic teaching in clinical settings"*, including *"how to teach faculty about dialogic teaching and learning, concretely implement it in their own practice, and engage more faculty"* (Kuper et al., 2019, p461).

There has been recent uptake of a call to increase the diversity of education and training materials, so that learners are exposed to more representative content that reflects the diverse population they will serve. One such example is the recent concerted effort to increase diversity and inclusion in dermatology educational materials. Dermatology training has historically lacked representation of, and exposure to skin diversity. Disparities in dermatologic care are related, in part, to a lack of training and medical education in the diagnosis of skin disease across different skin tones (Abduelmula et al., 2022; Ebede and Papier, 2006; Kamath et al., 2021). The presentation of skin disease differs across racial/ethnic groups, which may contribute to challenges in timely diagnosis and appropriate management.

- The dermatology curriculum at the University of Toronto Medical Doctorate (MD) Program was examined for the percentage of photographic representation of patients of color. Curriculum analysis revealed less than 7% of photographic images belonged to patients of color. A survey of 10 multiple-choice questions was administered to first- and third-year medical students to assess diagnostic accuracy and self-rated confidence in diagnosis of 5 common skin lesions in white skin and in skin of color. The survey results revealed a lack of confidence among students in diagnosing dermatologic conditions in skin of color. This project in collaboration with the medical students was an important first step in the diversification of dermatology education materials. Subsequently, the number of images with representation across skin types was increased in the dermatology curriculum in the University of Toronto MD program (Bellicoso et al., 2021).

The Opportunity

The basic principles of medical education in a clinical context have not changed. The major cornerstones to formulate a diagnosis require gathering information from a patient or caregiver (history taking), performing a physical examination, requesting further work up if needed (blood work, imaging, etc.) and developing a management plan. We will now discuss potential opportunities with few practical examples to incorporate various inclusive teaching strategies and suggestions on how to put them into practice.

History Taking

i.   An acute myocardial infarction (MI) or heart attack is always at the top of the differential diagnosis list in a patient presenting with acute retrosternal chest pain to the emergency room. However, the clinical presentation of a heart attack differs in men and women. There is a growing body of evidence suggesting that women with MI's do not present like men and women's symptoms may be labeled as anxiety or panic attacks or the diagnosis is missed in its entirety. According to a report published by the Canadian Heart and Stroke Foundation in 2018, early heart attack signs were missed in 74% of women (Heart and Stroke Foundation, 2018). When teaching learners about how to diagnose an acute MI, commenting on the atypical presentation in women, challenges of making this diagnosis in women and acknowledging the gender bias in history taking and diagnostic process can strengthen the learning process. This is itself a window for dialogue about gendered outcomes in acute care encounters.

ii.   While gathering medical information from patients or their family members, healthcare professionals can use inclusive language to role model history taking in a culturally safe manner. In the words of the Elder, Diane Longboat, a question phrased as "are there any practices from your culture or background that will help with your healing right now?" (Richardson et al., 2021) will add specific purpose to the medical history taking process.

iii.   Race and ethnicity have long been scored as independent risk factors for cardiovascular disease, with recent discussion about the biases contained in the risk calculators and treatment decision algorithms (Igoe, 2021; Vyas et al., 2020; Xu et al., 2022). The issues associated with algorithm bias are explored in further detail in Chapter 3. Various research-based scoring systems to ascertain the 10-year risk of cardiovascular disease in order to determine management plans for primary and secondary prophylaxis either do not take race or ethnic background into account or if they do, the concept of race is not representative of the current patient population. Most of the cardiovascular research in North America and the western world was completed with a patient population that was not as diverse as today's population. Lack of inclusive practices in patient recruitment in research studies also contributes to the lack of ethno-racial data. Recently, the American College of Cardiology collaborated with the American Heart Association to innovate the heart disease risk calculator (Prevention Guidelines Tool, 2018) and added inclusive choices from race and ethnicity perspectives. Highlighting the limitations of evidence-based medicine and lack of inclusive patient recruitment practices in various historical ground breaking research works is another way of incorporating equity principles in medical education and the broader clinical setting.

Physical Examination

i.   Assessment of vital signs (pulse, blood pressure, oxygen saturation, and temperature) is an essential start to any physical examination. In the current COVID-19 Pandemic, the assessment of oxygen saturation through pulse oximetry guided physicians in making decisions about admission to hospital and therapeutic choices. In a patient with no known lung disease, an oxygen saturation of less than 92% on room air likely requires an admission to hospital to provide oxygen. Use of dexamethasone therapy is indicated in hospitalized COVID-19 patients who require oxygen and respiratory support (Horby et al., 2021). However, recent research has provided information on how racial and ethnic biases may impact accuracy of pulse oximetry and raised concerns about providing patient-centered care in this context. The *"occult hypoxemia in Asian, Black, and non-Black Hispanic patients with COVID-19 was associated with significantly delayed or unrecognized eligibility for COVID-19 therapies among Black and Hispanic patients"* (Fawzy et al., 2022). Occult hypoxemia is defined as oxygen saturation in arterial blood samples of less than 88% in the setting of concurrent pulse oximetry oxygen saturation of 92-96% (Fawzy et al., 2022). Acknowledging occult hypoxemia when assessing patients with suspected or confirmed COVID-19 infection with learners may help clinicians in making informed patient-centered management plans.

ii. The Fitzpatrick Skin Type is the universally accepted descriptive classification of skin tone used in dermatologic practice. Originally described in 1975, it is based on the propensity of the skin to burn in the sun (Fitzpatrick, 1988). It is now used as a means of describing skin color and ethnicity (Table 2.1). Its conflation with ethnicity is widely criticized, but remains in use due to the lack of a widely accepted alternative (Ware et al., 2020).

Table 2.1 *Fitzpatrick classification of skin tone*

Type I	Light/Pale White - Always Burns, never tans
Type II	White/Fair - Usually burns, tans with difficulty
Type III	Medium White/Olive - Sometimes mild burns, generally tans to olive
Type IV	Olive to Moderate Brown - Rarely burns, tans to moderate brown easily
Type V	Brown to Dark Brown - Very rarely burns, tans very easily
Type VI	Very Dark Brown to Darkest Brown - Never burns, tans easily, deeply pigmented

Source: Fitzpatrick, 1988

For example, Fitzpatrick skin type V could be seen in a patient who is Hispanic, Black, or South Asian and as such is not informative about the patient's background. Skin tone is relevant to the assessment of skin disease because the presentation and incidence of conditions varies across different skin types. Inability to recognize these changes can lead to delay or misdiagnosis of skin disease and disparities in outcomes. As discussed previously, traditionally the patterns and presentation of skin diseases have been taught largely in white skin. Textbooks, atlases and medical literature reveal a lack of representation of patients with non-white skin (Abduelmula, et al., 2022; Bellicoso et al., 2021; Ebede and Papier, 2006; Kamath et al., 2021). This is problematic for clinical competence in the recognition of pathology and normative differences in non-white skin.

Clinical Vignette

A 2.5-month-old Black infant girl presents to the ER with congestion and runny nose. After assessing her respiratory status, the ER physician notes a series of linear hyper-pigmented horizontal lines across the infant's abdomen. The rest of the physical examination is unremarkable. The ER pediatrician asks the accompanying parent about the skin finding and the parent states they have been there since shortly after birth, and they are awaiting a dermatology consultation.

The ER pediatrician consults the suspected child abuse and neglect team, and reports concern for non-accidental injury given the marks. When the team arrives, the accompanying parent is tearful and surprised. They advise that the baby will not be able to go home and will be admitted for evaluation. The parent expresses that they have 2 other children at home and is extremely distressed. The following day, the dermatology consult service diagnoses the infant with *"transient pigmentary lines of the newborn"*, which is a condition mainly seen in babies with skin of color, is unrelated to abuse, and self-resolves between 3-6 months of age (Huang and Moolla, 2019).

Key Reflections: This case highlights how gaps in dermatology teaching, namely skin disease in non-white skin can adversely affect patients with skin of color. If the physicians involved had been aware of this condition that occurs in non-white infants, they may have recognized it and avoided unwarranted disruption and anxiety for the family. The infant would not have been hospitalized unnecessarily, and the potential cultivation of distrust for health care providers may have been avoided in this racialized family.

Diagnosis and Management Plan:

It is human to have bias. Healthcare providers are impacted by the historical and contemporary societal context. However, if they are not aware of their own implicit biases, this can impact their clinical work and may lead to premature diagnostic closure and ineffective management plans for their patients as highlighted in the clinical vignette below.

Clinical Vignette:

BF is a well-educated trained professional who is a hijab-wearing young black woman. She has childhood sickle cell disease. She was brought to the emergency department by her partner due to worsening abdominal pain and agitation for the last 48 hours. Her partner described her as not being herself. She was admitted with a diagnosis of a possible acute pain crisis with known sickle cell disease coupled with concerns about drug seeking behaviour by the on-call team. There was also discussion about a suspicion of possible domestic abuse. The review of the case with physical assessment at the patient's bedside by the staff physician was suggestive of a severe veno-occlusive crisis involving multiple organs. An urgent hematological and systemic workup is completed leading to a diagnosis of a serious medical concern. Immediate effective treatment with adequate pain control is instituted.

The dialogue with the on-call team afterwards provided an opportunity to reflect on how stereotyping and implicit bias can impact clinicians and may lead to premature diagnostic closure.

Key Reflections: There is a history of implicit bias among healthcare providers *"that black people are not as sensitive to pain"* (Meghani et al., 2012; Sabin, 2020) along with a strong perception and bias in our communities and societies that Hijab wearing women are oppressed and in need of saving (Hassouneh, 2017; Khan et al., 2022). These biases need to be acknowledged and addressed.

This case highlighted the importance of incorporating anti-black racism (Sabin, 2020), gendered islamophobia (Khan et al., 2022) and other forms of discrimination *"within existing anti-oppression and transformative learning teaching practices in medical education"* (Khan et al., 2022, p. E748). Furqan et al. (2022) argue that *"the medical community must consider the unique nature of Islamophobia and the ongoing harm that health care interactions may cause for both Muslim-identifying patients and health professionals"* (Furqan et al., 2022, p. E746).

Inclusion Strategies

Teaching Medical Curricula with an EDI Lens

> *"Medical educators see their roles as informative and formative: the transmission of knowledge to learners (to inform) and the placement of learners in settings to develop professional attitudes (to form), so that they become clinically and biomedically competent. However, if the next generation is to lead the reform of the health system so that it delivers health for all, then learners must become "agents of change"— that is, they must undertake **transformative learning**"* (Ambrose et al., 2014, p248)

The concept of transformative education is not new or novel. Transformative learning is not about memorizing and hoarding knowledge. Transformative learning is about transforming learners' educational experiences to enhance the way they understand and appreciate the world around them, their peers, and themselves. This transformation requires *learning* and *unlearning* by harnessing the abilities of the learners to question their own assumptions, perceptions, and biases. Learning and unlearning is often potentiated by having one's assumptions challenged for example, by a specific experience, or a "disorienting dilemma" (Kuper et al., 2019). Principles of transformative learning can be applied to clinical teaching to highlight constructs of equity, diversity, and inclusion (EDI) while delivering patient-centered care. However, in order to undertake transformative learning, we need transformative teachers.

Educational Practices to Promote Transformative Learning

The authors argue that transformative teaching practices need to be adopted to further strengthen the basic principles of clinical teaching. We will now discuss some educational practices associated with promoting transformative education and learning.

i.   **Storytelling:** (Charon, 2000; Charon, 2001)

Stories are *"narratives with a plot that knit events together"* allowing us to understand the deeper significance of an event. Stories are able to articulate and communicate facts as experiences, not as information. Patient's stories can be used to better understand their experiences of illness and care needs. In medical education, stories of patients and their caregivers are being increasingly used to educate healthcare professionals and to engage patients and their families to improve patient care. Organizations like the Institute of Healthcare Improvement (IHI) in the United States and the National Health Services in the United Kingdom are using patient stories to inspire Quality and Safety leaders. The Canadian Patient Safety Institute has a patient and stories webpage (www.patientsafetyinstitute.ca) designed to educate the general public and healthcare providers from a quality improvement perspective.

It is important to highlight that stories and narratives are different from case-based learning. Case Based Learning (CBL) is used to provide the scientific bases of learning about a disease, its manifestations, and skills required to make a diagnosis. Medical educators and teachers are very familiar with discussing patient cases for teaching and education; however, the use of stories and narratives lends a unique and contextual approach to a patient's experience. It is not only about a case of disease X but about a patient who is living with the disease X.

Clinical Vignette

Ms. Jane Doe has had type 1 diabetes for the past 18 years. She is on insulin. She has been admitted to hospital five times with diabetic ketoacidosis (DKA) in the last 11 months. Non-adherence with her medications is responsible for recurrent admissions with DKA.

Ms. Doe is a 25-year-old woman of South American descent. She has no fixed address and is currently living in a shelter. She dropped out of school at age 13 and is unable to read and write. As an adult, she was diagnosed with severe learning disability. This has impacted her employment abilities. She also has diabetic retinopathy with no vision in her left eye. She previously lived with her boyfriend in a rental apartment. Her boyfriend was her primary caregiver – he was paying for her insulin and helping with her injections. Sadly, he passed away a year ago in a road traffic accident. Due to financial difficulties, she was evicted from the apartment and was unable to afford her insulin. In one of her many hospital admissions, the social worker connected her with a compassionate drug plan. However, despite having access to insulin she is unable to inject an exact dose due to her learning disability and poor vision.

Key Reflections:

- It is extremely important to learn about the diagnosis and management of diabetic ketoacidosis.
- It is also common to find non-adherence with insulin as a cause of recurrent hospital admissions.
- The label of non-adherence is easy to place on a patient, however, exploring the details of Ms. Doe's story better accounts for the causes of non-adherence.
- The exploration of the contextual contributors enriches learners' educational experiences from a patient-centered perspective.

The nuances of Jane's story provide learners with a more fulsome understanding of EDI factors on a backdrop of social determinants of health. This holistic patient context is more likely to shape the development of a learner's professional identity into a more humanistic and reflective physician compared to the use of case summaries that are bereft of contextual factors.

> *Narrative medicine represents "clinical practice fortified by narrative competence - the capacity to recognize, absorb, metabolize, interpret, and be moved by stories of illness. It is medicine practiced by someone who knows what to do with stories"* - Rita Charon (Charon, 2001 p.1897; Charon, 2007 p.1265).

ii.   **Dialogic Teaching** (Kumagai and Naidu, 2015; Kumagai et al., 2018 ; Kuper et al., 2019; Woolf, 1985)

In dialogic teaching, the positional differences between pupil and teacher are suspended and instead the interaction takes the form of an egalitarian exchange of ideas that facilitates ongoing discussion and stimulates further critical thinking. Dialogue is an *"authentic exchange of ideas where participants bring their entire selves"* to enhance teaching and education experiences (Kuper et al., 2019). Kumagai and Naidu (2015) describe the differences between dialogue and discussion. Discussion focuses on cognitive processes and expresses one's perspective to arrive at a decision or to share information. A discussion— *"for example, around an inpatient ward team's consideration of the differential diagnosis in a patient—is goal oriented and chiefly cognitive. It appeals to a rational consideration of objective data and tends to preserve traditional differences in privilege, hierarchy, and power"* (Kumagai et al., 2018, p.1779). The teacher leads the discussion and holds the position of authority. In contrast, dialogues are *"experiential and affective, promoting new ways of understanding oneself and the world, new possibilities, and new questions"* (Kumagai and Naidu, 2015 p.284).

Dialogues focus on the subjective and encourage the sharing of authority, expertise, and perspectives between traditional teachers and learners (Kumagai and Naidu, 2015). Such interactions promote "*critical reflection and reflexivity"* (Kumagai and Naidu, 2015 p.283) by creating space for learners to question assumptions, perspectives, power dynamics, and structural inequities in medicine and in society more broadly. Dialogues require trust, respect, and acknowledgment of the power inherent in all interactions. Kuper et al. (2019) describe dialogues as occurring at *"moments of being [. . .] encountered in the presence of suffering and healing, death, and dying—that seem to focus one's perspective in a permanent way"* (Wear et al., 2015, p. 292). Dialogues are ideally prompted by encounters in the clinical environment and are usually done in parallel with discussions of clinical cases, to maintain professional and personal relevance. Dialogues can be used to enable the development of a *"humanistic, social justice orientation by promoting critical consciousness"* (Kumagai and Naidu, 2015; Kuper et al., 2019, p. 461).

Teachers need to identify moments when *dialogue* can happen, by slowing down and paying deliberate attention to specific moments in patient care and to the stories of their patients, peers and learners. Teachers may decide to share their own story too in order to form meaningful connection, to initiate *dialogue,* to improve educational experience and to enhance learning. This strategy of slowing down and paying deliberate attention is described by Wear et al. (2015) as "slow medical education". The perceived challenge or barrier in slowing down from the teachers' perspective is the lack of availability of time. Healthcare and patient care systems are designed to value efficiency, thus slowing down to promote dialogue can be perceived as inefficient. However, this perception of lack of time can be mitigated by identifying teachable moments and deliberately initiating a dialogue about EDI related topics in healthcare settings.

Key Takeaways: The Five A's

- *Acknowledge* the historical racism and discriminatory practices embedded in the foundation of medical education;
- *Appreciate* the evolving needs of the diverse communities we serve as healthcare providers, particularly for patients belonging to equity deprived groups;
- *Affirm* and assert the inalienable rights of pupils, patients, and peers from equity deprived groups;
- *Actively* develop, incorporate, and role model anti-racist curricula and practices in our learning, educational, and clinical spaces;
- *Advocate* to enhance awareness and to be a change maker at a structural level.

Conclusion

Deconstructing the history of medicine facilitates a greater understanding of the shifting paradigms of structural inequity, disease and illness, healthcare systems, and health inequities. In addition, understanding the underlying history that shapes the medical curriculum enables a critical examination of gaps with respect to reshaping medical education with an EDI lens. Historically whom, how, and what was taught in medicine has been steeped in structural racism, which breeds health inequities. In the journey to health equity for all, it is critical to teach with reflection, educate with anti-racist curricula, and maintain structurally safe clinical and learning spaces in order to shift the educational culture of medicine.

On a Parting Note...

My learners, I must acknowledge the inequities that exists in our academic world.

I know that racism and other oppressive behaviors exist in our clinical and learning spaces

I will help you learn and unlearn

As I myself continue to learn and unlearn

I will role model and try to teach anti-racist and anti-oppressive practices,

This I vow.

We are all responsible for changing the world, and together we can steer the change we seek.

U. Najeeb

References

Abduelmula, A., Akuffo-Addo, E., Joseph, M. (2022). The progression of skin color diversity and representation in dermatology textbooks. *J Cutan Med Surg*, 26(5), pp. 523-525.

Agarwal, S., Balakrishnan, A., Bryden, P., Fuller, F., Klein, J., Hamour, A., et al. (2021). "Uncloaking the Hidden Curriculum: Navigating Learner Mistreatment" workshop, University of Toronto, MD program [online]. Available from: https://meded.temertymedicine.utoronto.ca/sites/default/files/inline-files/2021AnnualLearnerExperienceReportFinal.pdf

Ahmad, N. J., & Shi, M. (2017). The Need for Anti-Racism Training in Medical School Curricula. *Academic Medicine: journal of the Association of American Medical Colleges*, 92(8), p. 1073.

Ambrose, A.J., Andaya, J.M., Yamada, S.,& Maskarinec, G.G. (2014). Social justice in medical education: strengths and challenges of a student-driven social justice curriculum. *Hawaii J Med Public Health*. 73(8), pp. 244-50.

American Heart Association. (2018). Prevention Guidelines Tool CV Risk Calculator [online]. Available from: https://static.heart.org/riskcalc/app/index.html#!/baseline-risk

Angelou, M. (1986). *All God's children need traveling shoes*. New York: Vintage Books.

Asiniwasis, R.N., Heck, E., Amir Ali, A., Ogunyemi, B., & Hardin, J. (2021). Atopic dermatitis and skin infections are a poorly documented crisis in Canada's Indigenous pediatric population: It's time to start the conversation. *Pediatr Dermatol*, 38(S2), pp. 188-189.

Bellicoso, E., Quick, S.O., Ayoo, K.O., Beach, R.A., Joseph, M., & Dahlke, E. (2021). Diversity in Dermatology? An Assessment of Undergraduate Medical Education. *Journal of cutaneous medicine and surgery*, 25(4), pp. 409–417.

Boatright, D., Ross, D., O'Connor, P., Moore, E., & Nunez-Smith, M. (2017). Racial Disparities in Medical Student Membership in the Alpha Omega Alpha Honor Society. *JAMA internal medicine*, 177(5), pp. 659–665.

Bryan, C.S., and Podolsky, S.H. (2019). Sir William Osler (1849–1919) — the uses of history and the singular beneficence of medicine. *N Engl J Med*, 381(23), pp. 2194-2196.

Bryan, C.S. (2021). Sir William Osler, eugenics, racism, and the *Komagata Maru* incident. *Proc Bayl Univ Med Cent*. 34(1), pp.194-198.

Canadian Patient Safety Institute. (2023). Patient Stories [online]. Available from: https://www.patientsafetyinstitute.ca/en/toolsResources/Member-Videos-and-Stories/Pages/default.aspx

CanMEDS Better Standards, better physicians, better Care (2022) available at URL https://www.royalcollege.ca/rcsite/canmeds/canmeds-framework-e [assessed 22 Nov 2022].

Charon, R. (2000). Literature and medicine: origins and destinies. *Academic Medicine: journal of the Association of American Medical Colleges, 75*(1), pp. 23–27.

Charon, R. (2001). Narrative Medicine: A Model for Empathy, Reflection, Profession, and Trust. *JAMA.* 286(15), pp. 1897–1902. https://doi.org/10.1001/jama.286.15.1897 .

Charon, R. (2001). Narrative medicine: form, function, and ethics. *Annals of Internal Medicine, 134*(1), pp. 83–87. https://doi.org/10.7326/0003-4819-134-1-200101020-00024.

Charon, R. (2007). What to do with stories: the sciences of narrative medicine. *Canadian Family Physician, Medecin de famille canadien, 53*(8), pp. 1265–1267.

Ebede, T., & Papier, A. (2006). Disparities in dermatology educational resources. *Journal of the American Academy of Dermatology, 55*(4), pp. 687–690.

Fawzy, A., Wu, T. D., Wang, K., Robinson, M. L., Farha, J., Bradke, A., Golden, S. H., Xu, Y., & Garibaldi, B. T. (2022). Racial and Ethnic Discrepancy in Pulse Oximetry and Delayed Identification of Treatment Eligibility Among Patients With COVID-19. *JAMA internal medicine, 182*(7), pp. 730–738. https://doi.org/10.1001/jamainternmed.2022.1906.

Fitzpatrick, T.B. (1988). The validity and practicality of sun-reactive skin types I through VI. *Archives of dermatology, 124*(6), pp. 869–871.

Fournier, C., and Smith, J. (2021). Indigenous Health Content in Postgraduate Medical Education: An Environmental Scan [online]. Available from: https://www.royalcollege.ca/content/dam/documents/about/health-policy/indigenous-health-content-postgraduate-medical-education-an-environmental-scan-e.pdf

Frank, J.R., Snell, L., Sherbino, J., editors. (2015). CanMEDS 2015 Physician Competency Framework. Ottawa: Royal College of Physicians and Surgeons of Canada.

Fuller, J., and Olszewski, M. M. (2013). Medical History in Canadian Undergraduate Medical Education, 1939-2012. *Canadian Bulletin of Medical History*, 30(2), pp. 199–209.

Furqan, Z., Malick, A., Zaheer, J., & Sukhera, J. (2022). Understanding and addressing Islamophobia through trauma-informed care. *Canadian medical association journal* 194(21), pp. E746–E747. https://doi.org/10.1503/cmaj.211298.

Goel, R., Nnorom, O., Kuper, A., Pham, T., McMurren, C., Owen, J., Balakrishna, A., Najeeb, U., and Kucharski, E. (2018). Cultural Safety and Anti-Oppression Lecture and Workshop Week 9 [online]. Available from: https://md.utoronto.ca/sites/default/files/2018-10-18%20Preclerkship%20Curriculum%20in%20Indigenous%20Health.pdf

Hassouneh, D. (2017). Anti-Muslim Racism and Women's Health. *Journal of women's health (2002)*, 26(5), pp. 401–402. https://doi.org/10.1089/jwh.2017.6430.

Heart and Stroke Foundation. *Heart and Stroke 2018 Heart Report: Ms.Understood* [online]. Available from https://heartstrokeprod.azureedge.net/-/media/pdf-files/canada/2018-heart-month/hs_2018-heart-report_en

Hess, L., Palermo, A. G., & Muller, D. (2020). Addressing and Undoing Racism and Bias in the Medical School Learning and Work Environment. *Academic medicine: journal of the Association of American Medical Colleges*, 95(12S Addressing Harmful Bias and Eliminating Discrimination in Health Professions Learning Environments), pp. S44–S50.

https://search.informit.org/doi/10.3316/informit.686664812822062 .

Horby, P., Lim, W. S., Emberson, J. R., Mafham, M., Bell, J. L., Linsell, L., Staplin, N., Brightling, C., Ustianowski, A., Elmahi, E., Prudon, B., Green, C., Felton, T., Chadwick, D., Rege, K., Fegan, C., Chappell, L. C., Faust, S. N., Jaki, T., and Landray, M. J. (2021). Dexamethasone in Hospitalized Patients with Covid-19. *The New England journal of medicine*, 384(8), pp. 693–704. https://doi.org/10.1056/NEJMoa2021436.

Huang, J., and Moolla, A. (2019). Transient pigmentary lines of the newborn. *Consultant*. 2019;59(4), pp. 124-125.

Igoe, K.J. (2021). Algorithmic bias in health care exacerbates social inequities — how to prevent it [online] March 12, 2023. Available from: https://www.hsph.harvard.edu/ecpe/how-to-prevent-algorithmic-bias-in-health-care/

Jones, D. S., Greene, J. A., Duffin, J., & Harley Warner, J. (2015). Making the Case for History in Medical Education: Fig. 1. *Journal of the History of Medicine and Allied Sciences*, 70(4), pp. 623–652.

Kamath, P., Sundaram, N., Morillo-Hernandez, C., Barry, F., & James, A. J. (2021). Visual racism in internet searches and dermatology textbooks. *Journal of the American Academy of Dermatology, 85*(5), pp. 1348–1349.

Khan, S., Eldoma, M., Malick, A., Najeeb, U., & Furqan, Z. (2022). Dismantling gendered Islamophobia in medicine. *Canadian Medical Association journal, 194*(21), pp. E748–E750. https://doi.org/10.1503/cmaj.220445.

Kumagai, A.K., & Naidu, T. (2015). Reflection, dialogue, and the possibilities of space. *Academic medicine: journal of the Association of American Medical Colleges, 90*(3), pp. 283–288. https://doi.org/10.1097/ACM.

Kumagai, A. K., Richardson, L., Khan, S., & Kuper, A. (2018). Dialogues on the Threshold: Dialogical Learning for Humanism and Justice. *Academic medicine: journal of the Association of American Medical Colleges, 93*(12), pp. 1778–1783. https://doi.org/10.1097/acm.0000000000002327.

Kuper, A., Boyd, V. A., Veinot, P., Abdelhalim, T., Bell, M. J., Feilchenfeld, Z., et al. (2019). A Dialogic Approach to Teaching Person-Centered Care in Graduate Medical Education. *Journal of graduate medical education, 11*(4), pp. 460–467. https://doi.org/10.4300/JGME-D-19-00085.1.

Lefkowitz, A., Kuper, A., and Najeeb, U. (2021). "Religious Discrimination in Medical Education" lecture and panel discussion, University of Toronto, MD program [online]. Available from: https://meded.utoronto.ca/medicine/events?id=15677.

Norris, M., Goguen, J., and Najeeb, U. (2022). "Making the CaRMS application more equitable and inclusive for Black and Indigenous applicants" Workshop in the International Conference on Residency Education Oct 29th, 2022, Montreal, Quebec, Canada ICRE 2022: Program Details - The International Conference on Residency Education (royalcollege.ca)

Meghani, S.H., Byun, E., and Gallagher, R.M. (2012). Time to take stock: a meta-analysis and systematic review of analgesic treatment disparities for pain in the United States. *Pain medicine (Malden, Mass.), 13*(2), pp. 150–174. https://doi.org/10.1111/j.1526-4637.2011.01310.x

Montréal: Medical Students' Society of McGill University. (2019). *Motion regarding the eponyms of Sir William Osler — motion relative aux éponymes de Sir William Osler.* Available from: https://mcgillmed.com/old-website/wp-content/uploads/2017/09/Resolution-Book-Fall-GA-2019-1.pdf

National Library of Medicine. "Father of Modern Medicine": The John Hopkins School of Medicine, 1889-1905. Available at: https://profiles.nlm.nih.gov/

spotlight/gf/feature/father-of-modern-medicine-the-johns-hopkins-school-of-medicine-1889-1905

Osler, W. (1979). Chauvinism in medicine. *Pediatrics (Evanston)*, *63*(4), pp. 627–627.

Persaud, N., Butts, H., & Berger, P. (2020). William Osler: saint in a "White man's dominion". *CMAJ*. *192*(45), pp. E1414–E1416.

Richardson, L., Funnell, S, Anderson, M., Little, L., Fréchette, D., Di Gioacchino, L. et al. (2021). Indigenous Health in Specialty Postgraduate Medical Education [online]. Available from: https://www.royalcollege.ca/content/dam/documents/about/health-policy/indigenous-health-in-specialty-pgme-education-guide-e.pdf

Royal College of Physicians and Surgeons of Canada. (2022). Indigenous Health [online]. Available from: https://www.royalcollege.ca/rcsite/health-policy/indigenous-health-e

Sabin, J.A. (2020). Insights: How we Fail Black Patients in Pain [online]. Available from: https://www.aamc.org/news-insights/how-we-fail-black-patients-pain

Sharda, S., Dhara, A., and Alam, F. (2021). Not neutral: reimagining antiracism as a professional competence. *CMAJ*, 193(3), pp. E101-E102

Statistics Canada. (2022). *Canada in 2041: A larger more diverse population with greater differences between regions* [online]. Available from: https://www150.statcan.gc.ca/n1/daily quotidien/220908/dq220908a-eng.htm

Stone, L., & Gordon, J. (2013). A is for aphorism - 'Wherever the art of medicine is loved there is also a love of humanity'. *Australian family physician*, *42*(11), pp. 824–825.

Twain, M. (1999). *The Wit and Wisdom of Mark Twain: A Book of Quotations*. Mineola, NY: Dover Publications, Thrift Editions

University of Toronto, Temerty Faculty of Medicine Academic Strategic Plan [online]. Available from: https://temertymedicine.utoronto.ca/sites/default/files/2018-Academic-Strategic-Plan.pdf

Vyas, D. A., Eisenstein, L. G., Jones, D. S. (2020). Hidden in plain sight - reconsidering the use of race correction in clinical algorithms. *The New England journal of medicine*, *383*(9), pp. 874–882. https://doi.org/10.1056/NEJMms2004740.

Wald, H.S., McFarland, J., and Markovina, I. (2019). Medical humanities in medical education and practice. *Medical teacher*, *41*(5), pp. 492–496. https://doi.org/10.1080/0142159X.2018.1497151

Ware, O.R., Dawson, J.E., Shinohara, M.M., and Taylor, S.C. (2020). Racial limitations of Fitzpatrick skin type. *Cutis, 105*(2), pp. 77–80.

Wear, D., Zarconi, J., Kumagai, A., and Cole-Kelly, K. (2015). Slow medical education. *Academic medicine: journal of the Association of American Medical Colleges, 90*(3), pp. 289–293. https://doi.org/10.1097/ACM.0000000000000581.

Westby, A. (2020). Time to Phase Out Caucasian, University of Minnesota Department of Family Medicine and Community Health [online]. Available from: https://med.umn.edu/familymedicine/news/time-phase-out-caucasian

White-Davis, T., Edgoose, J., Brown Speights, J.S., Fraser, K., Ring, J.M., Guh, J., and Saba, G.W. (2018). Addressing Racism in Medical Education; An Interactive Training Module. *Family medicine, 50*(5), pp. 364–368.

Woolf, V. (1985). A sketch of the past. In: Schulkind J, editor. *Moments of Being 2nd ed.* San Diego, CA: Harcourt Press; pp. 61–159.

Xu, J., Xiao, Y., Wang, W. H., Ning, Y., Shenkman, E. A., Bian, J., & Wang, F. (2022). Algorithmic fairness in computational medicine. *EBioMedicine*, 84, 104250. https://doi.org/10.1016/j.ebiom.2022.104250.

Yale, S., Tekiner, H., & Yale, E. S. (2021). Reimagining the terms Mongolian spot and sign. *Cureus,* 13(12), e20396. https://doi.org/10.7759/cureus.20396.

Chapter 3
The Ways of Teaching Medicine:
Whisperings of the Silent Curriculum

Irina Mihaescu, MD, Caroline Giroux, MD

❖

"Making the hidden visible and the implicit explicit — and positive — can help create a culture reflecting medicine's core values"
—Lehmann et al., 2018

❖

Abstract: The silent curriculum has a significant effect on the culture of medicine, yet it is often overlooked. It consists of unspoken rules that guide attitudes and behaviors among physicians, and constitutes a powerful socialization process that takes place beyond official academic lessons. The chapter examines how this hidden curriculum and unconscious biases within medical education can shape attitudes and behaviors in healthcare professionals, and ultimately influence patient care. It discusses ways to recognize the impacts of the silent curriculum on medical training and practice, and explores strategies for addressing these impacts while creating more open and equitable relationships between providers and patients. Vignettes will be used to facilitate understanding of how the silent curriculum surfaces in clinical practice.

Keywords: *formal curriculum, hidden, inequity, informal, rule, silent curriculum, socialization, third space, wellbeing*

Introduction

The silent curriculum includes "a set of unwritten rules, social and cultural values, expectations and assumptions" (Yazdani et al., 2020), and is arguably more influential than the formal curriculum with regards to the professional identity formation of physicians. While the volume of formal teaching material is extensive, particularly in the age of explosive digital information, Hafferty and colleagues (2015) suggests that the parallel silent curriculum is in fact responsible for most of the material that is learned in medical schools. This may relate to the fact that the silent curriculum spans a range of key facets of professional development and the space extends well beyond that of formal teaching, extending to professional ethics, spiritual issues, social issues, clinical skills and cultural issues (Yazdani et al., 2020). While formal teaching sessions can be decisively altered in response to inaccurate or new information, the everyday spaces in which students learn about acceptable values and behaviour in medical life can be slow to respond (Leong, 2019). In addition, tension can arise due to contradictions between the formal curriculum material and the intangible material promulgated through the silent curriculum.

Given the tensions between the parallel curricula, the medical learning environment can be full of contradictions with unintended consequences (Yazdani et al., 2020). Sometimes these consequences are positive, such as when positively modeled supervisor behaviour is emulated by a trainee. At other times, the consequences can be negative and quite deleterious, including unhealthy competition amongst trainees caused by interrogative teaching styles, working longer hours than is healthy or sustainable, and avoiding certain specialties or places in medicine due to attitudes and beliefs about a particular specialty (Shanafelt and Noseworthy 2016). In these latter instances, the formal curriculum espouses teamwork, advocates for wellness and self-care as professional responsibilities, and makes no distinction between the relative value of specialties, yet the reality is the opposite, thus the hidden messages in the silent curriculum may carry more weight than that which is explicitly taught in "the classroom".

In medical ecosystems, much of these negative consequences are perpetuated through the intermediary of "shame and blame", an outdated organizational strategy that is not effective, nor provides for long-term success (Boehm et al., 2019). The difference between what is intended to be taught, through explicit teaching whether in the classroom, in the textbook, on the exam or in other formal teaching forums, versus what is being emulated, is found in "the third space" of the silent curriculum. The silent curriculum is also used synonymously with the hidden curriculum, to distinguish from the explicitly taught or formal curriculum (see Chapter 2).The third space is the place where we cannot clearly identify one right and one wrong answer (Maniotes, 2005). The concept comes from multi-ethnic households where offspring have difficulties choosing between the two cultures in which they grew up. These offspring may be unsure of where they fit in because they identify with multiple cultural identities. In addition, the identities that they "look" like are not always the identities they most identify with. This intersection of identities is where people let "their real selves show" (Whitchurch, 2008).

The third space in the hidden curriculum consists of all the intermediary beliefs, biases, and attitudes that people unconsciously transmit. In the context of medicine, this can include that doctors are unconsciously thought of as male and nurses as female genders, that people of color are in supportive roles, but not the decision makers and leaders, and that someone who looks young cannot possibly be a doctor and must be a student (Mahood, 2011).

In addition, much of medical education is about fitting in and doing what others have done before in order to be successful. Medicine has historically been a very hierarchical and conservative environment, where conformity is valued and physicians generally maintain silence on witnessed injustices and disagreeable experiences in order to survive an environment that is demanding and stressful. In this setting, physicians may not stop to question concerning messages and observations; instead they absorb the informal ways as they become enculturated in the profession and stop "seeing" the road signs. Medical sociologist Frederic Hafferty (Hafferty and Franks, 1994) gave an example that people grow up knowing there is a posted, formal speed limit and an "informal" speed limit. There is how fast the posted signs say you should drive versus how fast you could drive without getting fined. In this way, Hafferty suggested we grow up knowing that there can be differences between the formal rules and the ways things actually work (American Association of Medical Colleges, 2019).

The socialization forces of medicine are so strong and ritualized that physicians may not consider the hidden messages and influences they have adopted or are transmitting to learners and staff physicians (Gaiser, 2009). The authors contend that the unconscious and conscious desire to fit into the medical ecosystem and appease those of senior rank in the hierarchy becomes one of the main drivers of perpetuated biases on the background of the implicit biases each physician carries. In the most ideal scenario, physicians are not only aware of their own implicit or unconscious biases, they also make a point of meaningfully checking their conduct and practice for the influence of these biases in their interactions with patients and peers of backgrounds relevant to these biases.

According to the Harvard Project Implicit (1998), unconscious bias and cognitive errors are common among physicians and can lead to a variety of diagnostic and relational issues. Cognitive bias is defined as a systematic pattern of deviation from rationality that affects decision making, resulting in inaccurate judgments or conclusions (Beck, 1979). In the medical field, cognitive biases can cause physicians to make incorrect diagnoses due to misinterpreting data or making assumptions about patient behavior. This diagnostic bias (Graff et al., 2022) occurs when physicians jump to conclusions too quickly before gathering all the facts needed for an accurate diagnosis. This could be due to factors like confirmation bias, a form of "cherry-picking," where they look only for evidence that confirms their initial hypothesis while neglecting evidence that contradicts their hypothesis, or anchoring bias, where they rely heavily on one piece of information while disregarding others (Graff et al., 2022), or algorithmic bias that generates biased outcomes through systematic errors along the course of an algorithm (e.g., data collection, model design, analysis, application) (Huang et al., 2022; Igoe, 2021; Xu et al., 2022).

Algorithm bias is particularly relevant in the context of the equity discourse given the fundamental questions that underlie clinical algorithms: what healthcare outcomes are societally important and why? Who should benefit from improved outcomes (Igoe, 2021)? Sources of algorithm bias may begin as early as the design and data collection stage from which prediction rules are built, thus influencing the algorithm at every stage. For example, it is estimated that Caucasians make up roughly 80% of data collected in the field of genomics and genetics, thus algorithms built on this data may result in skewed scores for underrepresented groups as seen with the Framingham Heart Score, which better predicts cardiovascular risks for White patients (Igoe, 2021).

Automation does not eradicate the issue of algorithm bias, thus artificial intelligence is subject to the same biases if sociocultural biases are not accounted for in the design. Obermeyer and colleagues (2019) study provides a case in point. They examined a healthcare risk-prediction algorithm used on more than 200 million people in the United States and identified racial bias; they note that removing bias from the algorithm would more than double the number of Black patients eligible for a program that provides additional care to the highest risk patients. Their study did not name the algorithm or identify its developer but instead focused on illuminating the issue and working with the algorithm developer to recalibrate it. Powers (as cited in Igoe, 2021) notes that "there will probably always be some amount of bias, because the inequities that underpin bias are in society already and influence *who* gets the chance to build algorithms and for *what purpose*". Automation is not devoid of bias. For this reason, precision medicine and the artificial intelligence it rests on need to be cautiously examined at each design stage to avoid perpetuating further inequity (Genevieve et al., 2020; Igoe, 2021; Xu et al., 2022).

When biases manifest on a relational level (i.e., relational biases), it may result in stereotyping patients or colleagues during interpersonal interactions. Relational biases can also lead to poor communication and relationships with patients, families, and other medical professionals. Stereotyping patients based on race, gender, or class could lead to different physicians providing different levels of care for the same patient. Physicians may also favor certain colleagues over others for promotions and recognition, leading to an uneven distribution of rewards and favoritism.

Challenging unconscious biases requires dismantling the status quo around oppression and White privilege (Okun, 2022). To do this, it is critical to look at the ways in which institutionalized racism has shaped healthcare systems in order to begin to undo the harm it has caused. This includes examining the ways in which access to resources is unequally distributed, policies that perpetuate racial inequalities, and cultural competency training for medical providers. It also requires dismantling implicit bias by actively challenging our assumptions and biases. Only through this combination of self-reflection and systemic examination can there be action on equity and a shift towards a more equitable healthcare system.

As noted previously, the silent or hidden curriculum is a set of unspoken rules that guide attitudes and behaviors (Yazdani et al., 2020). It is a powerful socialization process that takes place beyond official academic lessons. Hafferty et al. (2015) describe the hidden curriculum as anything outside of "the formal dimensions of learning". It is like a subtext made of underground narratives, with some of those narratives being counterproductive. The formal curriculum and the hidden curriculum sometimes contradict each other, as the actions or practice do not match the words. A physician may state and project to a person that they are open minded, but then unconsciously go to great lengths to avoid certain types of patients or colleagues (such as transgender, Indigenous, or foreign graduates).

This type of avoidance is not necessarily something to be ashamed of or embarrassed about. It is a natural evolutionary process rooted in tribalism and fear of the "other". It is a survival blueprint where another person's differing mannerisms, ideals, and projections about the world may be threatening to our own. However, it is something physicians need to be aware of in themselves. Physicians should continuously ask themselves when these natural implicit biases are influencing more than just their natural tendency to lean towards survival, and instead impacting a larger professional ecosystem around them (Marcelin et al., 2019). Much of what we think about other people or ourselves is colored by intermediary beliefs and cultural blueprints which may prove to be inaccurate on taking the time to learn more about the "other. In as many differences we can find, we can also discover as much commonality (Graff et al., 2022).

Implicit and explicit biases are often rooted in inexperience with the "foreign" other. This makes it a physician's responsibility to recognize their own implicit biases and the unintended messages they may be projecting on their professional microcosm, so as to then slowly dismantle these projections with curiosity and courage. Often this dismantling begins with a conversation.

Any inquiry into the hidden curriculum starts with understanding the formal and intended curriculum. It also helps to reflect on the null curriculum. The null curriculum is that which is taught through omission and may transmit the message that the topic is not important given its omission (Cahapay, 2021; Hafferty et al., 2015). Thus, the null curriculum can perpetuate inequity through the absence of representative material. This is evident on considering the issue of minority erasure for certain groups in medicine, raising the continued question: how can you count if you are not acknowledged? For example, 2SLGBTQ+ health has historically not been acknowledged in most formal medical curricula, which are largely cisgenderist and heteronormative (Bauer et al., 2009; Butler et al., 2019). This exclusion shapes the professional competency of physicians educated with this null curriculum.

At the clinical training level, the exclusionary null curriculum may be superseded by a silent curriculum that imparts further bias by way of transphobia and homophobia. In this context, the null curriculum of exclusion shapes both the provider and the patient: the physician does not have adequate exposure to develop the skills necessary to provide queer positive care while queer patients continue to experience erasure and the related burden of minority stress. Queer physicians and learners may experience the double tension of recognizing the equity gaps in their education and training while at the same time being complicit in the system.

The null curriculum is also evident in part when we examine the epidemic of physician burnout, physician mental health challenges, and the struggles with perfectionism, imposter syndrome, and otherness in physicians and physician trainees. It is only recently that medical schools and residency training programs began to formally teach about these occupational hazards of the profession. Similarly, physician associations have undertaken the task of burnout and physician wellness relatively recently.

The "compulsive triad" (i.e., doubt, feelings of guilt, and an exaggerated sense of responsibility) of the physician personality and the occupational hazards this can incur (Gabbard, 1985) are increasingly being discussed. This propensity towards compulsiveness leads to worsening of the quality of health of physicians, and thus, the healthcare they provide to patients. The compulsive triad in personality also predisposes physicians to higher rates of suicide and major depressive disorder than the general population (Swensen and Shanafelt, 2020). While medical associations have recently begun to survey the prevalence of physicians' psychological and psychiatric morbidity, curriculum inroads have been slow.

Over time, much of what was initially formalized and codified goes subterranean, becoming unexamined, routinized, and taken for granted. Thus, some aspects of explicit learning can become subconscious over time. This "subterranean" process occurs with both clinical skills and the social aspect of medicine (Hafferty and O'Donnell, 2015). It becomes the foundation for professionalism and accreditation standards for medical learners. It is in this subterranean space that we role model and socialize new trainees into the medical profession.

The Issues

❖

"Every word spoken, every action performed or omitted, every joke, every silence, and every irritation imparts values"
—Mahood, 2011

❖

Adverse Messaging through the Silent Curriculum

The silent curriculum can be a fertile ground for bias and inequity. It escapes the scrutiny of the profession because it is not in full view. According to Kalter (2019), "hidden curriculum messages in medicine abound, including notions like surgery is too hard for women, it's okay to talk down to nonphysician staff, and certain specialties trump others." The hidden curriculum has exerted significant sequelae on practice in that in certain specialties, such as the surgical specialties, historically the silent messaging helped convey the notion that "learning how to do a physical exam is more important than learning how to communicate with patients" (Brooks, 2015). Fortunately, much headway has been made in regard to the primacy of communication in the physician-patient encounter.

With implicit biases come implicit expectations: to sacrifice your own health for a life of service, to ignore cognitive dissonance when the implicit is antithetical to the explicit curriculum, and to make evidence-based medicine the principal dogma (Brooks, 2015). Other expectations include repressing emotional experiences and putting on a stoic face, as medical culture often emphasizes stoicism (Brooks, 2015). It is often in this invisible space that exposure occurs to mistreatment (perceived or otherwise), inequities, scapegoating, profiling, structural violence, and racism (Joseph et al., 2021).

Mistreatment in the learning environment can show up in many ways, especially when considering the informal curriculum on diversity, equity, inclusion, and accessibility. It also tends to breed disparate views about whether such mistreatment is valid or not. A faculty member may see a part of the informal, tacit curriculum as necessary, even crucial to the development of a trainee's professional competence, while the trainee may interpret this interaction as bullying or overly aggressive and unnecessary. An example of this is the use of the Socratic method by staff, where the intended impact may be to help the trainee learn or perform under pressure, especially when it happens in the presence of peers, but the trainee may see its use as outdated and irrelevant to the modern learning environment.

Much has been said about how to approach learners for formative and quantitative feedback. It is important to continue these conversations, but it is also wise to remember that context is a pivotal part of understanding the hidden curriculum. No matter the "validity" of the perception of mistreatment, a learning environment that is felt to be unsafe will not aid the development of the very physician competencies we aim to develop.

Educational elements such as high-stakes testing, class rankings, and chief residents may have some benefits to trainees being socialized into the norms of medicine, but these elements may also have some unintended consequences. It is precisely these unintended consequences that need to be unearthed from the silent curriculum so as to reshape the conversation and the environments in which they occur into one of inclusivity, safety and structural competence.

Some of the direct and indirect unintended consequences that can result from the silent curriculum include: psychological distress in both clinicians and trainees, increased risk of burnout and suicide among practicing physicians and physicians-in-training, suboptimal learning during medical training, and negative impact on patient care due to the adverse psychological impact on clinical staff (Yazdani et al., 2020; Holmes et al., 2015).

Pause and Reflect

The conflict arising from the discrepancy between the silent curriculum and the formal curriculum can create some distress in both medical learners and practicing physicians. If this is not expressed properly, it risks contributing to physician burnout (Mohanty et al., 2019) and even suicide (Stehman et al., 2019), as the tension created by the misalignment between the system and the physician's core values becomes untenable.

1. In your institution what are the specific "third space" gaps that cause cognitive dissonance, and where do the mismatched messages appear to be coming from?
2. What duties cause you emotional or spiritual distress? Can you name the core value(s) they go against?
3. How can this be addressed and resolved?
4. What duties or aspects of your work have given you the most fulfilment? What would it look like to scale this up?

The Opportunity

❖

"If knowledge is power, knowing what we don't know is wisdom"
—Adam M. Grant, 2021

❖

Opportunities to Give Voice to the Silent Curriculum

Brooks (2015) shared that "while studying for boards, I learned that the race of the patient was often a hint to his or her disease". This could lead to potentially serious patient outcomes (such as a missed diagnosis or inappropriate management), not only from the racist assumption, but from the contribution of confirmation and/or anchoring bias. The consequence is a further exacerbation of health inequities and reinforcement of the dynamic of structural violence. While patient demographics are important, overemphasizing race at the expense of other factors (e.g., family history, physical exam findings, lab investigations, social determinants of health) perpetuates a diagnostic bias (Amutah et al., 2021).

Uncovering the hidden curriculum within the medical learning environment takes some patience and fundamental skills in reflection. It is also never a completed process, nor is there a perfect, sustainable solution to the problems inherent in this invisible curriculum. By its very nature, over time, the gap between what is formally known and explicitly stated, and what is informally taught and/or observed, will go subterranean, as previously described.

This process also occurs when we make mistreatments visible and implement initiatives to combat the effects of the silent curriculum. Eventually, these initiatives of calling out mistreatments will also go subterranean and become a positive component of the silent cultural curriculum. Thus, the process of moral enculturation in medicine that constitutes the silent curriculum can be unveiled and transformed into a more explicit enculturation into the medical realm (Olthuis and Dekkers, 2003). Reflective skills and being comfortable with some degree of discomfort is also necessary in order to shift mistreatment and other adverse elements of the silent culture into the visible realm and thus develop meaningful solutions (Huber et al., 2020). In the absence of this, adverse elements remain powerful through silence and continue to cause internal distress.

By making elements of the silent curriculum increasingly visible over time, this can be built into the positive hidden medical culture. Social norms which were once formalized become subconscious processes from where physicians unconditionally operate and guide their workdays. Organizations and medical teams would benefit from making these processes conscious again on a regular basis, lest they become routine and unexamined. Using the Pareto principle (i.e., for many outcomes, roughly 80% of consequences come from 20% of causes) in this regard may be helpful, as 80% of our difficulties often come from 20% of our processes, whether formal or informal (University of California Berkeley, 2022). The Pareto principle also works the other way, in that 80% of the benefits and fulfillment that physicians experience at work or in their personal lives derives from 20% of their activities – i.e., the relationships, patterns, and projects they find to be rewarding (Swensen and Shanafelt 2020). If physicians can identify the 20% of their work practices that most help them, they can notionally bolster their professional satisfaction and potentially decrease the risk of disengagement in the other 80% of their work and home life.

The different layers of the silent curriculum arising from different work environments add complexity to the issue. The silent curriculum might have variations depending on country, speciality, cohort, or institution (academic or clinical setting) and it is important to be systematic as we look at the silent culture of a specialty in particular, or at a specific training site.

Revealing the hidden costs of an unexamined curriculum

Try some of the following exercises to reveal the hidden costs of an unexamined curriculum in medicine from the perspective of medical leaders, trainees, residents, and staff. This exercise can be done at intervals of every few years to capture the shifting nature of invisible dynamics, impacts, and unintended consequences of the academic and clinical environment.

1. List the top 10 things you learned in medical school that you were likely not supposed to learn (Dent et al., 2021; Dosani, 2010).

2. Organize a gathering to promote reflection from faculty and students. For example, ask each person to comment on how to dress, tools needed, who speaks first, or how to introduce self. Then compare the answers from the faculty and student group qualitatively. This delineates the different expectations and unintended impact of the tacit curriculum on trainees, and also serves to highlight how formalized learning becomes tacit and subterranean (subconscious) with time, immersion, and repeated experience.

3. Take a narrative medicine approach by creating time and space (a healing group) where students and/or faculty can come together and share EDI-related experiences with or without the use of prompts. Narrative medicine aims to create meaning through storytelling in medicine by reflecting on our cases and discussing them with others in a creative capacity. It can involve modalities such as making poems, writing a narrative article, or writing out reflections on the clinician's or patient's experiences, or both.

4. Reflect on workarounds (Seaman and Erlen, 2015) where the "right" way seems inefficient and remote. For example, figuring out how to chart or do something else in the electronic medical record (EMR) when the EMR is not working properly or efficiently (even if this "workaround" is not the correct process). What is the unintended impact of seeing these workarounds being role-modelled and left unexamined over time?

5. Reflect in a group on micro-ethical challenges, such as:
    - Do I laugh at a dehumanizing joke?
    - Do I stay quiet about my heritage?
    - Do I express my concern when a faculty member misbehaves or is aggressive?
    - Do I take time off to recharge?

6. Reflect on what is missing in current medical education. What is in the null curriculum, and would patients be concerned that the formal curriculum fails to discuss or teach these absent topics?

7. Use appreciative inquiry to discover the unintended beneficial effects of the invisible curriculum. Appreciative inquiry looks at what things are currently working, and why they are working. Recognizing the many things that clinicians and educators already do well, alongside all the things that are less positive, can become a positive yet hidden social force that utilizes and supports people's strengths. In turn, this promotes the application of these strengths to build positive social change and social capital.

Professional Vignette

Rana experienced a positive challenge to her unconscious cognitive biases when she first met the new psychiatry chair at the institution where she worked. The new chair was very animated and spoke passionately. He stated his opinions about professionalism without being subtle. He confronted Rana at one point during their first meeting and said that professionalism is an "inherently racist" concept in that implicit biases about how a physician should look, dress, interact with, and respond to their patients and other colleagues color much of the professionalism standards of the past. However, Rana had learned to prioritize professionalism in her own clinical practice and when dealing with other clinicians. Professionalism was mandatory training in her residency program, which had included much discussion about how to safeguard your reputation against any harm because the Canadian medical field is "small". Her education had also emphasized how professionalism meant you looked and behaved a certain way, and never once got tearful with a patient. She learned that a psychiatrist should not show any emotion because they need to be a "blank canvas" that the patient colors with their own impressions and ideas or symptoms.

Rana had subconsciously accepted these values and was surprised to have such an engaging and animated meeting with the head of the psychiatry department. Her expectation of these meetings through the years was that they were performative rituals with no real connection or passion being transmitted. Her implicit bias was that people in medical leadership are stoic, stick to the "company line", follow routinized scripts, look slightly bored, check off their list that they have had a conversation with her about the prescribed topics (such as wellness, EDI, etc.), but then really don't engage or relate in a way that builds camaraderie, collegiality, or a desire to work together.

Thus, they may be championing EDI initiatives or other initiatives, but their real feelings about the subject are subterranean and not explicitly stated in their mannerisms or even in their language. This was in stark contrast to Rana's meeting with the new chair, where she was surprised to see the opposite of what she was expecting. Instead of a functional, performative meeting, it was an engaging, energizing meeting where Rana felt she really got to know the chair in a more personal way, his passions, and what he really thought about EDI initiatives.

Professional Vignette Analysis

Rana's experience highlights the importance of unconscious cognitive biases, and how these can be challenged by medical leaders in a positive way. Rana was surprised to encounter an animated and passionate psychiatry chair who openly voiced his opinion about professionalism being an inherently racist concept. This situation provides insight into the hidden curriculum for physicians, which often teaches them to prioritize professionalism above all else. It demonstrates how implicit biases can be reinforced through years of socialization and education (Project Implicit, 1998).

In a study by Brown et al. (2020), professionalism was perceived as being negatively impacted by the hidden curriculum and seen as an imposition from senior faculty to control students. Students believe medical identity formation begins prior to medical school, in a process known as "anticipatory socialization", a previously unstudied identity transition. Students felt covert institutional agendas negatively impacted their identity, pushing them further from the identity their institution was encouraging them to acquire. Key messages for educators include the need to explore the hidden curriculum through dialogue with students.

Rana's situation also highlights the contrast between traditional medical leadership roles, where leaders are expected to be stoic and performative, versus a more engaging and energizing approach that builds camaraderie and collegiality. Medical leaders have the power to challenge unconscious cognitive biases and create an environment in which all voices are heard, respected, and embraced. By creating such a culture, medical leadership can foster an inclusive atmosphere that celebrates diversity of thought, background, and experience. Furthermore, by setting an example of open dialogue and respect for different perspectives, medical leaders can inspire and empower their colleagues and those in their care.

Hybrid Professional and Clinical Vignette

A surgical resident physician, Tyler, had been working in a program for several months and had noticed a significant power dynamic between the attending surgeons and the residents. The attending surgeons often spoke down to the residents, belittling their skills and knowledge, and making them feel as though they were not competent. Paradoxically, their academic teaching sessions emphasized issues such as the professional expectation of self-care, learner mistreatment and psychological safety, links between surgical error and surgeon fatigue, as well as emphasizing the inverse link between burnout and quality of care, particularly for minoritized patients. Tyler found it difficult to reconcile the formal teaching content with the bedside and supervisory manner of the attending surgeons. Although joy in work, team engagement and wellness were emphasized, there were no concrete social supports and Tyler found senior staff often warned them against letting "too many people" know about their internal lives as it could be used against them. The impact of "reputation" on his career was reiterated frequently. When Tyler brought up his various concerns to his supervisor, he was told to just "toughen up" and that "this is what residency is all about."

Tyler grew up in a mixed family, where half his family was heavily reliant on each other, and their social gatherings were at the center of his family's health and vitality. The family often did things together and saw themselves as one large functioning unit, having come from a collectivistic culture. When Tyler wanted to get married to his fiancée, his father refused several elements of the wedding, citing that the "wedding was not about him or his fiancée at all, but rather about the family and an opportunity for community gathering."

Tyler grew up learning that he was not the center of his life, but that, rather his community was. This was in explicit contrast to the messages he was now unconsciously and blatantly told on his rotation, where individualism and independent survival in service to "reputation" and safeguarding against any potential hurts and undermining were at the center of the decisions that his staff were making day to day. Unconsciously, not knowing much about the colonizing forces that have influenced patterns of perfectionism and individualism in this culture, he absorbed these messages. To fit into the new medical ecosystem, he felt he had to emulate his supervisors.

On his next clinical rotation, Tyler found himself taking care of several patients who were experiencing long-term side effects from a recent virus that had affected many people's health and vitality. These patients were requesting time off from work due to fatigue, and, although not visible clinically, they complained of cognitive fatigue and inability to sustain long-term detailed attention required for their work day. Tyler found himself frustrated and annoyed with these patients. He unconsciously began to belittle them about not having the "strength to get through it". He began counselling them on how they can also push through their discomfort, in the same way that he had been cultured to throughout medical training.

In one clinical encounter, a female patient expressed concern that she "would never get better", and how she missed her family ecosystem who were overseas. Tyler found himself rolling his eyes and telling her to "toughen up" and that she, the patient, could not expect things to just be "handed to her" and she must "work for it".

On later reflection, he realized that he had not only replayed the same dynamic as he experienced with his surgery supervisors, but he had also done so without even realizing. He found himself feeling discouraged, wondering what other negative messages he had unconsciously absorbed and was projecting on others. He found himself feeling guilt over his seeming loss of compassion and wondered whether he was burning out or whether this was just the expected outcome of becoming efficient in his profession.

Hybrid Professional and Clinical Vignette Analysis

Tyler's situation highlights the significance of the relational context within the hidden curriculum of medical training, and how "collateral learning" takes place. Collateral learning, conceptualized by John Dewey (Zigler, 2001), describes the accidental learning that occurs both inside and outside of the classroom. Collateral learning is the lesson students walk away with from the accidental experience with the lesson rather than the intent of the instructor.

The attending surgeons' behavior demonstrates how power dynamics within the medical hierarchy can lead to mistreatment of residents. The attending surgeons were in a position of power and responsible for shaping the work culture of the program. However, they had implicitly absorbed the message that the residents were not deserving of support for their health and wellbeing. Instead, the supervisors belittled the residents' skills and knowledge, warned against letting "too many people" know about their internal lives, and reinforced an individualistic, "tough" mentality with regards to medical situations. These teachings appeared to be in direct contrast to Tyler's previous understanding of community support and collective functioning, which he had experienced growing up.

In addition, the supervisor's dismissal of Tyler's concerns reinforced the toxic culture of "working through it" and accepting the status quo in medical training. This culture perpetuates the idea that residents must endure mistreatment as a rite of passage to becoming a physician, rather than recognizing the importance of supportive environments for learning and growth. The hidden curriculum, in this case, was harmful to Tyler and to the culture of the program. As a resident, Tyler was in a position of relative powerlessness. He was expected to follow the implicit rules of the program, even when those rules were detrimental to his health and the health of his patients.

When caring for his patients, Tyler unconsciously adopted the values taught to him by the attending surgeons, which was to push through any obstacles and be strong for the sake of one's reputation. He then passed on these values to the female patient who expressed concern over her health issues. He subsequently experienced cognitive dissonance over his lack of compassion in response to the patient. He recognized that his actions were not in keeping with his desire to be compassionate with his patients.

This situation demonstrates how oppressive power dynamics operating in medical education can lead to detrimental outcomes for patients if the healthcare provider is unable to recognize their own cultural biases. It also highlights how Tyler's understanding of community and collective functioning was replaced with a more individualistic mindset, which he then passed on to his patients without proper consideration, ultimately diminishing their wellbeing.

In order for healthcare providers to practice a holistic, patient-centered form of care, they must recognize their own cultural biases and understand the importance of an individualized approach when providing health services. Understanding how one's own values influence how they interact with patients can help foster a more open and equitable relationship between provider and patient. Ultimately, this vignette demonstrates the need to address oppressive power dynamics in medical education, to ensure that providers are providing care that is beneficial and respectful of patient wellbeing.

Medical educators must also recognize the impact of the hidden curriculum on shaping attitudes and behaviors in medical training. It is crucial to create supportive learning environments that prioritize the well-being of trainees and address power dynamics within the medical hierarchy. This involves providing mental health support and addressing issues related to mistreatment. By recognizing and addressing the hidden curriculum, medical training programs can ensure that the culture of medicine is one of compassion, empathy, and respect for all healthcare professionals.

Did you know?

Lehmann, Sulmasy and Desai (2018) noted that more than half of medical students experienced disconnects between what they were explicitly taught and what they perceived from faculty members' behaviors.

Key Takeaways

- The medical learning environment can be full of contradictions with both positive and negative unintended consequences.
- The "third space" of the silent curriculum consists of all the intermediary beliefs, biases, and attitudes that clinicians unconsciously transmit through medical education and practice.
- Unconscious bias and cognitive errors are common among physicians, and can lead to a variety of diagnostic and relational issues.
- By becoming more aware of their biases, medical professionals can make a conscious effort to reduce or eliminate them.
- The silent curriculum can be a fertile ground for biases and inequities because it is not in full view; therefore, it escapes the scrutiny of the profession.
- Discovering the silent curriculum within the medical learning environment takes some patience and fundamental skills in reflection.
- Reflective skills and being comfortable with some degree of discomfort are both necessary to make mistreatments in the invisible culture/curriculum visible and thus come up with solutions.

Conclusion

The work of the hidden curriculum is about making the subconscious impact of learning conscious, and about implementing regular formalized reflection on an informal but powerful curriculum. The hidden curriculum is the key socializing force that shapes professional identity formation. This is precisely why it is critical not to overlook the critical role of relational context such as hierarchy as a key force within the invisible curriculum.

When physicians demonstrate bias towards patients, peers or learners, the hierarchy may prevent learners from naming what they've witnessed. Furthermore, the learner may absorb the modelled behaviour as part of their socialization into the profession. Thus, the hidden curriculum is also a powerful socializing force because of the inherent hierarchy of training and education. By the same taken, a physician demonstrating equity-responsiveness in their interactions stands to positively shape learners and peers to adopt a similar ethos. This is where the silent curriculum is most powerful: in its infectiousness when positive messages are conveyed, emulated, and absorbed for replication, thus ideally building a critical mass of equity responsive clinical staff.

Within the larger EDI framework, the hidden curriculum highlights the importance of understanding and validating the impact of actions, words, and nonverbal cues, rather than merely focusing on the intention behind them. What people walk away with and, thereby, what is actually taught, may be very different than what was intended to be taught. It would be prudent for medical organizations to remind themselves of this unconscious force that propels the medical environment to either sink or swim. It is also vital to critically evaluate the formal curriculum in order to identify any distortion created by the influence of the hidden curriculum. Like the concept of the "shadow" in Jungian psychology (Jung, 1958), the hidden curriculum might lead to distortions and acting-out (such as racism, sexism, and other forms of mistreatment to self or others) if not recognized and integrated.

So, like archeologists, physicians and educators should aim to unearth the hidden, and select which artefacts are worth keeping, displaying, and studying. Amplifying the whispers of the silent curriculum is long overdue. In the absence of this, there will continue to be an intention-action gap in the curriculum, leading to further dissonance, particularly in the context of equity, diversity and inclusivity issues.

On a Parting Note...

It is not without fear that we become whole, but when we live alongside it, and invite it in, like old friends for tea.

© Irina Mihaescu, 2020

References

Amutah, C., Greenidge, K., Mante, A., A.B., Munyikwa, M., Surya, S.L., Higginbotham, E., Jones, D.S., Lavizzo-Mourey, R., Roberts, D., Tsai, J. and Aysola, J. (2021). Misrepresenting Race – The Role of Medical Schools in Propagating Physician Bias. *N Engl J Med*, 384, pp.872-878.

Bauer, G.R., Hammond, R., Travers, R., Kaay, M., Hohenadel, K.M., Boyce, M. (2009) '"I don't think this is theoretical; this is our lives": How erasure impacts health care for transgender people'. *Journal of the Association of Nurses in AIDS Care*, 20, pp. 348–361.

Beck, A.T., Rush, A.J., Shaw, B.F. and Emery, G. (1979). *Cognitive Therapy of Depression*. New York: The Guilford Press.

Boehm, K.S., McGuire, C., Boudreau, C., Jenkins, D., Samargandi, O.A., Al-Youha, S. and Tang, D. (2019). The Shame-Blame Game: Is It Still Necessary? A National Survey of Shame-based Teaching Practice in Canadian Plastic Surgery Programs. *Plast Reconstr Surg Glob Open* [online], 7(2). Available from: https://pubmed.ncbi.nlm.nih.gov/30881847/

Brooks, K., (2015). A Silent Curriculum. *JAMA*, 313(19), pp.1909-1910.

Brown, M.E., Coker, O., Heybourne, A. and Finn, G.M. (2020). Exploring the hidden curriculum's impact on medical students: professionalism, identity formation and the need for transparency. *Med Sci Educ*, 30, pp.1107-1121.

Butler, K., Yak, A., and Veltman, A. (2019) "Progress in medicine is slower to happen": Qualitative insights into how trans and gender nonconforming medical students navigate cisnormative medical cultures at Canadian training programs', *Academic Medicine*, 94(11), pp. 1757-1765.

Cahapay, M.B. (2021). A systematic review of concepts in understanding null curriculum. *International Journal of Curriculum and Instruction*, 13(3), pp.1987-1999.

Dent, J.A., Harden, R.M. and Hunt, D. (2021). *A Practical Guide for Medical Teachers*. Milton: Elsevier Canada.

Dosani, N., (2010). The top 10 things I learned in medical school (but wasn't supposed to!). *Plenary Session: The hidden curriculum exposed: perspectives of learners and educators*, unpublished.

Gabbard, G.O. (1985). The role of compulsiveness in the normal physician. *JAMA*, 254(20), pp.2926-2929.

Gaiser, R.R. (2009). The teaching of professionalism during residency: why it is failing and a suggestion to improve its success. *Anesth Analg,* 108(3), pp.948-954.

Geneviève, L. D., Martani, A., Shaw, D., Elger, B. S., and Wangmo, T. (2020). Structural racism in precision medicine: leaving no one behind. *BMC medical ethics,* 21(1), 17. https://doi.org/10.1186/s12910-020-0457-8.

Graff, S., Oppfeldt, A.M., Gotfredsen, M. and Christensen, B. (2022). [Diagnostic bias]. *Ugeskr Laeger* [online], 184(38). Available from: https://pubmed.ncbi .nlm.nih.gov/36178180/

Hafferty, F.W. and Franks, R. (1994). The hidden curriculum, ethics teaching, and the structure of medical education. *Acad Med,* 69, pp.861-71.

Hafferty, F.W., Gaufberg, E.H. and O'Donnell, J.F. (2015). The role of the hidden curriculum in "on doctoring" courses. *AMA Journal of Ethics,* 17, pp.130-139. https://doi: 10.1001/virtualmentor.2015.17.2.medu1-1502.

Hafferty, F.W. and O'Donnell, J.F. (2015). *The Hidden Curriculum in Health Professional Education.* Hanover: Dartmouth College Press.

Holmes, C.L., Harris, I.B., Schwartz, A.J. and Regehr, G. (2015). Harnessing the hidden curriculum: a four-step approach to developing and reinforcing reflective competencies in medical clinical clerkship. *Adv Health Sci Educ Theory Pract,* 20(5), pp.1355-1370.

Huang, J., Galal, G., Etemadi, M., & Vaidyanathan, M. (2022). Evaluation and mitigation of racial bias in clinical machine learning models: Scoping review. *JMIR medical informatics,* 10(5), e36388. https://doi.org/10.2196/36388.

Huber, A., Strecker, C., Hausler, M. Kachel, T., Hoge, T. and Hofer, S. (2020). Possession and Applicability of Signature Character Strengths: What Is Essential for Well-Being, Work Engagement, and Burnout? *Applied Research in Quality of Life,* 15, pp.415-436.

Igoe, K.J. (2021). Algorithmic bias in health care exacerbates social inequities — how to prevent it [online] March 12, 2023. Available from: https://www.hsph. harvard.edu/ecpe/how-to-prevent-algorithmic-bias-in-health-care/

Joseph, O.R., Flint, S.W., Raymond-Williams, R., Awadzi, R. and Johnson, J. (2021). Understanding Healthcare Students' Experiences of Racial Bias: A Narrative Review of the Role of Implicit Bias and Potential Interventions in Educational Settings. *Int J Environ Res Public Health* [online], 18(23). Available from: https://www.ncbi.nlm.nih.gov/pmc/articles/PMC8657581/

Jung, C. (1958). *The Undiscovered Self: The Dilemma of the Individual in Modern Society.* London: Penguin Books.

Kalter, L. (2019). Navigating the hidden curriculum in medical school [online]. Available from: https://www.aamc.org/news-insights/navigating-hidden-curriculum-medical-school

Lehmann, L.S., Sulmasy, L.S. and Desai, S. (2018). Hidden Curricula, Ethics, and Professionalism: Optimizing Clinical Learning Environments in Becoming and Being a Physician: A Position Paper of the American College of Physicians. *Annals of Internal Medicine* [online]. Available from: https://www.acpjournals .org/doi/10.7326/M17-2058

Leong, R., and Ayoo, K. (2019). Seeing medicine's hidden curriculum. Canadian medical association journal, 191, pp.E920-1. https://doi: 10.1503/cmaj.190359.

Mahood, S.C. (2011). Medical education: Beware the hidden curriculum. *Can Fam Physician*, 57(9), pp.983-985.

Maniotes, L.K. (2005). *The transformative power of literary third space* [unpublished]. PhD thesis, School of Education, University of Colorado.

Marcelin, J.R., Siraj, D.S., Victor, R., Kotadia, S. and Maldonado, Y.A. (2019). The Impact of Unconscious Bias in Healthcare: How to Recognize and Mitigate It. *The Journal of Infectious Diseases*, 220(2), pp.S62-S73.

Mohanty, D., Prabhu, A. and Lippmann, S. (2019). Physician burnout: signs and solutions. *J Fam Pract*, 68(8), pp.442-446.

Nundy, S., Cooper, L.A. and Mate, K.S. (2022). The quintuple aim for Health Care Improvement. *JAMA*, 327(6), p.521. doi.org/10.1001/jama.2021.25181.

Obermeyer, Z., Powers, B., Vogeli, C., and Mullainathan, S. (2019). Dissecting racial bias in an algorithm used to manage the health of populations. *Science (New York, N.Y.)*, 366(6464), pp.447–453. https://doi.org/10.1126/science.aax2342.

Okun, T. (2022). *(divorcing) White Supremacy Culture: Coming Home to Who We Really Are* [online]. Available from: https://www.whitesupremacyculture.info/

Olthuis, G., & Dekkers, W. (2003). Medical education, palliative care and moral attitude: some objectives and future perspectives. *Medical education*, 37(10), 928–933. https://doi.org/10.1046/j.1365-2923.2003.01635.x.

Project Implicit. (1998). *Welcome to Project Implicit* [online]. Available from: https://www.projectimplicit.net/

Seaman, J.B. and Erlen, J.A. (2015). Workarounds in the Workplace: A Second Look. *Orthop Nurs*, 34(4), pp.235-240.

Shanafelt, T.D. and Noseworthy, J.H. (2016). Executive leadership and physician well-being: Nine organizational strategies to promote engagement and reduce burnout. *Mayo Clin Proc*, 92, pp.129-146.

Stehman, C.R., Testo, Z., Gershaw, R.S. and Kellogg, A.R. (2019). Burnout, Drop Out, Suicide: Physician Loss in Emergency Medicine, Part I. *West J Emerg Med*, 20(3), pp.485-494.

Swensen, S. and Shanafelt, T. (2020). *Mayo Clinic Strategies to Reduce Burnout: 12 Actions to Create the Ideal Workplace*. New York: Oxford University Press.

University of California Berkeley, (2022). *Explaining the 80-20 Rule with the Pareto Distribution* [online]. Available from: https://dlab.berkeley.edu/news/explaining-80-20-rule-pareto-distribution

Williams, E.S., Rathert, C. and Buttigieg, S.C., 2019. The Personal and Professional Consequences of Physician Burnout: A Systematic Review of the Literature. *Medical Care Research and Review*, 77(5), pp.371-386.

Whitchurch, C. (2008). Shifting Identities and Blurring Boundaries: The Emergence of
Third Space Professionals in UK Higher Education. *Higher Education Quarterly*, 62(4), pp.377-396.

Xu, J., Xiao, Y., Wang, W. H., Ning, Y., Shenkman, E. A., Bian, J., & Wang, F. (2022). Algorithmic fairness in computational medicine. *EBioMedicine*, 84, 104250. https://doi.org/10.1016/j.ebiom.2022.104250.

Yazdani, S., Andarvazh, M.R. and Afshar, L. (2020). What is hidden in hidden curriculum? a qualitative study in medicine. *J Med Ethics Hist Med*, 13(4), pp.1-11.

Zigler, R.L. (2001). John Dewey, eros, ideals, and collateral learning: Toward a descriptive model of the exemplary teacher. *Philosophy of Education Archive* [online], pp.276-284. Available from: https://www.philofed.org/_files/ugd/803b74_59cf14ab3612412282eb4151db7ad456.pdf

Chapter 4
Peace, Order and Good Governance in Medicine: Medical Leadership and Structural Competence

Zainab Abdurrahman, MD, Mariam Abdurrahman, MD

❖

"The function of freedom is to free someone else."
—Toni Morrison, 1979

❖

Abstract: This chapter explores the concept of structural competence and the role of medical leadership in responsible healthcare. Medical leadership is examined as a function and a structure through which to create an equity-responsive environment. As a structure, medical leadership is responsible for the organization and operation of medical establishments and institutions. As a functional entity, medical leadership strongly shapes the activities of physicians and the tone of the climate in which physicians function. The role of staff diversity in addressing the physician-population diversity gap is explored in so far as it shapes the professional climate, patient care experiences and patient outcomes. The chapter concludes with an exploration of opportunities for EDI momentum in medicine.

Keywords: *equity, equity gap, equity-seeking, health equity, medical leadership, minoritized, Quintuple Aim, responsible healthcare, structural competence*

Introduction

The core ethos of the medical field is to do no harm. This is operationalized in various ways, along a spectrum from preventing or minimizing risk to restoring health, minimizing the effects of ill health, providing palliation and ultimately a good death where possible. However, the tenet of doing no harm has not always held true in the field. In fact, the history of medicine is anything but benign as illustrated in Chapter 1.

The same broader societal failures in equity, diversity, and inclusion have replayed themselves in the medical field, a microcosm of society that is at times a backdrop to societal ills, whilst at other times complicit, or at the forefront of social injustice. Yet medicine is also a strong vanguard for the vulnerable, a societal conscience and a source of momentum for the systemic ills that subjugate various equity-deprived groups. Physicians are schooled in both the science and humanism of medicine. The curriculum is set by medical leaders at various levels, with each education and training program being unique in its own way. The journey from medical student to qualified physician is a long one that requires the right medical leadership at the stern, leadership that is:

- attuned to and prescient of the shifting societal healthcare needs on a local to national and global level;
- aware of what came before (i.e., the history of medicine) and therefore shapes the present landscape of medicine so as to exercise a wise mind to that which is unfolding in current events and thus, better predict that which is to come;
- committed to operating structurally competent institutions such that they bridge the equity gap that exists in the populations served by the institutions they lead;
- responsive to the environmental and societal footprint of healthcare in an age of declining resources and expanding wealth gaps; and
- accountable for the actions and needs of its institution, faculty and learners so as to position them in a path that generates non-malfeasance and true beneficence.

The role of medical leadership is dynamic, extensive, and profound in its purpose and spectrum of effect. These responsibilities require a state of structural competence in the education and training institutions that shape physicians' professional identity. Structural competency calls on medical leaders and healthcare professionals to recognize the ways in which our societal fabric (institutions, neighborhood conditions, market forces, public policies, and healthcare delivery systems) collectively shape symptoms and diseases, resulting in health inequities (Hansen and Metzl, 2017; Metzl and Hansen, 2014; Metzl and Hansen, 2018). As physicians and leaders, structural competence requires us to mobilize in order to correct inequalities as they manifest in physician-patient interactions and beyond the clinic walls (Metzl and Hansen, 2014; Metzl and Hansen, 2018).

The professional identity of physicians is shaped by the silent curriculum which sources its feed from key areas including medical leadership and the shape they give the institutions in which medicine is delivered, institutional/organizational culture, patient safety culture, and the formal curriculum. As such, the role of medical leadership cannot be emphasized enough, whether in academic or non-academic settings. In academic settings, the silent curriculum draws from the formal curriculum in so far as the representativeness or diversity contained in the teaching materials and the "tone" of the formal curriculum in terms of how minoritized and marginalized patients are portrayed.

The question of competence in relation to the curriculum set by medical leaders has recently been a subject of discussion due to the mismatch between the patients depicted in audiovisual aids relative to the spectrum of patients that physicians see in practice. The equity of educational materials has already been explored in detail in Chapter 2. Setting curricular topics in terms of diseases and systems is not enough. In fact, a competent curriculum must also include representative content so that learners are familiar with the spectrum of normative and pathologic presentation across ethnoracial, age, gender and other social groups.

There have been notable equity, diversity and inclusion (EDI) failures in medicine that stem from a lack of representative material in the medical curriculum and discriminatory attitudes perpetrated through reference materials such as guidelines and diagnostic algorithms. Shameful diagnostic errors have arisen where normative differences were pathologized, for example conclusions of child abuse before the recognition of racially normative hyperpigmentation patches that were also inappropriately termed "Mongolian spots".

Medical leaders also need to commit to faculty, student and staff diversity as a proxy for patient care experiences and outcomes. In fact, staff diversity is a critical aspect of addressing disparities and health outcomes for equity-seeking groups (Jackson, 2014; Page, 2008; Simonsen and Shim, 2019; Smith et al., 2022). There is evidence that diversity is associated with better patient outcomes, as well making financial sense for institutions and the broader healthcare system (Gomez and Bernet, 2019; LaVeist and Pierre, 2014). Hence, competence in EDI issues can be used as a prognostic tool in improved patient and provider outcomes; this is explored further in Chapters 10 to 13.

Structural competence inherently implies an EDI-informed environment. However, educational and clinical institutions are yet to reach this state. The reality is that institutions struggle to go beyond branding to intention and commitment, and from thereon to action. The intention-action gap is evident in institutions that pursue equity, diversity, inclusion, indigenization and accountability as "niche" projects to be tackled as part of the organizational scorecard rather than an operational standard. Shifting from the outside ripples of branding towards a core of commitment and action requires the dedication of medical leaders.

As will be covered over the course of this book, the elevation of equity as a patient and provider due makes sense as it is intimately tied to patient safety, provider wellbeing and satisfaction, health human resource stability and is financially intelligent for the healthcare system at all levels (Gomez and Bernet, 2019; LaVeist and Pierre, 2014; Jackson and Gracia, 2014; Page, 2008; Simonsen and Shim, 2019; Smith et al., 2022). There has been further work of recent examining the Aims of health improvement. Nundy, Cooper, and Mate (2022) propose that in fact, the Quadruple Aim should be revised to the Quintuple Aim to account for the essential role of health equity. From the health provider standpoint, equity for patients requires concurrent EDI work within the ranks of the medical establishment itself.

The Issues

Diversity Barriers in Medical Leadership

There has been a depth of literature focused on the glass ceiling. Traditionally this term has been applied to the invisible barriers faced by women in their workplaces in their quest for career advancement (Chaffins et al., 1995; Davidson and Cooper, 1992; Purcell et al., 2010 pp. 705-717). In the context of diversity and medicine, the more appropriate analogy would be the force fields that exclude physicians of diverse sexual orientation, cultural practices, and races from the trajectory of privilege that traditionally rises up the leadership ladder. In short, it is difficult to go up if you cannot get into the building. For example, this was the case at Queen's University medical school in Kingston, Ontario, Canada, in 1918 when the university implemented a ban on Black medical students which it enforced until the mid-1960s. The ban was not officially rescinded until 2018 (Aiken, 2018). In addition, as part of the original Indian Act in Canada, Indigenous people lost their "Indian status" if they achieved a professional degree such as law or medicine or even simply by obtaining any university degree (Crey and Hanson, 2009).

Prior to discussing medical leadership progression, it is pertinent to consider the entry level. Although the entry level is medical school, the precursor points of undergraduate study and experiential opportunities are differentially accessible to various applicant groups, with racialized and economically marginalized groups having the least access at the "pre-med" and medical school entrance level as will subsequently be discussed.

At the medical school entry point, in spite of seemingly meritorious albeit competitive standards of entry, the front door is in fact selective and many who knock with the same qualifications do not gain entry. Thus, the pathway to being a medical doctor demonstrates multiple equity barriers that commence well before medical school entry itself (Rodriguez et al., 2015). The process has many parallels to other healthcare professions, and the findings and lessons may be generalizable. Given the access barriers at the entry level and the resultant lack of diversity in the entry level positions, we cannot expect to achieve a truly diverse leadership group.

Pause and Reflect: What do the numbers mean?

The racial composition within the Canadian medical student population differs from that observed in the Canadian population. Although 6.4% and 7.4% of the Canadian population aged 15-34 years old identified as Black and Indigenous, only 1.7% of medical students identified as Black and 3.5 % as Indigenous (Khan et al., 2020).

- What is your gut reaction when you see these numbers?
- What evidence around you informs your thoughts about these observed population differences?
- How many Black and Indigenous peers did you have in your medical school class? Have you ever had a conversation with them about the relative differences in their presence in medicine versus the general population?
- If you feel that the composition of medical learners should reflect that of the general population, how would you go about addressing the diversity gap? At what level would you choose to intervene if you are a medical leader?

Data shows that the diversity within Canadian medical students does not reflect the diversity of the Canadian population. In a 2020 cross-sectional study, Khan and colleagues compared the composition of the Canadian medical student body to their general population counterparts of similar age (15–34-year-old age bracket in the 2016 census data). In addition to the numbers cited in the reflective exercise above, 62.9% of the medical students surveyed indicated that their household incomes were over $100,000 compared to only 32.4% of Canadians. They were also noted to have higher rates of physician parents compared to the general population. Similar findings from the United States shows that those who identify as Black, Hispanic, or Native American were underrepresented in the 10 healthcare professions examined which include doctors, nurses and physiotherapists, among other healthcare professionals. (Salsberg et al., 2021).

In Canada's 2016 national census, about 22% of the Indigenous population achieved a university level degree compared to 45% of the non-Indigenous population (Statistics Canada, 2016). In contrast, about 28% of the Black population achieved a university level degree in comparison to 33% of non-Black women and 27% of non-Black men. There was also an increased likelihood of completion of trades or apprenticeship education in

Indigenous people at 26% compared to the rest of the population at 16% (Statistics Canada, 2021). This demonstrates the decreased diversity already within those eligible to be in the medical school applicant pool.

Tuition costs also play a role in access to higher education. The cost of tuition for medical school, which is unregulated in some Western nations, discourages those who are of lower income brackets from considering application. Kwong and colleagues (2002) showed that increasing unregulated medical tuition fees over the 1997 to 2000 period in Ontario, Canada, coincided with a decline of medical students from households with income less than $40,000 per annum, from 22.6% to 15%. Other medical school application requirements often include, but are not limited to the completion of the Medical College Admission Test (MCAT), and typically volunteer work demonstrating interest in medicine. This has been the norm for several years now, but these requirements already stratify and place several at a disadvantage.

The cost of the MCAT is not insignificant, currently standing at $330 USD in 2022. Of note, there are reduced fees for those whose combined family income is below certain pre-set limits in the USA and Canada. This registration fee does not account for the cost of the materials to study for the MCAT including books, practice tests, and for some an MCAT preparation course which cost significantly more than the exam itself. As such, MCAT scores are not entirely a direct correlation with examinee talent or skill but rather, reflect the differential access to preparatory materials and differential levels of discretionary income in pursuit of a medical education (Lucey and Saguil, 2020). Furthermore, the effect of stereotype threat likely shapes the performance of racialized students on aptitude test. Steele and Aronson (1995) theorize that racialized individuals may underperform on aptitude tests as a result of fear that their performance may confirm a negative societal stereotype about their race.

Stereotype threat is thought to a contributing factor in the gender and minority gaps in academic presence, performance and pursuit of opportunities. The consequences of structural racism on MCAT scores and medical school admissions is being more closely examined (Lucey and Saguil, 2020; Rodríguez et al., 2022). Rodríguez et al. (2022) describe the phenomena of academic redlining in which students from underrepresented backgrounds are systematically excluded from entry into medicine using standardized test hard cut-offs, such as the MCAT. Taken together, these facts reflect further evidence that a seemingly objective process and items as benign as test scores are influenced by social determinants and thus reflect the inequitable distribution of opportunity.

These multifactorial sources of homogeneity within the medical ranks begin upstream and maintain the pipeline of diversity in medicine at a trickle. This is unlikely to change unless there is a change from the top-down within the medical establishment. Medical leadership sets the undergraduate and postgraduate medical education eligibility criteria, entry standards, the application process, and are therefore in the utmost position to shape the structures that allow for diversity. The system is unlikely to change if medical leaders are unable to appreciate these factors. If there is no change, there will be ongoing perpetuation of the enduring systemic and structural racism that has been built into medicine (Nguemeni et al., 2022).

The very basics of being "seen" is an issue that triggers much discomfort. Canada, in particular, has been resistant to the collection of race-based data at so many levels including within healthcare, healthcare outcomes, educational systems, and other areas in which data and knowledge could be used to effect changes that bridge the equity gap (Bryant et al., 2011; Menezes et al., 2022; Munroe, 2022). Some have asserted the following: "the logic is simple: if we don't even notice race, then we can't act in a racist manner" (Nobel, 2012). Racial data is difficult to attain for medical students, residents, and practicing physicians as this is not traditionally recorded. Most studies are voluntary surveys to elicit this information. A fundamental principle to any problem solving is to first define the extent of the problem. How can an issue be addressed if there is no quantification of the issue at hand?

Without data to establish the extent of the problem, it is difficult to fully demonstrate the consequences of the deeply entrenched structural racism in Canada. For example, in countries that collect race-based data such as the United Kingdom (UK) this data collection has led to change on a policy level. Specifically, in the UK, this led to the creation of the Public Sector Equality Duty which "was designed to shift the onus from individuals to organisations, placing for the first time an obligation on public authorities to positively promote equality, not merely to avoid discrimination" (Equality and Human Rights Commission, 2011).

The lack of such policy or data collection in Canada was well demonstrated at the start of the COVID-19 Pandemic when the elevated case fatality rate of the disease was observed for certain ethnic and racialized populations, but the data was not being well captured (Thompson et al., 2021). Front line health workers and social agencies had to raise the alarm, but the healthcare system should have been able to see this trend quickly and adjusted the approach in response (Allen et al., 2021). The availability of this data would have allowed for more targeted approaches and earlier therapeutic interventions against the deadly virus. The irony here was that healthcare systems administrators and those in leadership typically wish to see objective data on which to base decisions but could not react quickly enough to devise an approach to this situation because the data was not being captured. The bottom line is well reflected in the title of McKenzie's (2020) paper: "if you are not counted you cannot count on the pandemic response."

Finally, there is ample evidence that professional licensure bodies, medical leadership associations and various upper levels of medical leadership have even lower levels of diversity than within the broader profession, let alone the richer diversity of the general population. Despite the increase in female applicants and some pioneering efforts towards increasing diversity in medical education and training programs, the core of the leadership in most medical institutions are White men (Ruzycki et al., 2021). One study reviewed over 3000 healthcare leaders from over 100 institutions in Canada and found that about 50% were female while under 10% were perceived to be racialized (Sergeant et al., 2022). In addition, racism has been cited as one of the contributors to the lack of diversity in healthcare leadership (Livingston, 2018). Hence, it is clear that the medical field cannot rely on the current approaches to healthcare leadership to provide diverse leadership and in turn downstream effects of such leadership (Soklaridis et al., 2022) which importantly include: patient care experiences, patient safety, burnout, and health human resource stability.

The Opportunity

Leadership Development: What are the Opportunities to Lead with Equity in Medical Leadership?

Sponsorship, mentorship and coaching are critical ingredients in the leadership journey. Sponsorship or the quality of being tapped on the shoulder and instrumentally supported in pursuing leadership is a powerful fuel that can drive self-actualization within the medical leadership ranks. Further success may entail ongoing coaching to further one's personal and professional development, recognize one's potential and continue to move towards realizing that potential, while mentorship allows an experienced person to guide, support and nurture the mentee through various journeys, whether directly related to leadership or other aspects of professional growth and development. Early identification of a mentor is essential. Most, if not all, CEOs likely had sponsorship, formally or informally utilized leadership coaches or life coaches as well as various mentors who have played a key role in getting them to where they are today. The case for mentorship has been well demonstrated in various healthcare and medical education literature (Ayyala et al., 2019; Schrubbe, 2004).

Mentorship is essential in any professional career, but once again differential access plays a role. With access to good mentorship relationships, individuals are able to develop new skills, access new opportunities, and experience growth on many levels. Mentors may also have access to the various rooms where key discussions about opportunities occur. Sponsors and mentors can open doors that help promote success in key times of negotiation when it may be difficult to exert the same level of influence independently. Now, consider being in a position of having had little to none of these resources and trying to navigate the medical leadership ranks with others engaged in a similar journey but who have access to all these resources!

The lack of access to mentors and networks were cited as common barriers to minority advancement (McCarty et al., 2005). Underrepresented minority resident physicians were also shown to be less likely to establish a relationship with mentors although the importance of a mentorship relationship was realized in most residents (Ramanan et al., 2006). Other studies showed similar results for gender, specifically looking at women (Shen et al., 2022).

Mentorship alone is not sufficient for leadership progression. Ayyala et al. (2019) note that "sponsorship, in addition to mentorship, is critical for successful career advancement". Sponsorship is a critical ingredient for underrepresented groups as many spaces traditionally occupied by the dominant majority are yet to view non-dominant voices as voices of belonging. Thus, sponsorship has much to add in the career advancement and leadership journey as sponsors are defined by having influence, power and access to routes that shape advancement. High stakes career advancement requires sponsorship; mentorship alone is unlikely to be sufficient to influence outcomes at high stakes levels like the corporate suite.

Sponsorship may yield some surprising responses, particularly when the would be sponsor and intended recipient are yet to recognize a shared view about the recipient's potential and trajectory of professional self-actualization. Consider the relatively early to mid-practice physician who has not considered that they could or would advance as far as the sponsor's perception of their potential. Where does the sponsor start the conversation? What if the sponsor's background and duration of privilege hampers the ability to establish a rapport that resonates with the recipient? Should the sponsor consider using a cis culture broker to the recipient in order to initiate the conversation and shift to a shared understanding of perceived potential and desired goals? Perhaps it is more effective for the sponsor and recipient to begin by examining the recipient's own journey to date, obstacles encountered on that journey and the recipient's views on what limits or promotes further leadership development. Similarly, reflecting on the sponsor's own journey to their level of privilege jointly will likely create a deeper space for mutual reflection, a safe space for inquiry and thereby further build rapport.

Assumptions are often made that underprivileged individuals just need to be tapped on the shoulder to jump at opportunity and that the individuals would want to create a legacy of opening doors. However, this can be far off the mark if a rapport and thoughtful conversation are not initiated such as suggested above. The delicate balance between thoughtful sponsorship and perceptions of being a checkmark for diversity impart a responsibility on the sponsor's part to devise a collaborative and nuanced journey of exploration and potentiation with the recipient. Thus, being a sponsor for equity elevation and restoration is a task of equal parts coach, power broker, leadership whisperer, soothsayer and combined armchair psychologist and historian. These are stimulating issues for a sponsor to consider as part of this crucial and delicate aspect of shifting medicine to look more like the diverse population it serves.

❖

Tap, tap, tap, comes the would be sponsor……no response.
Tap, tap, tap, tap, *and still no response.*
How much harder can I tap?
Why can't she hear the tapping?
Why haven't I tapped her on the shoulder before?
Why am I able to see her now, where before I could not?
Why do I see and the others do not? How do I go about opening eyes and opening minds amongst my governing brethren?
After all, it is well past time.
Past time to relinquish the keys and open the doors apace
For it is time she claimed her space
For we shall make good on this race and bestow others with a tap, tap, tap.
And they shall hear the tapping, and they shall believe they are sought.

— Mariam Abdurrahman, 2022

❖

Professional Vignette

Dr. Carstairs is an internist and newly appointed diversity officer for his division in a large metropolitan hospital affiliated with a local medical school. The hospital is located in a busy urban location that serves a culturally diverse population, including a large South Asian community. He is excited about his new role as his work with Medecin Sans Frontiers has created an abiding commitment to bridging the equity gap.

As part of his diversity office programming, Dr. Carstairs has identified that the division lacks diversity in the medical leadership ranks which he finds concerning as his staff is quite ethnoculturally and gender diverse. He decides to erect a leadership development group that will kick off an antiracism and anti-oppression campaign. He sends invitations out to the physicians in division. When the group meets, he observes that only two physicians are from underrepresented groups. He is disappointed to observe that the turnout is low, the engagement muted, and he is doing most of the talking.

He sends out a survey for anonymous completion by the division and is pleased to receive many more responses than the number who attended the first meeting. He is surprised to receive feedback to the effect that his ideas were viewed as being questionable given his perceived lack of credibility as an ally. Comments that stood out in the free entry section of the survey included: "I am not sure why we need this committee; the department is running fine.....why can't we just do clinical work, education and training? Let's leave all this EDI politics out of department business please, it's so tiresome, too many "sensitive" people....This working group is already biased as the head, the secretary and the campaign lead are all White....You haven't consulted but you are making plans to help us advance in leadership? Do you even know why a minority physician like me has not applied for leadership roles in this department?......How can you know what leadership hurdles I face when you've never walked in my shoes?" He was most surprised to learn that his appointment as diversity officer is perceived with disquiet because he is seen as a privileged White male who dually holds a role as the division co-lead. He is not sure where he went wrong and how to reset the course.

Vignette Analysis

Dr. Carstairs conundrum is not uncommon. The fact that he quickly identified an equity and representation problem which informed the mandate of the working group is extremely reassuring. Based on the feedback received, it is quickly evident that some staff members were not attuned or aware that EDI is a problem, whilst a few who are aware do not think this is something that constitutes a problem. Staff members who recognized that there is a problem were not receptive to following along. Very simply put, the staff were signalling that *not for us without us*. It is probably instructive to reflect on any prior attempts to bridge EDI gaps in the department. It may well be that the lack of consultation in exploring the context around the problem and lack of idea sharing resulted in a perception of a "poster campaign to check the boxes".

In this scenario, it would be important to capture the desire to engage and be engaged as evident in the survey responses. Although well intentioned, this scenario repeats one that replays itself in many settings where traditional power structures are utilized in attempted problem solving. Given that the leadership equity gap was likely fostered by historic cis White male privilege, it is unlikely to be well received in this context. To prevent inertia, the working group should be an egalitarian and representative one that begins by asking what the experience, barriers and facilitators are for leadership growth before the group meets to discuss the background information, establish a mutually agreeable task list and prioritize the group's activities. Some degree of "pre-work" is often required in order to understand the scope of the problem and engage others in a shared sense of urgency that there is in fact a problem before a working group can then be struck to work on bridging the EDI gap.

We have now explored the chief issues, gaps and opportunities for action in medical leadership and the fabric of the medical establishment. The question is how to shift the system we know so well to one that fosters equity, diversity and inclusion at its core, and thus approaches the structural competence required to deliver responsible healthcare. The subsequent section will explore inclusion strategies, recognizing that there is no best or right answer, and that action is required at various levels, from internally within the field to intersectorial work.

Inclusion Strategies: How do we Build a Structurally Competent System?

❖

Responsible healthcare…..what is that?

❖

As previously defined, structural competence is the recognition and action on the ways in which institutions, neighborhood conditions, market forces, public policies, and healthcare delivery systems shape symptoms and diseases (Metzl and Hansen, 2014; Metzl and Hansen, 2018). Structural competence is the ideal state for medical education and training institutions, healthcare facilities and the broader infrastructures that constitute the fabric of society. This occurs when the health workforce and medical leadership reflects the diversity of the general population.

Politics, racism and socioeconomic status shape health status. Furthermore, it is well recognized that marginalization, racism and exclusion are notable factors in access to care, the quality of care received, and the lack of diversity in healthcare leadership (Metzl and Hansen, 2018; Gomez and Bernet, 2019; LaVeist and Pierre, 2014; Jackson and Gracia, 2014; Page, 2008). We also know enough to recognize that the interaction between these domains distributes risks inequitably across various groups. As such, healthcare is not a bedside phenomenon. Rather, responsible healthcare requires mobilization in order to correct inequalities as they manifest both in physician-patient interactions and beyond the clinic walls (Hansen and Metzl, 2017; Metzl and Hansen, 2018), as well as in the interpersonal dynamics and structure of the medical institutions from top down and across all ranks of the health education, training and clinical workforce. Are we ready to do this?

We are in fact primed and ready to chart the course as medical leaders. If we consider the four broad domains that interact to shape a state of structural competence (see Figure 4.1), the inroads for action are plentiful and range from quick wins to ongoing concerted action.

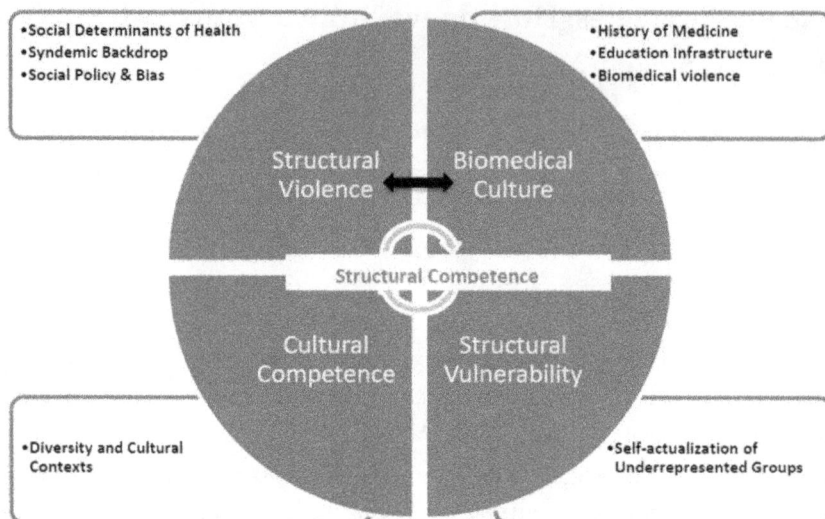

Figure 4.1. *Building a culture of health through structural competence. Competence (and its failure) arises through a nuanced interaction of four domains each of which shape the power structures in which patients, pupils and providers interact*

Figure 4.1 highlights intersectorial and internal avenues for thoughtful and concerted action. This is an exciting point in time. We now know enough about the relationships between the social impacts of identities (i.e., genderism, racism, transphobia etc.), health and disease patterns, and structural factors to begin acting on this knowledge in a more premeditated manner. In fact, this moment presents an unprecedented opportunity to begin training physicians for structural interventions (Farmer et al., 2006; Hansen and Metzl, 2017). For medical education and training leaders, this means a curriculum shift that is informed by contextual factors. Hansen and Metzl (2017) call for a shift towards the provision of more comprehensive healthcare such that students, trainees, and faculty engage with community organizations, non-health sector institutions (e.g., schools, corrections, housing), and policy makers to promote patient and community health.

The ability to pivot away from a context-devoid approach is strongly supported by the recognition of the effects of sociopolitical and economic factors interacting synergistically at multiple levels to collectively limit opportunity, generate poor health status and excess disease amongst populations experiencing marginalization (Farmer et al., 2006; Hansen and Metzl, 2017; Singer et al., 2017). Furthermore, training medical students, trainees and faculty in structural interventions will raise their awareness and mutual appreciation of the role social forces play on the interpersonal dynamics and structure of the medical institutions. It can foster increased understanding and commitment to addressing the systemic inequities that affect minoritized learners, staff and faculty.

In essence, when medical leadership steers a paradigm shift in education, training and institutional ethos, it stands to enrich learners, staff and faculty who can in turn administer that lifesaving breath to each other and to patients. The business case for this could not be stronger when one reconsiders the previous discussion of safe clinical spaces where patient experience, patient safety, professional wellbeing, and a critical staffing mass all interact favourably with the bottom line. Arguably, the Quintuple Aim can only be realized through this seismic but exciting and achievable shift. Institutionally, the intention and commitment to EDI needs to be translated into the structure and function of the institution through the commitment of medical leaders who inspire and are inspired by their staff, learners and patients.

The approach to achieving structural competence is a long road with a multipronged approach across many levels and multi-sectorial stakeholders (Adjo et al.; Farmer et al., 2006; Stewart et al., 2020). Stakeholders need to be committed to the time, effort, and more immediate investment the process would require to unfold. This is not an easy task, and token or superficial efforts will only waste already constrained resources, therefore embarking on the process requires firm commitment to the process of change. Some have stated that this process "requires a major disruption to culture and institutional practices that mask centuries of structural racism embedded within complex academic systems" (Smith et al., 2022). However, allowing the status quo to continue unchecked goes contrary to the commitment to do no harm as ultimately patients suffer the effects of inequitable clinical spaces directly when patients are themselves minoritized and indirectly when their healthcare provider(s) belong to minority groups that are subject to the ill effects of being othered.

At the individual practice level, there is a substantial knowledge gap amongst healthcare professionals when it comes to addressing bias in order to achieve structural competency (Ricks et al., 2022). There are several frameworks that have been suggested and being utilized at this time (Adjo et al., 2021; Alarcon et al. 2022; Deliz et al., 2020; Lin et al., 2017; Marja and Suvi, 2021). There are any number of recommended approaches to managing bias and a dense literature on their relative merits to inform healthcare providers and various institutions in their journey (Bisbey et al., 2021; Botelho and Lima, 2021; Homan et al., 2020). The key feature to the approaches is that they are dynamic, multipronged and require ongoing evaluation to ensure that goals are being achieved (Arruzza and Chau, 2021; Chae et al., 2020). No one size fits all and each system has to identify their deficiencies and prioritize the areas to be addressed.

At the pre-entry point to a potential career in medicine, high school programs should consider opportunities to increase the diversity of students taking subjects such as sciences, technology, engineering, math (STEM), humanities and music. Furthermore, undergraduate students should receive instrumental support in the pursuit of formative extracurricular activities such as volunteer experiences so that they can also grow, begin to recognize their potential and acquire a competitive edge in their applications for those who subsequently desire a STEM career or other competitive career.

At the entry point to medical education, leading with equity would result in changes that facilitate the recruitment of a diverse student pool that more closely resembles the local population. Efforts should be made to provide financial support to applicants from low-income brackets so that application fees and tuition fees are not prohibitive. Increasingly it is recognized that lived experience may in fact supersede academic rankings and the highest MCAT score. Faculty involved in the selection process, whether application review or interview, should routinely attend implicit bias training.

Finally, medical education materials should reflect the diversity of humanity, with textbooks showing medical conditions in various shades of skin and the cultural shades of symptom presentation. Structural and cultural sensitivity should be ingrained in the curriculum, including awareness of the local history of the institution. The curriculum should also incorporate other ways of knowing such as oral histories and storytelling. Storytelling and oral histories are a part of many cultures as the spoken word predates the written word. Storytelling has been used to share the history of many Indigenous peoples globally to teach morals and cultures (Hare, 2011; McKeough, 2008), as well as to teach the impact of colonialism (Edosomwan and Peterson, 2016). Storytelling also provided a method for marginalized groups to share the tales that colonial history did not document.

Storytelling has been used for resistance against colonialism and to preserve culture and history (Sium and Ritskes, 2013). It is also used to teach children about the world, societal expectations, and morality. These varied and compelling uses of storytelling suggest that it should be utilized more in the medical curriculum to teach about the patient experience and to ground education in contextual factors that enrich the understanding of the syndemic factors at play in disease. Stories from diverse cultural backgrounds should be included as a method of building cultural competence, instilling cultural humility and teaching active listening.

Traditional recruitment methods have not been adequate in bringing forward a truly diverse applicant pool (Davenport et al., 2022). Those who may not think that a medical career is even an option for them need to see themselves in those in the medical field. Targeted recruitment strategies are required at the applicant stage, but the seed can be planted long before this stage. School teachers and guidance counsellors should be aware of the need for diversity to be reflected in all areas and perhaps medical schools should be actively linked to their communities to provide opportunities for shadowing and educational drop-ins.

In Canada, the expansion of programs such as the Communities of Support at the University of Toronto across all universities (with or without a medical school) was undertaken to provide support and mentorship through the medical school application process. The success of this program is further evidence that communities and agencies need to be involved to address the issue of diversity in medicine (Saddler et al., 2021). The expansion of similar programs will lead to improved diversity as well as linking universities with their communities in a more closely aligned fashion.

On entry into medical school, there are multiple ways in which equity, diversity, inclusion, indigenization and accountability can be infused into the curriculum. Although not exhaustive, Table 4.1 demonstrates some such examples of leading with equity in medical education. It may be beneficial to give careful consideration to the prospect of rotations or longitudinal projects in social justice.

Table 4.1. *Examples of leading with equity in Medical Education.*

Areas of Diversification	Examples
Case Based Learning	Employ diverse genders and sexual orientation Show common presentations in various skin tones Standardized patients should also reflect the diversity within the population Showcase racial differences in presentation of healthcare problems (Uzelli Yilmaz et al., 2022)
Language	In discussion of patients and family units. Avoid using traditional cis gendered nomenclature e.g., 'mother and father' for parental figures or caregivers
Approach to Counseling	Discussion of dietary approaches to include the importance of asking about the patient's traditional foods and their components so that any dietary advice can be given in the appropriate context

As medical students and trainees progress in their studies, they also explore their leadership potential. There are significant differences in the leadership opportunities afforded to various minorities in medicine; further discussion about this is available in the racism, identity politics and gendered discussions in Chapters 5-10. Ideally a variety of leadership development support and mentorship are made available, and various routes and styles of leadership are explored. This includes leadership styles that are more focused on soft power, distributive leadership, collaboration, and consensus building, rather than more autocratic and centralized styles. It may also be helpful to undertake reviews of the pathways that led current leaders to where they are today. Consider Figure 4.2 as a guide for this review.

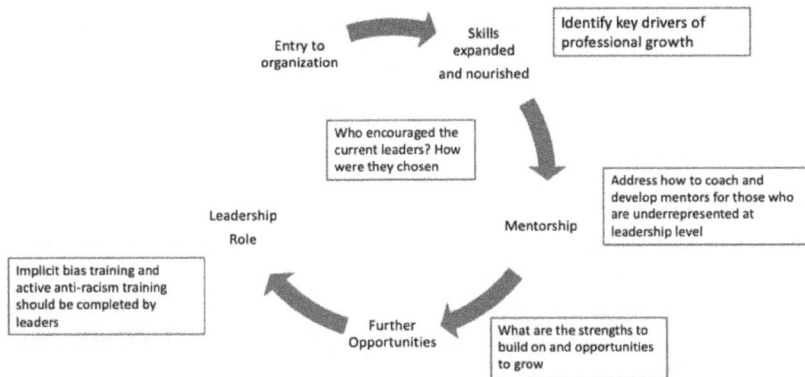

Figure 4.2 *An Example of a Leadership Pathway Audit highlighting various stages for appraisal and potential areas of growth.*

Key Takeaways

- Medical leadership and the medical climate are far from benign as they harbor centuries of structural bias embedded within complex academic, clinical and regulatory systems.
- Responsible healthcare is the key accountability for medical leadership.
- Responsible healthcare rests on creating and maintaining structural competence within the medical establishment and broader medical field.
- Training physicians in structural interventions can facilitate health equity impacts beyond the clinic walls.
- Multifactorial sources of homogeneity within the medical education, training and leadership ranks begin upstream and maintain the pipeline of diversity at a trickle.
- There have been notable EDI failures and thus, less than responsible healthcare stemming from a lack of representative curricular material and bias perpetrated through the reference materials used over time in medical education. Curricular representativeness is a matter of physician competence.
- The business case for diversity and equity for both providers and patients alike is undeniable and favours the bottom line in an age of diminishing resources.

- Shifting to structural competence in medicine and healthcare will entail a seismic but achievable and necessary shift in order for the profession to truly *do no harm*.

Conclusion

Medical leadership constitutes the chief organizing hub of the medical field, establishing and synchronizing education, training, regulatory requirements and the administration of healthcare as it dispenses its key accountability of responsible healthcare. As demonstrated over the course of the chapter, there has been much growth and maturation in this complex system, however there are still some outstanding EDI gaps for the patients, learners and physicians at the centre of the system.

Although the equity gaps for patients and providers from traditionally underrepresented groups represent a broader failure of society, they also represent a failure of medical leadership. Paradoxically, shifting towards the structural competence required for responsible healthcare is good practice- it is an investment that pays as it is tied with improved care experiences, improved patient outcomes and enhanced professional satisfaction, all of which move us closer to the Quintuple Aim. Subsequent chapters will again identify the enrichment and system benefits that arise from a diverse and inclusive health workforce practicing in an equitable environment.

The task of shifting towards structural competence may appear daunting but the time is now; in fact, the time is well past, and the opportunities are limitless. The most exciting feature of medical leadership today is the fact that it is dynamic and innovative, with the capacity to bridge the equity gap. There are any number of low hanging fruits, from intervening at the pre-entry and entry points into medical education to recognizing and addressing the inequitable access to opportunity within the trajectory from medical training to practice years when physicians are primed and ready to grow, advocate and realize their potential as healthcare leaders. There is no better time than now to begin creating more virtuous social cycles, starting with medical leadership.

On a Parting Note...

'We see you, Black woman leader, your tree so tall and strong'

They chant this at me while sitting on my gnarled exposed roots

'Come mentor our future, these young saplings need you'

But where is my mentor on this journey

I may have grown against the odds but my tree has no leaves

My branches are bare, withered, and hardened

Nourish me so I can nourish others

Show kindness

So I can share of a tale of growth with you rather than a tale of growth despite you

©Zainab Abdurrahman, 2022

References

Adjo, J., Maybank, A. and Prakash, V. (2021) 'Building inclusive work environments', *Pediatrics*, 148 (Supplement 2). p. 9. https://doi.org/10.1542/peds.2021-051440e.

Alarcon, B.O., O'Connor, L., Rowan, S., Henson, B.S., Doan Van, A.E., Simeteys, P. and Watanabe, M.K. (2022). 'Bringing structural competency to the forefront of dental education'. *Journal of Dental Education, 86*(9), pp.1083-1089.

Aiken, R. (2018). *Senate repeals 1918 'colour ban' on Black medical students*, November 2, 2018 [online]. Available from: https://www.queensjournal.ca/story/2018-11-02/news/senate-repeals-1918-colour-bar-on-black-medical-students/

Allen, U., Collins, T., Dei, G.J., Henry, F., Ibrahim, A., James, C., Jean-Pierre, J., Kobayashi, A., Lewis, K., McKenzie, K. and Mawani, R. (2021). 'Impacts of COVID-19 in racialized communities'. Royal Society of Canada.

Arruzza, E. and Chau, M. (2021). 'The effectiveness of cultural competence education in enhancing knowledge acquisition, performance, attitudes, and student satisfaction among undergraduate health science students: A scoping review', *Journal of Educational Evaluation for Health Professions*, 18, p. 3. https://doi.org/10.3352/jeehp.2021.18.3.

Ayyala, M.S., Skarupski, K., Bodurtha, J.N., González-Fernández, M., Ishii, L.E., Fivush, B. and Levine, R.B. (2019). 'Mentorship is not enough: exploring sponsorship and its role in career advancement in academic medicine', *Academic Medicine, 94*(1), pp. 94-100.

Botelho, M.J. and C.A. Lima. (2020). 'From Cultural Competence to Cultural Respect: A Critical Review of Six Models', *Journal of Nursing Education, 59*(6), pp. 311-318.

Bisbey, T.M., Kilcullen, M.P., Thomas, E.J., Ottosen, M.J., Tsao, K. and Salas, E. (2021). 'Safety culture: An integration of existing models and a framework for understanding its development', *Human factors, 63*(1), pp. 88-110.

Bryant, T., Raphael, D., Schrecker, T., Labonte, R. (2011) 'Canada: A land of missed opportunity for addressing the Social Determinants of Health', *Health Policy*, 101(1), pp. 44–58. https://doi.org/10.1016/j.healthpol.2010.08.022.

Chae, D., Kim, J., Kim, S., Lee, J. and Park, S. (2020). 'Effectiveness of cultural competence educational interventions on health professionals and patient outcomes: A systematic review', *Japan Journal of Nursing Science, 17*(3), p.e12326.

Chaffins, S., Forbes, M., Fuqua, H.E., Jr. and Cangemi, J.P. (1995) 'The glass ceiling: are women where they should be?', *Education*, [online] 115(3), 380. Available from: https://link.gale.com/apps/doc/A17039288/AONE?u=anon~c74a3177&sid=goog leScholar&xid=f864cfb5

Crey, K., & Hanson, E. (2009) Indian Status [online]. Available from: https://indigenousfoundations.arts.ubc.ca/indian_status/

Davidson, M. J., & Cooper, C. L. (1992). *Shattering the glass ceiling: The woman manager*. Paul Chapman Publishing.

Davenport, D., Natesan, S., Caldwell, M.T., Gallegos, M., Landry, A., Parsons, M. and Gottlieb, M. (2022). 'Faculty recruitment, retention, and representation in leadership: an evidence-based guide to best practices for diversity, equity, and inclusion from the council of residency directors in emergency medicine', *Western Journal of Emergency Medicine*, 23(1), p.62.

Deliz, J.R., Fears, F.F., Jones, K.E., Tobat, J., Char, D. and Ross, W.R. (2020). 'Cultural competency interventions during medical school: a scoping review and narrative synthesis', *Journal of General Internal Medicine*, 35(2), pp. 568-577.

Edosomwan, S. and Peterson, C.M. (2016). A History of Oral and Written Storytelling in Nigeria [online]. Available from: https://eric.ed.gov/ ?id=ED581846

Equality and Human Rights Commission. (2011). Public Sector Equality Duty [online]. https://www.equalityhumanrights.com/en/advice-and-guidance/public -sector-equality-duty

Farmer, P.E., Nizeye, B., Stulac, S. and Keshavjee, S. (2006). 'Structural violence and clinical medicine', *PLoS Medicine*, 3(10), p.e449.

Gomez, L.E., Bernet, P. 'Diversity improves performance and outcomes'. *Journal of the National Medical Association*. (2019). 111(4), 383-392. doi: 10.1016/j.jnma. 2019.01.006.

Hansen, H. and Metzl, J.M. (2017). 'New medicine for the US health care system: training physicians for structural interventions', *Academic Medicine: Journal of the Association of American Medical Colleges*, 92(3), p.279.

Hare, J. (2011). 'They tell a story and there's meaning behind that story: Indigenous knowledge and Young Indigenous Children's literacy learning,' *Journal of Early Childhood Literacy*, 12(4), pp. 389–414. https://doi.org/10.1177/1468798411417378.

Homan A.C., Gündemir S., Buengeler C., and van Kleef G.A. (2020). 'Leading diversity: Towards a theory of functional leadership in diverse teams', *J Appl Psychol*, 105(10), pp.1101-1128.

Jackson, C.S. and Gracia, J.N. (2014) 'Addressing health and health-care disparities: The role of a diverse workforce and the social determinants of health', *Public Health Reports*, 129(1_suppl2), pp. 57–61. https://doi.org/10.1177/003335 49141291s211.

Khan, R., Apramian, T., Kang, J.H., Gustafson, J. and Sibbald, S. (2020). 'Demographic and socioeconomic characteristics of Canadian medical students: a cross-sectional study', *BMC medical education*, 20(1), pp.1-8.

Kwong, J.C., Dhalla, I.A., Streiner, D.L., Baddour, R.E., Waddell, A.E. and Johnson, I.L. (2002). 'Effects of rising tuition fees on medical school class composition and financial outlook', *CMAJ*, *166*(8), pp. 1023-1028.

LaVeist, T.A. and Pierre, G. (2014). 'Integrating the 3Ds—social determinants, health disparities, and health-care workforce diversity', *Public Health Reports*, *129*(1_suppl2), pp. 9-14.

Lin, C.J., Lee, C.K. and Huang, M.C. (2017). 'Cultural competence of healthcare providers: A systematic review of assessment instruments', *Journal of Nursing Research*, 25(3), pp. 174-186.

Livingston, S. (2018). 'Racism Is Still a Problem in Healthcare's C-Suite: Efforts Aimed at Boosting Diversity in Healthcare Leadership Fail to Make Progress', *Journal of Best Practices in Health Professions Diversity*, [online] 11(1), 60–65. Available from https://www.jstor.org/stable/26554292

Lucey, C.R. and Saguil, A. (2020). 'The consequences of structural racism on MCAT scores and medical school admissions: the past is prologue', *Academic Medicine*, 95(3), pp. 351-356.

Marja, S.L. and Suvi, A. (2021). 'Cultural competence learning of the health care students using simulation pedagogy: An integrative review', *Nurse Education in Practice*, 52, p.103044.

McKenzie, K., (2020). 'Race and ethnicity data collection during COVID-19 in Canada: if you are not counted you cannot count on the pandemic response', In *Royal Society of Canada* Vol. 12 November.

McCarty Kilian, C., Hukai, D. and Elizabeth McCarty, C. (2005). 'Building diversity in the pipeline to corporate leadership', *Journal of Management Development*, 24(2), pp. 155-168.

McKeough, A., Bird, S., Tourigny, E., Romaine, A., Graham, S., Ottmann, J. and Jeary, J. (2008). 'Storytelling as a foundation to literacy development for Aboriginal children: Culturally and developmentally appropriate practices', *Canadian Psychology / Psychologie canadienne*, 49(2), pp. 148–154. https://doi.org/10.1037/0708-5591.49.2.148.

Menezes, A., Henry, S. and Agarwal, G. (2022). 'It's High Time Canada started collecting race-based performance data on medical training and Careers', *The Lancet Regional Health - Americas*, 14, p. 100326. https://doi.org/10.1016/j.lana.2022.100326.

Metzl, J.M., Hansen, H. (2014). 'Structural competency: theorizing a new medical engagement with stigma and inequality', *Social Science and Medicine*, 103, pp. 126–133.

Metzl J.M., Hansen, H. (2018). 'Structural Competency and Psychiatry'. *JAMA Psychiatry*, 75(2), pp.115-116. https://doi: 10.1001/jamapsychiatry.2017.3891.

Munroe, M., (2022). 'The Need for Race Based Data in Canada', *University of Toronto Medical Journal*, 99(3).

Nguemeni Tiako, M.J., Ray, V. and South, E.C., (2022). 'Medical schools as racialized organizations: How race-neutral structures sustain racial inequality in medical education — A narrative review', *Journal of General Internal Medicine*, pp. 1-8.

Nobel, C., (2012). 'The Case Against Racial Colorblindness", *HBS Working Knowledge* [online] Feb 13, 2012, Available from: https://hbswk.hbs.edu/item/the-case-against-racial-colorblindness.

Nobles, A., Martin, B.A., Casimir, J., Schmitt, S. and Broadbent, G., (2022). "Stalled progress: medical school dean demographics', *The Journal of the American Board of Family Medicine*, 35(1), pp. 163-168.

Nundy, S., Cooper, L.A. and Mate, K.S. (2022). 'The quintuple aim for Health Care Improvement', *JAMA*, 327(6), p. 521. https://doi.org/10.1001/jama.2021.25181.

Ontario Colleges. (2023). Paying for College: Tuition and Financial Assistance [online]. Available from: https://www.ontariocolleges.ca/en/colleges/paying-for-college

Page, S.E. (2008). *The difference: How the power of diversity creates better groups, firms, schools, and Societies.* Princeton, NJ: Princeton University Press.

Purcell, D., MacArthur, K.R. and Samblanet, S. (2010). 'Gender and the glass ceiling at work', *Sociology Compass*, 4(9), pp. 705–717. https://doi.org/10.1111/j.1751-9020.2010.00304.x.

Ramanan, R.A., Taylor, W.C., Davis, R.B. and Phillips, R.S. (2006). 'Mentoring matters: mentoring and career preparation in internal medicine residency training', *Journal of General Internal Medicine*, 21(4), pp. 340-345.

Ricks, T.N., Abbyad, C. and Polinard, E. (2022). 'Undoing racism and mitigating bias among healthcare professionals: lessons learned during a systematic review', *Journal of Racial and Ethnic Health Disparities*, 9(5), pp. 1990-2000.

Rodriguez, J. E., Campbell, K. M., & Adelson, W. J. (2015). Poor representation of Blacks, Latinos, and Native Americans in medicine. *Family medicine*, 47(4), pp. 259–263.

Rodríguez, J. E., Figueroa, E., Campbell, K. M., Washington, J. C., Amaechi, O., Anim, T., et al. (2022). Towards a common lexicon for equity, diversity, and inclusion work in academic medicine. *BMC medical education*, 22(1), 703. https://doi.org/10.1186/s12909-022-03736-6.

Ruzycki, S.M., Franceschet, S. and Brown, A. (2021). 'Making medical leadership more diverse'. *British Medical Journal*, p.373.

Salsberg, E., Richwine, C., Westergaard, S., Martinez, M.P., Oyeyemi, T., Vichare, A. and Chen, C.P. (2021). 'Estimation and comparison of current and future racial/ethnic representation in the US health care workforce', *JAMA Network Open*, 4(3), pp.e213789-e213789.

Saddler, N., Adams, S., Robinson, L.A. and Okafor, I. (2021). 'Taking initiative in addressing diversity in medicine', *Canadian Journal of Science, Mathematics and Technology Education*, 21(2), pp. 309-320.

Schrubbe, K.F. (2004). 'Mentorship: A Critical Component for Professional Growth and Academic Success', *Journal of Dental Education*, 68, pp324-328.

Sergeant, A., Saha, S., Lalwani, A., Sergeant, A., McNair, A., Larrazabal, E., Yang, K., Bogler, O., Dhoot, A., Werb, D. and Maghsoudi, N. (2022). 'Diversity among health care leaders in Canada: a cross-sectional study of perceived gender and race', *CMAJ*, 194(10), pp. E371-E377.

Shen, M.R., Tzioumis, E., Andersen, E., Wouk, K., McCall, R., Li, W., Girdler, S. and Malloy, E. (2022). 'Impact of mentoring on academic career success for women in medicine: a systematic review', *Academic Medicine*, 97(3), pp. 444-458.

Simonsen, K.A. and Shim, R.S. (2019). 'Embracing diversity and inclusion in psychiatry leadership.' *Psychiatric Clinics*, 42(3), pp. 463-471.

Sium, A., and Ritskes, E. (2013). 'Speaking truth to power: Indigenous storytelling as an act of living resistance.' *Decolonization: Indigeneity, Education & Society*, 2(1), pp 1-10.

Smith, S.G., Banks, P.B., Istrate, E.C., Davis, A.J., Johnson, K.R. and West, K.P. (2022). 'Anti-racism structures in academic dentistry: Supporting underrepresented racially/ethnically diverse faculty', *Journal of Public Health Dentistry*, 82, pp.103-113.

Soklaridis, S., Lin, E., Black, G., Paton, M., LeBlanc, C., Besa, R., et al. (2022). 'Moving beyond 'think leadership, think white male': the contents and contexts of equity, diversity and inclusion in physician leadership programmes', *BMJ leader*, 6(2), pp. 146–157. https://doi.org/10.1136/leader-2021-000542.

Stewart, A.J., Shim, R.S. and Trivedi, H.K. eds. 2020. *Achieving mental health equity*. Elsevier.

Statistics Canada. (2021). Data products, 2016 Census [online]. Available from: https://www12.statcan.gc.ca/census-recensement/2016/dp-pd/index-eng.cfm

Statistics Canada. (2021). Tuition fees for degree programs, 2021/2022 [online]. Available at: https://www150.statcan.gc.ca/n1/daily-quotidien/210908/dq210908 a-eng.htm

Steele, C. M., & Aronson, J. (1995). Stereotype threat and the intellectual test performance of African Americans. *Journal of personality and social psychology*, 69(5), pp. 797–811. https://doi.org/10.1037//0022-3514.69.5.797.

Singer, M., Bulled, N., Ostrach, B. and Mendenhall, E. (2017). 'Syndemics and the biosocial conception of health', *The Lancet*, 389(10072), pp. 941-950.

Thompson, E., Edjoc, R., Atchessi, N., Striha, M., Gabrani-Juma, I. and Dawson, T. (2021). 'COVID-19: A case for the collection of race data in Canada and abroad', *Canada Communicable Disease Report*, 47(7-8), p.300.

Uzelli Yilmaz, D., Azim, A. and Sibbald, M. (2022). 'The Role of Standardized Patient Programs in Promoting Equity, Diversity, and Inclusion: A Narrative Review', *Academic Medicine*, 97(3), pp. 459-468.

Part 2.
What is the Status Quo and What are the Issues?

Chapter 5
The Parity Smokescreen: The Gendered Experience of Wom*n in Medicine

Emma Gregory, MD, Noam Raiter, MD, Ana Hategan, MD,
Mariam Abdurrahman, MD

❖

"To call woman the weaker sex is a libel; it is man's injustice to woman"
—Mahatma Gandhi, 1930

❖

Abstract: There has been increased representation of women in medicine over time, leading some to believe that gender equity has been achieved. However, there is ample evidence that gender inequity is widespread for women and gender diverse physicians. This chapter explores systemic causes of gender inequity that are rooted in antiquated gender norms, roles, and relations, with a focus on women, as gender diversity will be covered more extensively in Chapter 6. Next, this chapter outlines examples of inequities experienced by gendered persons in medicine, including an exploration of the consequences at the physician, patient, institutional and systems level. Finally, evidence-based interventions to reduce gender inequity in medicine will be reviewed with the goal of inspiring further initiatives.

Keywords: *gender, gender equity, gender bias, gender discrimination, non-binary, women in medicine, transgender*

Introduction: A Brief History of Gender Inequity in Medicine

Gone are the days when physicians across North America were only, or most likely, to be White, heterosexual, and cisgender men. There has been improvement in the representation of equity-deserving groups in medicine, including women. However, this is a fairly recent change given that medicine has historically excluded gendered persons. This history of exclusion is heavily reflected in the chronicles of the female gender. In fact, many of the early practices of medicine very much relied on the male gaze and its patriarchal custody of women's minds and bodies, as exemplified by the origins of hysteria, the asylum committal of non-conforming women and resistance to women's entry into the profession (Jefferson et al., 2015; Newman et al., 2020; Starr, 1982). Nonetheless, the female gender's presence in the profession has evolved from the role of patient alone, to that of increasing professional representation. The historical absence of female clinicians has evolved over time from limited presence to broad presence in the profession, however representation from the broader gender diverse spectrum remains very low.

Despite the increased presence of women and gender diverse physicians in the profession, the traditional ways of recognizing and validating professional contributions have not kept apace. In fact, the meritocracy in medicine continues to be a gendered experience in spite of the near on par presence of women in the profession and the increased representation of non-binary physicians. The toll of continued gender bias and inequity bodes poorly for career satisfaction, physician wellbeing and in turn, clinical outcomes for patients (Baumhäkel, Müller, and Böhm, 2009; Berthold et al., 2008; CMA, 2018; Frank et al., 2013; Jefferson et al., 2013; Joseph et al, 201; Kang and Kaplan, 2019; Kim et al., 2005; Kruger et al., 2012; Ramirez et al., 2009; Smith et al., 2011; Tsugawa et al, 2017; Wallis et al., 2022).

The Rise of Women in Medicine

There has been a significant increase in the number of women medical trainees (which include medical students, residents, and fellows) and practicing physicians. For example, women reached gender parity in Canadian medical schools by 1995, and accounted for nearly 60% of first-year medical students from 2020 to 2021 (AFMC, 2020). Similarly, women accounted for nearly 60% of first-year residents from 2021 to 2022 (CAPER, 2021). The irony of celebrating gender parity in medicine in the 1990s is not lost on anyone. This is in direct contrast to the complete absence of women formally in medicine until the mid-1800s in some countries (Starr, 1982).

In 1972, Title IX of the Education Amendments law passed in the United States, which prohibited sex discrimination in federally-funded educational activities and programs (DOJ, 2021). Thereafter, the number of women in medicine exponentially increased (Starr, 1982). Yet there has not been a similar trajectory for gender diverse persons, and they remain conspicuous by their absence, as explored in detail in Chapter 6. Gender diverse persons have been historically excluded from medicine altogether, or made invisible due to fear of disclosure (DOJ, 2021; Madrigal et al., 2021). Given the paucity of research on gender diverse persons (Westafer et al., 2022), much of this chapter focuses on women's experiences.

Indeed, the lack of research on gender diversity in medicine is itself a reflection of gender inequity. Topics of gender bias and equity are often dominated by a binary discussion which reflects the extent of the problem as gender diverse trainees and physicians are rarely included (Westafer et al., 2022). Given the scarcity of the gender diverse perspective, one hopes that future research will expand to explore the lived experiences and perspectives of gender diverse physicians.

Professional Vignette

Early on in medical school, we had a morning dedicated to wellness lectures including one that caught my attention – "Women in Medicine." Even before I stepped foot into medical school, I was warned about the "old boys club." I feared I would have to give up my femininity in order to fit in. However, seeing these women physicians gave me hope that field was changing, and I could be part of that change. The first half of the discussion made me feel connected, revitalized, and inspired. That was until one woman peer asked, "Do you have advice on starting a family during residency?" One panelist answered, "With enough advanced planning, I had a child during my second year with nearly no repercussions from my program."

Another panelist jumped in and reminded us of the rates of infertility, miscarriage, and other pregnancy complications among women physicians. The first panelist sighed, softly saying, "Yes, I tried to have a second child, but I had several miscarriages. I guess the high stress and lack of sleep were just too much. I told myself I would try again, but I need full-time childcare to help me raise one child. I don't think it would be feasible to have more. That's just the price I paid for medicine." She meekly smiled and shrugged, and the other panelists nodded knowingly as if it was all so ordinary and expected that women must sacrifice themselves for medicine. After that discussion, I could not get the panelists' soft words and knowing nods out of my head.

Professional Vignette Analysis

Based on the experiences described in the vignette, the medical student was experiencing gender inequity although perhaps from an unwitting source – other women. Some of the questions that may have run through her head afterwards were: Why did the staff mention repercussions in the first place? Why do women physicians experience higher rates of infertility, miscarriage, and other pregnancy complications (Rangel et al., 2021)? Why could the staff not spend more time with her child? What would be the consequences if she did? Why should they accept that this is the best that women in medicine get? Surely, "that's just the price I paid" cannot be acceptable.

This chapter will illustrate the effect of the 'masculinity' of medicine as this has shaped and solidified gendered expectations about women in medicine and women as patients. These expectations have been so deeply normalized that some medical trainees and practicing physicians may not even realize their own degree of internalization and/or how they continue to perpetuate these messages. This unfortunately becomes part of the hidden or silent curriculum that is passed onto more junior trainees and physicians unless there are systems in place to challenge this messaging effectively. Keep this vignette in mind as the chapter successively explores some of the contributing factors to gender inequity in medicine, the lived experiences of gendered physicians, and the toll it takes on these physicians and their local ecosystem.

Pause and Reflect: What Do We (Not) Know about Gender Bias and Equity?

Assessing Perceptions, Presumption and Position

Similar to many equity-based topics, it is often helpful to take stock of what you *do* know before you start considering what you *do not* and what you would like to know. Below are several questions to help you think about gender bias and equity in medicine.

- What is my gender identity? How do I express it? Do I share it with others readily?
- Does my gender identity give me privilege? Why? Why not? Do my other social identities intersect with gender (e.g., age, sex, race/ethnicity)? How so?
- What have I been taught about gender to date? How have I been taught about this? Do I agree with what I have learned? Why? Why not?
- Am I comfortable discussing gender, gender bias, and gender discrimination in medicine with peers, colleagues, and patients? Why? Why not?
- What gender equity initiatives have I seen or experienced in medicine so far? Who is included in these initiatives? Who is missing? Why?
- What would I like to see changed in terms of gender equity in medicine? Why is this important to me? Who is most responsible for making these changes?

The Issues

Systemic causes of gender inequity in medicine

Given the male-female gender parity in medical school and residency programs in some countries, gender inequity in medicine cannot simply be reduced to a "numbers in the pipeline" argument anymore (Kang and Kaplan, 2019). Yet when individuals hear about ongoing gender inequity, some may still be quick to blame other factors such as work location, specialty choice, work hours, experience, and seniority (CMA, 2018). This outlook is not only reductive of the gendered experience in medicine, but it also ignores significant evidence that indicates systemic causes of gender inequity. In fact, many studies that provide evidence for systemic causes, such as in remuneration, do so because they have already controlled for these factors (CMA, 2018).

Some individuals may defend against the uncomfortable truth that medicine has historically maintained the status and power of cisgender men. Similar to other societal institutions, medicine has been rooted in a patriarchy that marginalized women trainees and physicians, allied health colleagues, and patients alike (Newman et al., 2020). It has done so by legitimizing, and therefore normalizing, biases based on socially-constructed gender norms, roles, and relations (Tricco et al., 2021). For example, physicians have historically reinforced a binary sex and gender through birth gender assignment based on sex, framed women as the "weaker" gender, and supported that they were best suited for marriage, child rearing, and homemaking, and not for work in "demanding" careers or positions (Newman et al., 2020).

Today gender bias and discrimination takes various forms by peers, colleagues, and patients at the individual, organizational, and systemic levels. For example, women are more likely to experience subtle biases such as assumptions that they are nurses or cleaners, and are also more likely not to be addressed by their professional title; women are also more likely to be asked for their credentials (Dellasega et al., 2020). Despite laws and policies, women may still experience overt sex- and gender-based verbal and physical harassment and violence in their learning and work environments (Dellasega et al., 2020). However, this chapter will focus on biases in policies and procedures that can lead to gender-based discrimination and can negatively affect work, livelihood, and wellbeing (CMA, 2018) as these are closely tied with important sequelae like burnout, patient care experiences and patient outcomes.

There has been much rhetoric about the role of cisgender men in perpetuating gender inequity in medicine, however this is not the full picture. In fact, it is recognized that women themselves also internalize gendered expectations, and perpetuate inequity against themselves, as well as other women and gender diverse persons (Byerly, 2018; Hui et al., 2020). While relatively little is known about the experiences of gender diverse persons in medicine, they challenge the existing narrative of gender norms, roles, and relations. As such, they are relegated to the utmost margins of gender identity, and are likely at greatest risk of gender bias and discrimination (Madrigal et al., 2021).

Gender as a Social Construct

A number of gender-related terminology that may be less familiar to some individuals have been used so far. Thus before further reviewing examples of gender inequity in medicine, a glossary of common gender-related terms and definitions have been provided in Table 5.1 as well as in the subsequent chapter on 2SLGBTQ+ identities (Chapter 6) and the EDI Lexicon. These terms are not universal. They are fluid across time and space, and they do not have one best or correct definition. Their meaning may differ according to those that coined them, institutionalized them, reclaimed them, and/or individually or communally relate to them.

This chapter does not focus on "sex," which is a human-made classification system based on attributes such as "chromosomes, gene expression, hormone levels and function, and reproductive/sexuality anatomy" (CIHR, 2020). Instead, the focus is on "gender," which is another human-made classification system based on attributes such as "socially constructed roles, behaviours, expressions, and identities of girls, women, boys, men, and gender diverse people" (CIHR, 2020). As such, "gender is not something we are born with, and not something we have, but something we do–

something we perform" (Eckert and McConnell-Ginet, as cited in Lippi et al., 2020). Despite many cultures across time and space having a variety of gender identities, Eurocentric cultures (implicitly regarding European cultures as preeminent) often still consider gender to be binary, and thus further marginalize gender diverse persons (Yarbrough, Kidd, and Parekh, 2017).

Table 5.1. *Glossary of gender-related terms in alphabetical order.*

Term	Definition
Cisgender	A person who conforms to sex-/ gender-based societal expectations; also considered a person whose sex assigned at birth matches their gender identity; also considered gender normative; not someone who is transgender
Cisgenderism	Within the sex/gender binaries, it is the assumption that every person is cisgender; also considered the assumption that every person must conform to sex-/gender-based societal expectations; also considered the subjugation of a person or group that is not cisgender
Gender	A system of classifying persons according to socially expected attributes, e.g., constructed roles, behaviours, expressions, and identities; often constructed as a binary framework
Genderism	Within the gender binary, it is the assumption that every person must conform to gender-based societal expectations; also considered the subjugation of a person or group based on their gender
Gender bias	Refers to a person or group receiving different treatment based on their real or perceived gender identity
Gender discrimination	Refers to a person or group receiving disadvantaged treatment based on their real or perceived gender identity
Gender expression	How a person expresses their gender identity
Gender identity	How a person identifies their own gender
Gender norms	Within the gender binary, these refer to ideas of how boys/men and girls/women should appear, communicate, and behave in society
Gender roles	Within the gender binary, these refer to the roles and responsibilities that are assigned to boys/men and girls/women at home, work, and in society

Term	Definition ...*continued*
Gender relations	Within the gender binary, these refer to relationship dynamics between boys/men and girls/women which can lead to inequities in power
Nonbinary	A person whose gender identity is beyond the gender-binary; can include identities such as being agender, genderqueer, gender fluid, or gender nonconforming, among others
Transgender	A person whose gender identity differs from societal expectations of masculinity or femininity; also considered a person whose sex assigned at birth does not match their gender identity; not someone who is cisgender
Transphobia	An irrational fear or hatred of persons who are, or are perceived to be, transgender

Sources: (CIHR, 2020; Cornell, 2020; EIGE, 2022; Langston, 2020; McMaster, 2015; Tricco et al., 2021).

Systemic Gender Inequity in Medicine

❖

*"Freedom cannot be achieved unless the women
have been emancipated from all forms of oppression."*
—Nelson Mandela, 2004

❖

Gendered medical trainees and practicing physicians disproportionately experience gender bias in medicine. Gender inequities experienced by women are well-described in areas such as training, employment, academics and leadership, advancement, remuneration, retention, and safety (Tricco et al., 2021). While inequities experienced by gender diverse persons are yet to be well studied, there are emerging reports of similar experiences to women, including having few concordant mentors, underfunding of relevant research, and bias against faculty promotion (Sánchez et al., 2015). There are also reports of unique experiences such as transphobia, being misgendered, fear of disclosure, and fear of job or license loss (Westafer et al., 2022).

Gender Inequities Faced by Women in Medicine

Gender inequities are likely to follow women in medicine from training through to practice, as summarized in Table 5.2. (Adesoye et al., 2017; Barch and Yee, 2011; Buell et al., 2018; CMA, 2019; Fnais et al., 2014; Fridner et al., 2015; Jagsi et al., 2016; Jena et al., 2015; Kralj, 2019; Levine et al., 2013; Merman et al., 2018; Sambunjak et al., 2006; Silver et al., 2017; Tockey and Ignatova, 2018; Travis et al., 2013; Trix and Psenka, 2003; Witteman et al., 2019). The "numbers in the pipeline" issue has become one of a leaky pipeline that is pushing women out of medicine (Kang and Kaplan, 2019). Indeed, women are more likely to leave academic medicine earlier and at a faster rate than men (Jena et al., 2015).

As early as medical school, women may still be encouraged by practicing physicians in supervisory and other roles to pursue specialties based on gendered expectations. While some individuals argue that these recommendations merely reflect what is known about work-life balance in some specialties, the recommendations are often proffered as unsolicited advice. It may be assumed that women want to start a family in residency or early career, and so they are discouraged from pursuing "demanding" specialties in favour of primary care (Levine et al., 2018). This in itself is a paradox as primary care is no less rigorous or demanding than other specialities, and in fact there are elevated rates of burnout in primary care.

Women made up only 30% of surgical specialists in Canada in 2019, and were severely underrepresented in cardiac (8.7%), neuro (10.6%), and cardiothoracic (10.7%) surgery (CMA, 2019). When women are underrepresented in certain specialties, this results in a dearth of women mentors and sponsors available to more junior trainees and physicians (Sambunjak et al., 2006; Travis et al., 2013). Limited mentorship and sponsorship opportunities can also impact specialty choice, academic and leadership opportunities, and career advancement (Sambunjak et al., 2006; Travis et al., 2013).

In terms of applications, business studies have found that women are less likely to apply to positions unless they meet 100% of the hiring criteria (Tockey and Ignatova, 2018). In comparison, men are more likely to apply when they meet just 60% of the criteria, thus increasing their chances of being considered for a position (Tockey and Ignatova, 2018). Women are also often hired based on previous experience (Barch and Yee, 2011), perhaps contributing to the practice of self-screening themselves out of applying. Whereas men are often hired based on future potential (Barch and Yee, 2011), perhaps contributing to men's self-assurance in applying to positions with less skills and experience.

In academic medicine, women are underrepresented in research, publications, presentations, and senior academic ranks. For example, women principal investigators were less likely to receive funding for prestigious grants compared to men (Witteman et al., 2019). When explored more closely, researchers found that women's evaluations were "less favourable," despite the objective quality of their grant proposals (Witteman et al., 2019). Women are also less likely to be editors-in-chief and editorial board members of esteemed international medical journals, and they have lower rates of scientific publishing (Amrein et al., 2011; Fridner et al., 2015). Therein lies the diversity-innovation paradox in that novel contributions by women receive increased scrutiny and lower uptake than those by cisgender White men. Although diversity breeds innovation, underrepresented groups that diversify organizations and make novel contributions paradoxically have less successful careers in the organizations (Hofstra et al., 2020).

Women are also less likely to receive awards from medical societies, with some societies having had limited or nil women recipients (Silver et al., 2017). They are less likely to be senior authors on medical guidelines, and are underrepresented on these committees generally (Merman et al., 2018). They are less likely to be chosen as speakers at grand rounds and less likely to be introduced by their titles, especially when introduced by men (Buell et al., 2018; Files et al., 2017). They may also engage in administrative, leadership, education, and advocacy roles that are undervalued by not being included on their curriculum vitae, in work or academic reviews, or in organizational news (Hunter et al., 2022).

Physicians often advance in academic medicine based on a variety of factors including successful grant applications, the number of trainees they supervise, the number of scientific publications (including impact factors of journals and citations), as well as other forms of recognition (e.g., awards, presentations) (Hunter et al., 2022; Tricco et al., 2021). Considering the areas in which women are disadvantaged, it is not surprising that women receive less supportive reference letters for faculty positions, and are less likely to be promoted to full professors, chairs or deans (Carnes et al., 2015; Jena et al., 2015; Tricco et al., 2021).

One might think that women "stick it out" for financial remuneration, but they are expected to make 20% to 40% less on average than men based on national and global physician gender pay gap studies (Cohen and Kiran, 2020; Dacre et al., 2020; Kralj, 2019; WHO, 2022). As will be reviewed later on, women tend to spend more time with psychosocially complex patients, which hinders them in the fee-for service types of remuneration model (Jefferson et al., 2013; Kruger et al., 2011; Smith et al., 2011), however the pay gap persists in settings that use other remuneration models. Women are also more likely to work in underpaid specialties such as primary care, family medicine, pediatrics, and psychiatry (CMA, 2018). Even in men-dominated specialties that tend to be well-compensated such as surgical specialties, women are paid less for the same work and women tend to perform procedures that pay less (Dossa et al., 2019).

Furthermore, women trainees and physicians are more likely to experience sexual harassment compared to men (Fnais et al., 2014; Jena et al., 2015). At the same time, they are less likely to report these incidents in part due to fear of negative consequences socially and professionally (Jagsi, 2018). For example, in Jena et al.'s 2015 survey of American clinician-researchers, 30% of women experienced sexual harassment in learning or work environments, 40% rated it as severe, and nearly 50% felt that reporting it negatively impacted their careers.

Women trainees and physicians are also more likely to experience gender discrimination. For example, in a 2016 survey of American physician mothers, over 65% reported experiencing gender discrimination at work, and over 35% reported experiencing maternal discrimination related to being pregnant, on leave, or breastfeeding (Adesoye et al., 2017). Maternal discrimination is even more problematic given that there are gendered expectations that women trainees and physicians should still take on most household and caregiving duties even when they have physician spouses (CMA, 2021; Jolly et al., 2014).

Table 5.2. *Impacts of gender inequity on women in medicine.*

Areas in medicine	Impact of gender inequity
Academia	• Fewer successful grant applications • Fewer scientific publications • Less likely to be senior guideline authors • Fewer professional awards • Fewer rounds/presentations
Advancement	• Lower academic ranking
Employment	• Not considered on future potential • Less likely to apply to open positions • Receive weaker reference letters
Remuneration	• Lower average income
Retention	• Higher and faster rates of attrition
Safety	• Sexual harassment • Gender discrimination • Maternal discrimination
Training	• Siloed in primary care specialties • Underrepresented in surgical specialties • Limited mentorship and sponsorship

Sources: Levine et al., 2013; CMA, 2019; Sambunjak et al., 2006; Travis et al., 2013; Barch and Yee, 2011; Tockey and Ignatova, 2018; Trix and Psenka, 2003; Witteman et al., 2019; Fridner et al., 2015; Merman et al., 2018; Silver et al., 2017; Buell et al., 2018; Kralj, 2019; Jena et al., 2015; Fnais et al., 2014; Jagsi et al., 2016; Adesoye et al., 2017.

Clinical Vignette

I was on call as a medical student with a resident physician in the emergency room when a young adult named "Skylar" popped up next on the board. I remembered that names in quotation marks tend to be a patient's preferred name; however, their given name appeared to be a woman's name– "Hailey." When we entered the room, the resident physician jumped right in and called the patient Hailey without appearing to realize. A look of irritation swept across Skylar's face– "I go by Skylar, and I would appreciate it if you use this name." The resident physician shrugged, "Yeah, sure. Sorry." Skylar also identified that they were non-binary and used they/them/their pronouns. When asked which pronouns we use, the resident physician said, "I'm not sure that matters. We're here to talk about you." Skylar had the same look, and then turned to me. "Oh, uhm, sure. I guess I prefer she/her? To be honest, I don't think about it much." There was that look again.

As the resident physician continued, Skylar grew progressively irritated, looking away, pursing their lips, tapping their foot, and only responding "nope," "yeah," and so on. When we were wrapping up, our staff passed by – "Hey, you ready to review?" The resident physician stood up and left the room without me. Skylar and I sat in uncomfortable silence. We could hear the resident physician reviewing outside. "Yeah, her name's Hailey or Skylar or whatever … she said she wants help, but she clearly doesn't want to be here … she doesn't look that sick. I think she's fine to go … We can probably just discharge her, right?" The staff said, "Sounds good" and off they went. More looks. Shaking their head, Skylar said, "Why do I even bother? Doctors are all the same. If anything, they make me feel worse. I'm better off going home. Thanks for nothing." I did not know how to respond in that moment. I did not like how the resident physician spoke about Skylar, but I did not know what to say to either of them. So I said nothing, and waited for the resident physician to return.

Clinical Vignette Analysis

We can likely each imagine ourselves in the shoes of anyone in this situation – the medical student's, the resident's, the staff's, and Skylar's. Some may be quick to blame the resident physician in this scenario, but both the medical trainee and the practicing physician were complicit in enacting gender bias against Skylar who identified as non-binary. For example, the resident physician did not use Skylar's chosen name, providing pronouns was unexpected and even rebuffed, Skylar was misgendered and this was not corrected, therapeutic rapport was lost early on, and Skylar did not appear to have their needs met. In addition, while the medical student identified their pronouns as she/her/hers and Skylar identified theirs as they/them/theirs, we do not know the other staff members' gender identities. We may already have a preconceived notion of the gender identities of the resident and the staff, which may, ironically, also reflect gender bias.

As reviewed in this chapter, gender equity tends to focus on the experiences of women which can come at a cost to gender diverse persons. We must all attend to the gendered expectations we have of others, our role in perpetuating biases even if we face them ourselves, as well as our part in advocating for equity. As with the medical student in this scenario, it is important to question our complicity as silent bystanders as it is increasingly evident that silence is itself a potential source of violence.

Pause and Reflect

An Exercise in Self-Reflection: What is our Role in Gender Bias and Equity?

Anyone is capable of engaging in gender bias whether consciously or not, and it is important for us to consider our role in the issue and potential solutions. Below are several prompts to facilitate reflection on your lived experiences of gender bias and equity in medicine.

- Can you recall a time when you experienced, engaged in, or witnessed gender bias (e.g., against you, peers, colleagues, patients, or caregivers) in medicine?
- What were some of the gendered expectations that you think contributed to the biases at that time? How do you think these were learned?
- How did the situation affect you? How did it affect others? For example, if it happened to a patient, do you think it impacted the care they received?
- Did you or anyone else recognize what happened and challenged it? If yes, what was done? What was the response? If not, why do you think so? What were the barriers?
- Knowing what you know now, would you act or want others to act any differently in the future? What do you think would be most helpful to achieve this change?

The Consequences of Gender Inequity in Medicine

Having reviewed examples of gender inequity in medicine, it is also important to consider its effect more systematically at the individual, institutional, and systems levels. Gender equity is a human rights issue at its core. It has resounding impacts on physicians, patients, and communities.

The Impact on Physician Wellness

In 2021, the Canadian Medical Association (CMA) surveyed nearly 4000 resident physicians and practicing physicians, including 60% who identified as women, on items related to health and wellbeing. In comparison to men, women were more likely to report burnout (59% vs. 43%); moderate to severe anxiety (27% vs. 19%); depression (50% vs. 43%); lifetime suicidal ideation (38% vs. 32%); and, worsened mental health since the coronavirus disease (COVID-19) pandemic (64% vs 52%). It is well-known that women continue to experience disproportionately higher rates of burnout in medicine compared to men (Shanafelt et al., 2022).

In terms of work itself, lack of schedule control, poor remuneration, barriers to advancement, and decreased professional fulfillment can increase the risk of burnout (Shanafelt et al., 2015). Household and caregiving duties can also heighten the risk of burnout, and women often spend more hours on these duties compared to their spouses (Jolly et al., 2014; Robinson, 2003). Gender bias and discrimination, especially towards expectant or current mothers, is also associated with increased risk of burnout (Adesoye et al., 2017). When burnout goes unaddressed, it can confer risk for mental health such as depression (Menon et al., 2021).

The impact of household and caregiving duties on women physicians' mental health during the COVID-19 pandemic cannot be overstated (Matulevicius et al., 2021). Women took on increased household responsibilities, caregiving for children, parents, or other family members, as well as home-schooling children. As a result, they were more likely than men to leave medicine or reduce their clinical, academic, leadership, or other roles (Matulevicius et al., 2021). For those who left medicine, it will be interesting to see how many return to the workforce now that schools have reopened and there is increased availability of adult and childcare.

As a recurring gap in the literature, many surveys only ask respondents for sex identity, and it is only recently that they began asking for gender identity too (CMA, 2021). Even when gender diverse trainees and physicians comprise a subgroup of a general physician sample, their numbers are often too small to allow for additional subgroup analyses (CMA, 2021). Westafer et al. (2022) recently interviewed transgender and gender expansive physicians in the United States and identified common experiences of emotional distress secondary to transphobia, as well as societal expectations for these physicians to be part of a binary gender framework.

Patient-centered Care and Clinical Outcomes

In terms of patient-centered care, studies have shown that women spend more time with patients; use more empathetic communication; engage in more preventative care; provide more psychosocial support; and, are more likely to follow clinical guidelines (Baumhäkel, Müller, and Böhm, 2009; Berthold et al., 2008; Frank et al., 2013; Jefferson et al., 2013; Kim et al., 2005; Kruger et al., 2012; Ramirez et al., 2009; Smith et al., 2011). Medicine patients admitted under women physicians have lower rates of readmission and mortality (Tsugawa et al., 2017), and surgical patients whose surgeries were performed by women physicians had lower rates of mortality, thirty-day complications, and readmission (Wallis et al., 2022). These two studies also accounted for factors that could have otherwise impacted clinical outcomes.

Other studies have shown that sex discordance between physicians and patients has been associated with poorer outcomes specifically for women patients treated by men physicians. For example, it has been associated with women patients being less likely to discuss sensitive health issues such as mental and sexual health with men physicians (Glauser, 2018). It has also been linked to worse therapeutic rapport, lower likelihood of correctly identifying a medical condition as high severity, and lower certainty of diagnosis (Gross et al., 2008). When patients do not feel like they can trust their physician, this can also impact treatment adherence which, in turn, can further affect clinical outcomes (Gross et al., 2008).

It is also important to consider that the time and effort that women physicians choose to put into providing patient-centered care can come at a cost to their health and wellbeing. For example, "going the extra mile" can result in increased workload, excessive documentation, poor compensation, and poor work-life balance, which also relates to burnout (CMA, 2021). There is risk of further gender bias as patients and colleagues (e.g., peers, allied health, administrative assistants) may come to expect women physicians to provide a certain level of care unlike men (Byerly, 2018). This is also dangerous because, if women deviate from these gendered expectations, patients and colleagues may be more critical towards them, and patient may yield regulatory college complaints from patients, which then exacerbates an already taxing gendered cognitive load. The confluence of these factors places women physicians at increased risk of patient dissatisfaction and internalized drive to continue to deliver this level of service even as they begin to experience the personal toll of these expectations.

There is a lack of data on the care experiences and outcomes of patients receiving care from gender diverse physicians. However, racially and ethnically diverse patients provided care by concordant physicians report higher levels of trust, satisfaction, and likelihood of treatment adherence (Cooper et al., 2006; LaVeist and Nuru-Jeter, 2002). It is expected that other marginalized patient groups may also benefit from concordance with their physicians (Sánchez et al., 2015).

Community Health and Workforce Sustainability

Women health care leaders continue to positively influence public health and policy, which has important practical implications for marginalized groups (Downs et al., 2014). Historically, women physicians have supported access to care for lower income persons, women and children, but they are also strong advocates for other marginalized groups now (Downs et al. 2014). Similarly, sexual and gender diverse physicians have been found to spend more time in research, education, and advocacy roles related to concordant communities (Sánchez et al., 2015).

Gender inequity also threatens the sustainability of the physician workforce in general, including those caring for marginalized communities. For example, burnout is in part related to gender discrimination, and burned-out physicians are at higher risk of attrition and perpetuation of implicit and explicit biases towards marginalized patients (Adesoye et al., 2017; Dyrbye et al., 2019; West et al., 2018). Attrition rates financially cost the health system and patients care suffers as burned-out physicians are more likely to change practices, reduce their hours, and retire earlier (Dewa et al., 2014). The leaky pipeline for gendered physicians is likely to have negative downstream effects on the concordant communities they serve.

The Opportunity

Opportunities for Gender Equity in Medicine

As explored in this chapter, gender equity in medicine is critical to improving physician wellbeing, promoting patient-centered care, and sustaining the workforce. Knowing this, the focus must include eliciting the sources and mechanisms of gender inequity, concurrent with exploring potential solutions. Opportunities to advance gender equity are most effective in areas such as mentorship, career flexibility, remuneration, and protection from harassment and discrimination (Tricco et al., 2021).

Building Gender Equity for Women in Medicine

Recent literature indicates that advocating for organizational and systemic interventions is likely to be more effective in achieving gender equity than primarily relying on individual interventions (Kang and Kaplan, 2019; Westafer et al., 2022). Kang and Kaplan (2019) note that while all humans have implicit biases towards others, implicit bias training alone is poorly associated with positive outcomes (e.g., changing people's attitudes), and it sometimes results in negative outcomes (e.g., more discriminatory behaviour) towards marginalized groups. Instead, shifting the focus to designing, implementing, and evaluating organizational and systemic interventions provides greater opportunities to create meaningful change for people of all gender identities (Kang and Kaplan, 2019).

Mentorship for gender concordant trainees and physicians includes one-to-one, two-to-one, and group mentorship models (Farkas et al., 2019). With fewer women in senior academic and leadership positions, opportunities for mentorship are not always easy to find (Carnes et al., 2015; Jena et al., 2015). Given that mentorship from seniors allows juniors to form the connections and frameworks they need for ongoing success, opportunities must be cultivated within workplaces (Farkas et al., 2019). All three models have been shown to be effective at improving outcomes for junior trainees and physicians. For example, they help junior physicians develop clinical and research skills, obtain leadership positions, as well as contribute to career satisfaction and retention (Farkas et al., 2019).

Career flexibility is also a strategy to promote gender equity and improve physician wellbeing. Many organizations have since implemented policies and programs such as extended parental leave and work-from-home options (Shauman et al., 2018). However, there is still work to be done in ensuring equitable access to these options, and decreasing stigma that can be associated with using them. For example, Shauman et al.'s 2018 study surveyed faculty members in order to assess common barriers to career flexibility. Respondents reported the following deterrents: lack of reliable information on program eligibility and benefits; workplace norms and stigma; concerns for how participation may negatively impact their peers; and the potential negative impact on their career prospects.

Evidently, improving career flexibility requires more than simply offering these types of policies and programs. Additional suggestions include providing education to ensure that all staff and learners are aware of policies and programs, increasing the number of medical residency positions to allow scheduling flexibility, and building allyship among physicians to normalize leaves as an expected occurrence (Villablanca et al., 2013). For example, in Villablanca et al.'s 2013 study at the University of California, Davis, researchers implemented an intervention to educate physicians on available options for career flexibility. Positive outcomes for all physicians, but particularly for women, included increased understanding of resources, improved attitudes towards the policies, and decreased cited barriers to career flexibility.

Improving remuneration for women physicians is another strategy to promote gender equity. For example, Catenaccio et al.'s 2022 study showed that most medical specialties studied reported lower starting salaries for women compared to men. The effect of equalizing starting salaries was modelled and shown to significantly improve the ten-year earning potential of early career physicians. In practice, various medical organizations across North America have implemented initiatives to reduce the gender pay gap. For example, the John Hopkins University School of Medicine includes the pay gap as an essential mission of the institution, reviews faculty salary and completes related analyses, interviews women physicians for their experiences, and has an oversight committee amongst other gender income parity initiatives. These combined initiatives were shown to decrease the pay gap by 0.7% after ten years of implementation (Rao et al., 2018).

Finally, protecting persons against gender-based harassment and discrimination is critical to supporting gender equity. The first step to addressing this type of harassment and discrimination is accepting the role that organizations play in allowing for these incidents to unfold (Choo et al., 2019). Systemic factors that cultivate an unsafe environment include unclear policies and reporting structures, minimal support and protection for targets of harassment, organizational reliance on formal complaints and lawsuits, an environment in which reporting may lead to punitive career impacts, minimal consequences for perpetrators, and absence of standardized approaches to ensure accountability (Choo et al., 2019). Changing culture and creating specific policies and practices to address these factors is critical to improving workplace culture and decreasing harassment and discrimination against gendered persons in medicine.

Inclusion Strategies

Inclusion Strategies for Achieving Gender Equity

Inclusion strategies should be nuanced and grounded in institutional operating standards. Developing and implementing programs and resources to support gender equity requires strong commitment from medical institutions. This section provides some ideas and resources to help the reader develop practices or programs that encourage the participation of gendered persons. The goal is to integrate diverse perspectives in organizational structures and decision-making processes. Addressing gender equity and diversity in medicine is a shared responsibility that calls for action at both the individual and system levels. The following equity building exercise reflects the complexities of attempting to redress the balance.

Pause and Reflect
What Do I Bring to this Issue?
• How often do my biological sex and my gender intersect with my professional role?
• What are the chief obstacles to career advancement for my female peers?
• How often am I compelled to defend the professional space I occupy?
• What is my responsibility when I observe gendered microaggressions?
What Can I Do to Contribute to Gender Equity Building?
• Follow the egalitarian principles that guide the medical profession
• Respond assertively when I witness these principles being ignored
• Make a personal commitment to recognize others as equals in my work or learning environment
• Cultivate respect, open mindedness, and transparent dialogue in relationships
• Advocate for gender equity and diversity to achieve equitable health outcomes
• Support my peers in meeting their individual and collective responsibilities to both their patients and colleagues

Table 5.3 outlines a few strategies for increasing gender equity and inclusivity in medical workplaces. Although some strategies may appear

too distal for organizational adoption, it is important to reflect on organizational and personal contributions to the issue.

Table 5.3. *Some strategies proposed for increasing gender inclusion toward reaching physician workforce equality*

Inclusion Strategies
• Look outside the inner circle, or the "typical candidates;" candidates brought before a search committee are often only as diverse as the search committee itself. • Nominate women physicians for awards • Sponsor women physicians for leadership opportunities • Invite women to speak nationally and internationally at medical events • Address women by title or academic rank • Acknowledge that implicit bias is present in everyone, and take steps to be intentional in decision-making to ensure unconscious biases are not the driving force in decisions • Acknowledge that women physicians are at higher risk for burnout and meaningfully address the root causes • Address the gap payment and advocate for pay transparency to ensure equal compensation for physicians with similar skills and credentials • Routinely conduct assessment of the equity of physician compensation arrangements by institutions that hire physicians

Key Takeaways

- Despite the increased representation of women in medicine over the past decades, gender inequity is widespread for women and gender diverse physicians.
- There are deeply entrenched systemic factors that underlie gender inequity, with these factors being rooted in hegemonic ideas of gender norms, roles, and relations.
- These systemic factors disadvantage gendered persons in medicine and impart widespread effects on their work, livelihood, and safety.
- Gender inequity can have negatives consequences for medical trainees' and practicing physicians' wellbeing, as well as for patient care and health systems.

- Opportunities to improve gender equity in medicine are extensive.
- It is essential to continue to invest in gender equity research that explores the lived experiences of women and gender diverse persons in medicine, and that informs evidence-based protocols that can best support gendered persons.

Conclusion

There has been a significant increase in the number of women and gender diverse medical learners and practicing physicians. However, this increased presence has not been matched by a resolution of gender inequity in salient areas such as career advancement, income and inclusivity amongst other gender related issues. Furthermore, the voice of gender diverse physicians is still largely underrepresented in the literature. Drawing on the perspective of women and gender diverse persons is critical in shaping safe clinical spaces for gender diverse patients whilst also improving the professional quality of life of women and gender diverse physicians.

Addressing gender bias and inequity in medicine is just and necessary if we are to foster a greater sense of solidarity and inclusion among physicians. This contributes to the sustainability of the healthcare system in terms of the retention of women and gender diverse physicians, particularly in academic settings. Although some organizations adopt a blind equality approach, this does not translate to the level of recognition and acceptance required to thrive and reach a fulsome professional potential for many women and gender diverse clinicians.

When front-line clinicians and medical leaders reflect the gender diverse population they serve, patients stand to have better experiences of care. Creating leadership development spaces and policy requirements for the inclusion of gender diverse leaders on boards and in the executive suite where key policies and decisions are made is an essential starting point. In so doing, we can begin to reflexively examine institutional policies and procedures through a lens of gender equity, thus moving medicine closer to the ultimate goal of decreasing the systemic factors that dispropor-tionately affect underserved and under-represented communities.

On a Parting Note...

Woman, they say fickle be thy nature, be you fair.

Yet here I stand today with the charge of your care.

Lend me your ear,

for I shall bend it with the story of my journey here

and pray that you have a care,

for the sacrifices I've laid bare

in order to climb this ladder of rungs so shaky.

Yet I trust in the one above and below my foothold,

to join hands, pulling and pushing at the fold.

For by that, we shall surely ascend together,

ever more bold in our foothold.

©Mariam Abdurrahman, 2022

References

Adesoye, T., Mangurian C., Choo E.K. et al. (2017) 'Perceived discrimination experienced by physician mothers and desired workplace changes: a cross-sectional survey,' *JAMA Intern Med*, 177(7), pp. 1033-6. https://doi.org/10.1001/jamainternmed.2017.1394.

Association of Faculties of Medicine of Canada (AFMC). (2020) *Canadian medical education statistics 2020: Section G. The AFMC undergraduate medical education enrolment (MD program) study – description* [online]. Available from: https://www.afmc.ca/sites/default/files/pdf/CMES/CMES2020-SectionG_EN.pdf.

Amrein, K., Langmann, A., Fahrleitner-Pammer, A. et al. (2011) 'Women underrepresented on editorial boards of 60 major medical journals,' *Gend Med*, 8(6): pp. 378-87. https://doi.org/10.1016/j.genm.2011.10.007.

Barsh, J. and Yee, L. 'Unlocking the full potential of women in the US economy,' McKinsey & Company, 1 April [online]. Available from: https://www.mckinsey.com/business-functions/organization/our-insights/unlocking-the-full-potential-of-women.

Baumhäkel, M., Müller, U., and Böhm, M. (2009) 'Influence of gender of physicians and patients on guideline-recommended treatment of chronic heart failure in a cross-sectional study,' *Eur J Heart Fail*, 11(3): pp. 299–303. https://doi.org/10.1093/eurjhf/hfn041.

Berthold, H.K., Gouni-Berthold, I., Bestehorn, K.P. et al. (2008) 'Physician gender is associated with the quality of type 2 diabetes care.' *J Intern Med*, 264(4), pp. 340-50. https://doi.org/10.1111/j.1365-2796.2008.01967.x.

Buell, D., Hemmelgarn, B.R. and Straus, S.E. (2018) 'Proportion of women presenters at medical grand rounds at major academic centres in Canada: a retrospective observational study,' *BMJ Open*, 8(1). https://doi.org/10.1136/bmjopen-2017-019796.

Byerly, S.I. (2018) 'Female physician wellness: are expectations of ourselves extreme?,' *Int Anesthesiol Clin*, 56(3): pp. 59-73. https://doi.org/10.1097/AIA.0000000000000197.

Canadian Institutes of Health Research (CIHR). (2020) *What is gender? What is sex?* [online]. https://cihr-irsc.gc.ca/e/48642.html

Canadian Medical Association (CMA), Federation of Medical Women of Canada (FMWC). (2018) *Addressing gender equity and diversity in Canada's medical profession: A review.* https://www.cma.ca/sites/default/files/pdf/Ethics/report-2018-equity-diversity-medicine-e.pdf.

Canadian Medical Association (CMA). (2019) *Number and percent distribution of physicians by specialty and gender, Canada 2019.* https://www.cma.ca/sites/default/files/2019-11/2019-06-spec-sex_0.pdf.

Canadian Medical Association (CMA). (2022) *CMA 2021 National Physician Health Survey* [online]. Available from: https://www.cma.ca/sites/default/files/2022-08/NPHS_final_report_EN.pdf

Canadian Post-M.D. Education Registry (CAPER). (2021) *G-5 First year trainees: Canadian citizens/permanent residents by field of post-M.D. training and gender – 2021-22.* https://caper.ca/sites/default/files/pdf/census-tables/2021.g-5.pdf.

Carnes, M., Bartels, C.M., Kaatz, A. et al. (2015) 'Why is John more likely to become department chair than Jennifer?,' *Trans Am Clin Climatol Assoc,*126: pp. 197-214.

Catenaccio, E., Rochlin, J.M. and Simon, H.K. (2022) 'Addressing gender-based disparities in earning potential in academic medicine,' *JAMA Network Open*, 5(2). https://doi.org/10.1001/jamanetworkopen.2022.0067.

Choo, E.K., Byington, C.L., Johnson, N.L. et al. (2019) 'From #MeToo to #TimesUp in health care: can a culture of accountability end inequity and harassment?,' *Lancet*, 393(10171), pp. 499-502. https://doi.org/10.1016/s0140-6736(19)30251-x.

Cohen, M., & Kiran, T. (2020). Closing the gender pay gap in Canadian medicine. *CMAJ: Canadian Medical Association journal = journal de l'Association medicale canadienne*, 192(35), pp. E1011–E1017. https://doi.org/10.1503/cmaj.200375.

Cooper, L.A., Beach, M.C., Johnson, R.L. et al. (2006) 'Delving below the surface: understanding how race and ethnicity influence relationships in health care,' *J Gen Intern Med*, 21(Suppl 1), pp. S21-7. https://doi.org/10.1111/j.1525-1497.2006.00305.x.

Cornell Law School Legal Information Institute. (2020). *Gender bias* [online]. Available at: https://www.law.cornell.edu/wex/gender_bias

Dacre, J., Woodhams, C., Atkinson C., Laliotis, I., Williams, M., Blanden, J., et al. (2020). Mend the gap: the independent review into gender pay gaps in medicine in England [online]. Available from: https://e-space.mmu.ac.uk/627043/1/Gender_pay_gap_in_medicine_review.pdf

Dellasega, C., Aruma, J.F., Sood, N. et al. (2022) 'The impact of patient prejudice on minoritized female physicians,' *Front Public Health*, 10. https://doi.org/10.3389/fpubh.2022.902294.

Dewa, C.S., Jacobs, P., Thanh N.X., et al. (2014) 'An estimate of the cost of burnout on early retirement and reduction in clinical hours of practicing physicians in Canada,' *BMC Health Serv Res*, 14(1). https://doi.org/10.1186/1472-6963-14-254.

Capers, Q., 4th, Bond, D. A., & Nori, U. S. (2020). Bias and Racism Teaching Rounds at an Academic Medical Center. *Chest, 158*(6), 2688–2694. https://doi.org/10.1016/j.chest.2020.08.2073.

United States Department of Justice (DOJ). (2021) *Title IX* [online]. https://www.justice.gov/crt/title-ix

Dossa, F., Simpson, A.N., Sutradhar, R. et al. (2019) 'Sex-based disparities in the hourly earnings of surgeons in the fee-for-service system in Ontario, Canada,' *JAMA Surg*, 154(12), pp. 1134-42. https://doi.org/10.1001/jamasurg.2019.3769.

Downs, J.A., Reif, L.K., Hokororo A. et al. (2014) 'Increasing women in leadership in global health,' *Acad Med*, 89(8): p.1103-7.: https://doi.org/10.1097/ACM.0000000000000369.

European Institute for Gender Equality (EIGE). (2016) *Gender norms* [Online]. https://eige.europa.eu/thesaurus/terms/1194.

European Institute for Gender Equality (EIGE). (2016) *Gender roles* [online]. Available from: https://eige.europa.eu/thesaurus/terms/1209

Farkas, A.H., Bonifacino, E., Turner. R. et al. (2019) 'Mentorship of women in academic medicine: a systematic review,' *J Gen Inter Med*, 34(7), pp.1322-29. https://doi.org/10.1007/s11606-019-04955-2.

Files, J.A., Mayer, A.P., Ko, M.G. et al. (2017) 'Speaker introductions at internal medicine grand rounds: forms of address reveal gender bias,' *J Womens Health (Larchmt)*, 26(5), pp. 413-9. https://doi.org/10.1089/jwh.2016.6044.

Fnais, N., Soobiah, C., Chen, M.H. et al. (2014) 'Harassment and discrimination in medical training: a systematic review and meta-analysis,' *Acad Med*, 89(5), pp. 817-27. https://doi.org/10.1097/ACM.0000000000000200.

Frank, E., Dresner, Y., Shani, M. et al. (2013) 'The association between physicians' and patients' preventive health practices,' *CMAJ*, 185(8): pp. 649-53. https://doi.org/10.1503/cmaj.121028.

Fridner, A., Norell, A., Åkesson, G. et al. (2015) 'Possible reasons why female physicians publish fewer scientific articles than male physicians - a cross-sectional study,' *BMC Med Educ*, 15. https://doi.org/10.1186/s12909-015-0347-9.

Glauser, W. (2018) 'Medicine changing as women make up more of physician workforce,' *CMAJ*, 190(13), pp. E404-5. https://doi.org/10.1503/cmaj.109-5577.

Gross, R., McNeill, R., Davis, P. et al. (2008) 'The association of gender concordance and primary care physicians' perceptions of their patients,' *Women Health*, 48(2), pp. 123-44. Available at: https://doi.org/10.1080/03630240802313464.

Hofstra, B., Kulkarni, V. V., Munoz-Najar Galvez, S., He, B., Jurafsky, D., & McFarland, D. A. (2020). The diversity-innovation paradox in science. *Proceedings of the National Academy of Sciences of the United States of America*, 117(17), pp. 9284–9291. https://doi.org/10.1073/pnas.1915378117.

Hui, K., Sukhera, J., Vigod, S. et al. (2020) Recognizing and addressing implicit gender bias in medicine,' *CMAJ*, 192(42); p.E1269-70. Available at: https://doi.org/10.1503/cmaj.200286.

Hunter, J., Grewal, R., Nam, D. et al. (2022) 'Gender disparity in academic orthopedic programs in Canada: a cross-sectional study,' *Can J Surg*, 65(2), pp. E159-69. https://doi.org/10.1503/cjs.008920.

Jagsi, R. (2018) 'Sexual harassment in medicine - #MeToo,' *N Engl J Med*, 378(3), pp. 209-11. https://doi.org/10.1056/NEJMp1715962.

Jagsi, R., Griffith, K.A., Jones, R. et al. (2016) 'Sexual harassment and discrimination experiences of academic medical faculty,' *JAMA*, 315(19), pp. 2120-1. https://doi.org/10.1001/jama.2016.2188.

Jefferson, L., Bloor, K., Birks, Y. et al. (2013) 'Effect of physicians' gender on communication and consultation length: a systematic review and meta-analysis,' *J Health Serv Res Policy*, 18(4): p.242-8. Available at: https://doi.org/10.1177/1355819613486465

Jefferson, L., Bloor, K., Maynard, A. (2015) 'Women in medicine: historical perspectives and recent trends,' *British Medical Bulletin*, 114(1), pp. 5–15. https://doi.org/10.1093/bmb/ldv007.

Jena, A.B., Khullar, D., Ho, O. et al. (2015) 'Sex differences in academic rank in US medical schools in 2014,' 314(11): p.1149-58. https://doi.org/10.1001/jama.2015.10680.

Jolly, S., Griffith, K.A., DeCastro, R. et al. (2014) 'Gender differences in time spent on parenting and domestic responsibilities by high-achieving young physician-researchers,' *Ann Intern Med*, 160(5), pp. 344-53. https://doi.org/10.7326/M13-0974.

Joseph, M.M., Ahasic, A.M., Clark, J., Templeton, K. (2021) 'State of Women in Medicine: History, Challenges, and the Benefits of a Diverse Workforce,' *Pediatrics*, 148 (Supplement 2), p. e2021051440C.

Kang, S.K. and Kaplan, S. (2019) 'Working towards gender diversity and inclusion in medicine: myths and solutions,' *Lancet*, 393(10171), pp. 579-86. https://doi.org/10.1016/S0140-6736(18)33138-6.

Kim, C., McEwen, L.N., Gerzoff, R.B. et al. (2005) 'Is physician gender associated with the quality of diabetes care?,' *Diabetes Care*, 28(7), pp. 1594-8. https://doi.org/10.2337/diacare.28.7.1594.

Kralj, B. (2019) *Male FPs out-earn women FPs annually by over 30%: Ontario data*, Medical Post, 2 April [online]. https://drbobbell.com/male-fps-out-earn-women-fps-annually-by-over-30-ontario-data/

Kruger, J., Shaw, L., Kahende, J. et al. (2012) 'Health care providers' advice to quit smoking, National Health Interview Survey, 2000, 2005, and 2010,' *Prev Chronic Dis*, 9(E130). https://doi.org/10.5888/pcd9.110340.

Langston University. (2020) *Gender discrimination defined* [online]. Available from: https://www.langston.edu/title-ix/gender-discrimination-defined

LaVeist, T.A. and Nuru-Jeter, A. (2002) 'Is doctor-patient race concordance associated with greater satisfaction with care?,' *J Health Soc Behav*, 43(3), pp. 296-306. https://doi.org/10.2307/3090205.

Levine, R.B., Mechaber, H.F., Reddy, S.T. et al. (2013) '"A good career choice for women:" female medical students' mentoring experiences: a multi-institutional qualitative study,' *Acad Med*, 88(4), pp. 527-34. https://doi.org/10.1097/ACM.0b013e31828578bb.

Lippi, D., Bianucci, R., & Donell, S. (2020). Gender medicine: its historical roots. *Postgraduate medical journal*, 96(1138), pp. 480–486. https://doi.org/10.1136/postgradmedj-2019-137452.

Madrigal, J., Rudasill, S., Tran, Z. et al. (2021) 'Sexual and gender minority identity in undergraduate medical education: impact on experience and career trajectory,' *PLoS One*. 16(11). https://doi.org/10.1371/journal.pone.0260387.

Gandhi, G. (1930) *Woman's Status and Role in Society* [online]. Available from: https://www.mkgandhi.org/momgandhi/chap60.htm

Mandela, N. (2004) *Nelson Mandela International Day 18 July* [online]. United Nations. Available from: https://www.un.org/en/events/mandeladay/mandela_photo_gallery.shtml

Matulevicius, S.A., Kho, K.A., Reisch, J. et al. (2021) Academic medicine faculty perceptions of work-life balance before and since the COVID-19 pandemic,' *JAMA Netw Open*, 4(6). https://doi.org/10.1001/jamanetworkopen.2021.13539.

McMaster University Michael G. DeGroote School of Medicine. (2015) *Glossary of diversity-related terms* [online]. https://mdprogram.mcmaster.ca/students/diversity-affairs/diversity-affairs-resources/glossary-of-diversity-related-terms

Menon, N.K., Shanafelt, T.D., Sinsky, C.A. et al. (2020) 'Association of physician burnout with suicidal ideation and medical errors,' *JAMA Netw Open*, 3(12). https://doi.org/10.1001/jamanetworkopen.2020.28780.

Merman, E., Pincus, D., Bell, C. et al. (2018) 'Differences in clinical practice guideline authorship by gender,' *Lancet*, 392(10158): p.1626-8. https://doi.org/10.1016/S0140-6736(18)32268-2.

Negron, R. (2022) *rayo & honey* [online]. Available from: https://rayoandhoney.com/products/much-to-be-done-undone?_pos=1&_sid=8018081c1&_ss=r

Newman, C., Templeton, K. and Chin EL. (2020) 'Inequity and women physicians: time to change millennia of societal beliefs,' *Perm J*, 24(3): pp. 1-6. https://doi.org/10.7812/TPP/20.024.

Rao, A.D., Nicholas, S.E., Kachniarz, B. et al. (2018) 'Association of a simulated institutional gender equity initiative with gender-based disparities in medical school faculty salaries and promotions,' *JAMA Network Open*, 1(8). https://doi.org/10.1001/jamanetworkopen.2018.6054

Ramirez, A.G., Wildes, K.A., Nápoles-Springer, A. et al. (2009) 'Physician gender differences in general and cancer-specific prevention attitudes and practices,' *J Cancer Educ*, 24(2), pp. 85-93. https://doi.org/10.1080/08858190802664396.

Rangel, E.L., Castillo-Angeles, M., Easter, S.R. et al. (2021) 'Incidence of infertility and pregnancy complications in US female surgeons,' *JAMA Surg*, 156(10), pp. 905-15. https://doi.org/10.1001/jamasurg.2021.3301

Robinson, G.E. (2003) 'Stresses on women physicians: consequences and coping techniques,' *Depress Anxiety*, 17(3), pp. 180-9. https://doi.org/10.1002/da.10069.

Sambunjak, D., Straus, S.E. and Marusić, A. (2006) 'Mentoring in academic medicine: a systematic review,' *JAMA*, 296(9), pp. 1103-15. https://doi.org/10.1001/jama.296.9.1103.

Sánchez, N.F., Rankin, S., Callahan, E. et al. (2015) 'LGBT trainee and health professional perspectives on academic careers--facilitators and challenges,' *LGBT Health*, 2(4), pp. 346-56. https://doi.org/10.1089/lgbt.2015.0024.

Shanafelt, T.D., Gorringe, G., Menaker, R. et al. (2015) 'Impact of organizational leadership on physician burnout and satisfaction,' *Mayo Clin Proc*, 90(4), pp. 432-40. https://doi.org/10.1016/j.mayocp.2015.01.012.

Shanafelt, T.D., West, C.P., Sinsky, C. et al. (2022) 'Changes in burnout and satisfaction with work-life integration in physicians and the general US working population between 2011 and 2020,' *Mayo Clin Proc*, 97(3), pp. 491-506. https://doi.org/10.1016/j.mayocp.2021.11.021.

Shauman, K., Howell, L.P., Paterniti, D.A. et al. (2018) 'Barriers to career flexibility in academic medicine,' *Acad Med*, 93(2), pp. 246-55. https://doi.org/10.1097/acm.0000000000001877.

Silver, J.K., Slocum, C.S., Bank, A.M. et al. (2017) 'Where are the women? The underrepresentation of women physicians among recognition award recipients from medical specialty societies,' *PMR*, 9(8), pp. 804-15. https://doi.org/10.1016/j.pmrj.2017.06.001.

Smith, A.W., Borowski, L.A., Liu, B. et al. (2011) 'U.S. primary care physicians' diet-, physical activity-, and weight-related care of adult patients,' *Am J Prev Med*, 41(1), pp. 33-42. https://doi.org/10.1016/j.amepre.2011.03.017.

Starr, P. (1982) *The social transformation of American medicine: the rise of a sovereign profession and the making of a vast industry.* New York: Basic Books.

Tockey, D. and Ignatova, M. (2018) *Gender insights report: How women find jobs differently.* LinkedIn Talent Solutions [online]. Available from: https://business.linkedin.com/content/dam/me/business/en-us/talent-solutions-lodestone/body/pdf/Gender-Insights-Report.pdf

Travis, E.L., Doty, L. and Helitzer, D.L. (2013) 'Sponsorship: a path to the academic medicine C-suite for women faculty?,' *Acad Med*, 88(10), pp. 1414-7. https://doi.org/10.1097/ACM.0b013e3182a35456.

Tricco, A.C., Bourgeault, I., Moore, A. et al. (2021) 'Advancing gender equity in medicine,' *CMAJ*, 193(7), pp. E244-50. https://doi.org/10.1503/cmaj.200951.

Trix, F. and Psenka, C. (2003) 'Exploring the color of glass: letters of recommendation for female and male medical faculty,' *Discourse* Soc, 14(2), pp. 191-220. https://doi.org/10.1177/095792650301400227

Tsugawa, Y., Jena, A.B., Figueroa, J.F. et al. (2017) 'Comparison of hospital mortality and readmission rates for Medicare patients treated by male vs female physicians,' *JAMA Intern Med*, 177(2), pp. 206-13. https://doi.org/10.1001/jamainternmed.2016.7875.

Villablanca, A.C., Beckett, L., Nettiksimmons, J. et al. (2013) 'Improving knowledge, awareness, and use of flexible career policies through an accelerator intervention at the University of California, Davis, School of Medicine,' *Acad Med*, 88(6), pp. 771-7. https://doi.org/10.1097/acm.0b013e31828f8974.

Wallis, C.J.D., Jerath, A., Coburn, N. et al. (2022) 'Association of surgeon-patient sex concordance with postoperative outcomes,' *JAMA Surg*, 157(2), pp. 146-56. https://doi.org/10.1001/jamasurg.2021.6339.

West, C.P., Dyrbye, L.N. and Shanafelt, T.D. (2018) 'Physician burnout: contributors, consequences and solutions,' *J Intern Med*, 283(6), pp. 516-29. https://doi.org/10.1111/joim.12752.

Westafer, L.M., Freiermuth, C.E., Lall, M.D. et al. (2022) 'Experiences of transgender and gender expansive physicians,' JAMA Network Open, 5(6), p. e2219791. https://doi.org/10.1001/jamanetworkopen.2022.19791.

Witteman, H.O., Hendricks, M., Straus, S. et al. (2019) 'Gender bias in CIHR Foundation grant awarding,' *Lancet*, 394(10214), pp. E41-2. https://doi.org/ 10.1016/S0140-6736(19)31808-2.

Witteman, H.O., Hendricks, M., Straus, S. et al. (2019) 'Are gender gaps due to evaluations of the applicant or the science? A natural experiment at a national funding agency,' *Lancet*, 393(10171), pp. 531-40. https://doi.org/10.1016/S0140-6736(18)32611-4.

World Health Organization (WHO). (2022). The gender pay gap in the health and care sector a global analysis in the time of COVID-19 [online]. Available from: https://www.who.int/publications/i/item/9789240052895

Yarbrough, E., Kidd, J. and Parekh R. (2017) *Gender Dysphoria Diagnosis*. American Psychiatric Association, November [online]. Available from: https://www.psychiatry.org/psychiatrists/cultural-competency/education/transgender-and-gender-nonconforming-patients/gender-dysphoria-diagnosis

Appendix 5.1: Additional Resources

For readers who are interested in learning more about gender equity for women in medicine Table 5.4 provides examples of North American and other international women physicians' organizational mission statements and links to their sites for added information. For example, the American Medical Women's Association has launched a Gender Equity Task Force with the goal of achieving gender equity in healthcare specifically, and in society more generally.

Table 5.4. *Examples of North American & international women physicians' organizations*

Organization	Mission statement
Canada	
Federation of Medical Women of Canada (FMWC) https://fmwc.ca/about-us/goals/	"… committed to the professional, social and personal advancement of women physicians and to the promotion of the well-being of women both in the medical profession and in society at large."
Canadian Women in Medicine (CWIM) https://www.cwimorg.com/about	"… to help women in medicine thrive both professionally and personally. Through advocacy, mentorship and recognition we strive to achieve our goals of increasing the number of women in medical leadership roles and achieving a work environment that is safe and equitable."
United States	
American Medical Women's Association (AMWA) https://www.amwa-doc.org/about-amwa/	"To advance women in medicine, advocate for equity, and ensure excellence in health care."
American Medical Women's Association Gender Equity Task Force (AMWA GETF)	"…to accomplish gender equity as a fact of life in society, and to engage in activities, action and collaborations pursuant to this goal, beginning with the healthcare industry of which women physicians are one component."

Organization	Mission statement ...*continued*
American Medical Association Women Physicians Section (WPS) https://www.ama-assn.org/member-groups-sections/women-physicians/about-women-physicians-section-wps	"... seeks to influence and contribute to AMA policy and program development on issues of importance to women physicians, and to increase the number and influence of women physicians in leadership roles."
International	
Medical Women's International Association (MWIA) https://mwia.net/	"... an important voice and influence on issues of interest to medical women e.g., work-life balance, maternity leave, career progression, fighting discrimination and mentoring of young medical doctors and students."
Association of Women Surgeons (AWS) https://www.womensurgeons.org/page/AboutAWS	"... to inspire, encourage, and enable women surgeons to realize their professional and personal goals."

Chapter 6
Dispelling Erasure: 2SLGBTQ+ Identities in Medicine

Albina Veltman, MD, Tara La Rose, MSW, PhD

❖

"It is revolutionary for any trans person to choose to be seen and visible in a world that tells us we should not exist."
—Laverne Cox, 2015

❖

Abstract: Healthcare profession learners and providers who have a minority sexual orientation or gender identity face minority stress that can have a profound impact as they continue to face stigma and discrimination within healthcare professional programs and clinical settings. Individuals who identify as 2SLGBTQ+ still face significant barriers within the professional landscape they experience as physicians and healthcare providers. Similarly, there remain barriers with accessing appropriate and inclusive healthcare services for patients who are 2SLGBTQ+, often resulting in significant health inequities and disparities. This chapter will explore cisgenderism and heterosexism in medicine, the value of gender and sexual orientation diversity in the healthcare professions, and strategies to promote 2SLGBTQ+ positive spaces within healthcare settings and healthcare professions.

Keywords: *2SLGBTQ+, cisgenderism, diversity, equity, gender identity, homophobia, sexual orientation, transphobia*

Introduction

2SLGBTQ+ is an acronym for Two Spirit, Lesbian, Gay, Bisexual, Transgender, Queer, and represented by the + sign, other diverse minority sexual orientations and gender identities. Sexual orientation refers to how one thinks of oneself in terms of one's emotional, romantic, or sexual attraction, desire, or affection for another person. It is very important to note, however, that sexual behaviour is not always congruent with sexual orientation or identity. For example, a man who has sex with men may not identify as a gay or bisexual man, but rather, he may identify as a heterosexual man.

Gender identity is one's internal and psychological sense of oneself as male, female, both, or neither (The Center, 2006). It is important to note that gender identity is totally independent of sexual orientation. For example, regardless of whether someone identifies as cisgender, transgender, non-binary (or any other gender identity), they can identify as having any sexual orientation. Terminology with respect to diverse sexual orientations and gender identities continues to evolve and it can sometimes seem like quite a challenge to try to "keep up" with the latest terms being used. Please see the glossary at the end of this chapter and the EDI Lexicon chapter for further exploration of current commonly used terminology with respect to a diversity of sexual orientations and gender identities.

It is important to be cognizant of the fact that medicine in general (and this is perhaps most glaring within the specialty of psychiatry specifically) has a history of conflating 2SLGBTQ+ identities with mental illness (Veltman et al., in press). For example, the American Psychiatric Association (APA) removed the diagnosis of homosexuality from the Diagnostic and Statistical Manual of Mental Disorders (DSM), Second Edition (APA, 1968), in 1973 (after much debate and political/societal pressure to do so) (Bayer, 1981; Drescher and Merlino, 2007). However, despite many healthcare professionals who work with people who identify as transgender arguing that any diagnosis related to gender identity issues should also be removed from the DSM because its inclusion pathologizes transgender identities, the diagnosis of gender dysphoria remains in the current DSM-5-TR (APA, 2022). This historical pathologization of 2SLGBTQ+ identities contributes to the stigma and discrimination faced by people who identify as 2SLGBTQ+, affecting their mental and physical health as well as their access to appropriate and inclusive healthcare services (Hatzenbuehler and Pachankis, 2016).

While the DSM continues to include gender dysphoria in its list of mental disorders, the Manual of International Statistical Classification of Diseases and Related Health Problems (ICD-11) removed the term "transsexualism" which was previously included in the chapter on mental disorders, replacing it with the term "gender incongruence" (in a newly created chapter called "conditions related to sexual health") (ICD-11, 2019). Transgender activists and healthcare providers who work with trans-identified patients celebrated this change within the ICD-11 and saw this change as a great advance. By placing "gender incongruence" outside of the chapter on mental disorder, this helped to depathologize transgender identities while ensuring access to transition-related medical treatments for trans-identified individuals who wished to pursue these (Global Action for Trans Equality, 2020).

Statistics about the prevalence of 2SLGBTQ+ identities vary quite widely, based on the definitions used and how this type of identity information was collected in various studies. However, most studies worldwide estimate that between 2% to 16% of the population identify as 2SLGBTQ+ (Peter et al., 2021; Saewyc et al., 2007). It is important to recognize that the 2SLGBTQ+ population is a heterogeneous one, with the experience of each individual member of this community varying widely depending on numerous potentially intersectional factors, including ability, age, ethnoracial group, nationality, religion, socioeconomic status, geographical location, and other factors. However, what is common to sexual and gender minorities is that experiences of individual and systemic oppression can often threaten their health and wellbeing (Hatzenbuehler and Pachankis, 2016).

❖

"I believe that telling our stories, first to ourselves and then to one another and
the world, is a revolutionary act. It is an act that can be met with hostility,
exclusion, and violence. It can also lead to love, understanding, transcendence,
and community."
—Janet Mock, 2014

❖

Stigma and discrimination based on sexual orientation and/or gender identity have a tremendous negative impact on the mental health of 2SLGBTQ+ people (Moagi et al., 2021; Mongelli et al., 2019). Stereotypes and prejudices can have an impact on the way 2SLGBTQ+ people living with mental health issues are treated, both within the 2SLGBTQ+ community and within the healthcare system. People who identify as 2SLGBTQ+ who also happen to have mental health issues often experience a double stigma or dual alienation in which they feel they are not accepted within the mental health community because of their 2SLGBTQ+ identities and are also not accepted within the 2SLGBTQ+ community because of their mental health issues (Kidd et al., 2011; Veltman and La Rose, 2019). When an individual possesses additional traditionally marginalized identities (e.g., racialization, disability, immigration), experiences of stigma and alienation are often amplified and compounded (Veltman and La Rose, 2018).

In a Canadian study of 2873 trans and non-binary people aged 14 and over, 1 in 3 participants reported having considered suicide in the past year and 1 in 20 participants reported attempting suicide in the past year (The Trans Pulse Canada Team, 2020). In a large U.S. study (the largest survey to date of gender-variant and transgender people with an N = 6,450), 41% reported attempting suicide at some point in their lives (Grant et al., 2011). A recent meta-analysis (Wittgens et al., 2022) demonstrated that people who identified as lesbian, gay or bisexual had a higher risk for mental disorders than people who identified as heterosexual in all investigated diagnostic/symptom categories (i.e., depression, alcohol use disorder, anxiety disorders, and suicidality). The risk for depression and suicidality was higher in people who identified as bisexual compared with lesbians and gay people (Wittgens et al., 2022). It should be noted that there is nothing inherent in identifying as part of the 2SLGBTQ+ community that increases the risk for any of these mental health issues, but rather, it is the stigma and discrimination that people who identify as a sexual or gender minority face that leads to the increased risks (Reisner et al., 2015; Veltman and La Rose, 2019).

LGBT youth who come from highly rejecting families are more than three times as likely to have attempted suicide than LGBT peers who reported no or low levels of family rejection (Ryan et al., 2010). Many studies have demonstrated that risks for 2SLGBTQ+ youth can be reduced significantly by family acceptance and connection with other 2SLGBTQ+ youth (Hafeez et al., 2017; Price and Green, 2021; Taylor et al., 2020; Travers et al., 2012). Using and respecting trans-identified youth's chosen names has also been shown to reduce depressive symptoms, suicidal ideation and suicidal behaviour among transgender youth (Russell et al., 2018).

It is important for healthcare providers to understand that the marginalization and discrimination experienced by 2SLGBTQ+ people contributes to barriers in accessing health services (Mongelli et al., 2019; Smith et al., 2019; Steele et al., 2017). These barriers are compounded by healthcare providers often lacking the appropriate knowledge and skills around 2SLGBTQ+ health, having been ill-prepared by their healthcare professional training programs to care for individuals who identify as having a minority sexual orientation and/or gender minority (Chan et al., 2016; Coutin et al., 2018; Hana et al., 2021; Mackinnon et al., 2016; McPhail et al., 2016; Morrison et al., 2017; Nama et al., 2017; Obedin-Maliver et al., 2011; Rowe et al., 2017; Varley, 2022).

Many 2SLGBTQ+ people avoid traditional healthcare settings in order to try to shield themselves from mental or physical harm at the hands of potentially homophobic/transphobic healthcare providers (Bauer et al., 2014; James et al., 2016; Mahowald et al., 2020). In a large U.S. survey of trans-identified people, 28% reported delaying medical care for fear of discrimination and 50% reported having to teach their clinicians about transgender care (Grant et al., 2011). Negative experiences with healthcare professionals after disclosing a minority sexual orientation or gender identity (e.g., the healthcare provider being visibly uncomfortable, using harsh or abusive language, being physically rough or abusive during physical exams, or refusing to provide care) shaped future use of health services (Bauer et al., 2014; Mahowald et al., 2020).

Did You Know?

There are many healthcare disparities faced by people who identify as having a minority sexual orientation and/or gender identity:

- Patients who identify as 2SLGBTQ+ face many barriers in healthcare settings such as:
  - Discomfort or fear in disclosing their identity to their healthcare provider for fear of possible discrimination or bias
  - Healthcare provider ambivalence or discomfort related to inadequate education regarding 2SLGBTQ+ issues
  - Heterosexist or cisgenderist assumptions on forms or in interviews
  - Pathologization of 2SLGBTQ+ identities
  - Previous experiences or stories of "reparative" therapies
  - No opportunity for disclosure (providers are not asking the right questions)
- Patients who identify as 2SLGBTQ+ have an increased risk of depression, anxiety, and suicidality (especially if they are not accepted by their families, friends and colleagues)
- Increased vulnerability to mental health issues among 2SLGBTQ+ people is due to:
  - Loss of supports/rejection
  - Burden of keeping a secret identity
  - Bullying/violence
  - Discrimination/heterosexism/cisgenderism
  - Homo/bi/transphobia
  - Coming out process
  - Pathologization by the medical community
- Patients who identify as 2SLGBTQ+ are less likely to seek preventative healthcare, sometimes avoiding healthcare services until the issues are urgent/emergent

---

Reparative or conversion therapy (a range of pseudo-scientific treatments that aim to change a person's sexual orientation from homosexual to heterosexual or gender identity from transgender to cisgender) has been condemned by many professional organizations worldwide as unethical and harmful, while in some jurisdictions, such "therapy" has been made illegal. As an example, the American Psychiatric Association (APA) position statement on this issue includes the following: "Efforts to change an individual's sexual orientation or gender expression have been shown to be harmful and potentially deadly" (APA, 2020).

For transgender people, lack of access to gender affirming treatments such as both hormonal and surgical treatment (if desired by the person) can adversely impact their mental health (Almazan and Keuroghlian, 2021; Branstrom and Pachankis, 2019; Coleman et al., 2022; Tordoff et al., 2022). For healthcare providers who are providing care to transgender and gender diverse people, the World Professional Association for Transgender Health (WPATH)'s Standards of Care would be an important resource to review (Coleman et al., 2022). Many North American organizations and associations have released statements or policies that support the importance of access to gender-affirming care for transgender and gender variant people (American Psychiatric Association, 2018; American Psychological Association, 2015; Canadian Medical Protective Association, 2015; Veltman et al., in press).

The Issues

Cisgenderism and Heterosexism in Medicine

Cisgenderism and heterosexism remain prevalent issues in healthcare, both from the perspective of patients seeking care and also from the perspective of healthcare workers and healthcare professional students (Butler et al., 2019). Discrimination against 2SLGBTQ+ people, reflective of prevailing social attitudes, is present in incoming medical trainees (Burke et al., 2015). However, it has been demonstrated that increased student exposure to and favorable contact with 2SLGBTQ+ health issues and patients (including standardized patients) are associated with increased knowledge (Sanchez et al., 2006; Wahlen et al., 2020) as well as self-reported comfort (Sequeira et al., 2012) in the care of patients who identify as 2SLGBTQ+.

Aside from cultural safety and cultural humility skills that students who identify as 2SLGBTQ+ may bring to individual interactions with patients who also identify as part of the 2SLGBTQ+ community, increased diversity of students within medical school classes has been shown to benefit all students in the class (Niu et al., 2012). While the value of increasing the diversity of healthcare trainees (with respect to a wide range of issues including racial, socioeconomic, ability, sexuality, and gender diversity) is clear, it is also clear that navigating healthcare training while facing minority stress takes a toll on students from underrepresented groups who gain admission (Butler et al., 2019, Dyrbye et al., 2005; Hatzenbuehler, 2009; Meyer, 2003; Nama et al., 2017). Sexual-minority identified students (as compared to heterosexual students) are more likely to report harassment and isolation, higher stress levels, and less social support (Grbic and Sondheimer, 2014; Przedworski et al., 2015). In a study by Nama et al. (2017), 41.7% of medical students reported witnessing or experiencing anti-LGBT jokes, rumours and/or bullying by fellow medical students and/or members of the healthcare team. In the same study, it is noteworthy that while half of medical students who identified as LGBT shared their identity with all of their classmates, they were more likely to conceal this information from staff physicians.

Qualitative data about medical students who identify as a gender minority suggests that these students have to navigate a cisnormative medical culture in which throughout their education and training, it is almost never acknowledged that gender diverse people might be part of their patient population, classroom or their healthcare provider team (Butler et al., 2019).

Although institutional initiatives to mitigate the impact of minority stress on sexual and gender minority students may be valuable, such initiatives may not stop the perpetuation of bias through medicine's hidden or silent curriculum (Giffort and Underman, 2016). Curricular and cultural changes in medical education are both necessary to improve the wellbeing of 2SLGBTQ+ students and, ultimately, of 2SLGBTQ+ patients (Alexander et al., 2017; Giffort and Underman, 2016; Hollenbach et al., 2014; Varley, 2022). The silent curriculum is explored in detail in Chapter 3.

The process by which the existence of transgender and gender non-conforming people is precluded in healthcare has been termed "erasure" and described as taking place through both informational and institutional processes (Bauer et al., 2009). Trans-identified students' descriptions of curricula that assume all patients to be cisgender as well as a strict correlation between masculine gender and male sex, and between feminine gender and female sex, constitute informational erasure. An example of institutional erasure is demonstrated by trans-identified students' descriptions of institutional infrastructure that make related assumptions, such as by automatically assigning students to gendered locker rooms based on their legal gender markers (Butler et al., 2019).

Cisnormative and heteronormative medical cultures (in which cisgender and heterosexual identities are framed as normative) reinforce the continued ignorance of medical trainees regarding 2SLGBTQ+ individuals and their health needs, contributing to and perpetuating the healthcare inequities of sexual and gender minority patients seeking care (Alexander et al., 2017; Giffort and Underman, 2016; Mansh et al., 2015). Prevailing cisnormative and heteronormative medical cultures in medical schools is not unique to this context, given that research on the experiences of 2SLGBTQ+ students in multiple higher education contexts also demonstrates cisnormativity and heteronormativity as prevalent (Greathouse et al., 2018; Hollenbach et al., 2014). However, given the unique obligation of medical education institutions to consider how culture affects the care of vulnerable patients, it is important to examine the effects of this medical culture on students as well as on patients (Varley, 2022).

Pause and Reflect

Think back to an encounter with a patient who identifies as part of the 2SLGBTQ+ community.

How did this encounter make you feel? Were you uncomfortable or unsure of what questions to ask your patient related to their sexual orientation or their gender identity? Were you unsure about terminology related to various sexual/gender minority identities? Do you think that your patient felt comfortable enough to disclose their sexual/gender minority identity to you as a healthcare provider? If so, what helped them to feel comfortable to disclose this information? If not, are there things that you could do or say that would make a patient feel more comfortable to disclose their identity to you?

Please see Table 6.1 for some ideas about how to create and maintain a 2SLGBTQ+ Positive Space within your healthcare setting. Please see the Glossary of Terms at the end of the chapter to increase your knowledge of terminology related to various sexual and gender minority identities.

Table 6.1. *Creating and Maintaining a 2SLGBTQ+ Positive Space*

Creating and Maintaining a 2SLGBTQ+ Positive Space
- Use inclusive language in interviews and intake forms
- Reflect back the language used by your patient, including using their stated name and pronouns (which may be different than their legal name/pronouns)
- Do not make any assumptions about patient's sexual orientation or gender identity
- Display posters/pamphlets/signs that are inclusive of 2SLGBTQ+ people and issues
- Offer gender-inclusive bathrooms
- Post a non-discrimination policy that includes sexual orientation, gender identity and gender expression
- Accept and celebrate diversity

The Opportunity

The Value of Sexual and Gender Diversity in Healthcare

❖

"Homosexuality is immutable, irreversible and nonpathological"
— Abhijit Naskar, 2017

❖

Clinical Vignette

Paul is a 50-year-old man who identifies as gay. After his general practitioner (GP) retired 3 years ago, he found himself without a family doctor. Before the GP's retirement, Paul (who is generally in good health), drove to Toronto, Canada, to see his GP (a 2.5 hour drive each way) from the small town community where he and his partner, Dylan, live. Paul made the decision to keep his Toronto GP after moving out of the city in order to receive healthcare that he describes as "gay positive".

Since his GP's retirement, Paul has considered on a number of occasions the idea of signing on to a new primary care practice if the opportunity ever arose closer to his current town; he has decided against this idea for now due to his concern about the potential new doctor's "attitude" towards Paul's sexual identity/sexual orientation. Paul has stated that the "small town doctors" respond negatively to his preferred sexual practices and to the fact that he and Dylan are in an open relationship. Both Dylan and Paul have engaged in open, casual sex within the gay/MSM (men who have sex with men) community since the late 1980s. Both men are HIV-negative and engage in safe sex practices. Paul has also expressed concerns about the potential for a lack of confidentiality in a small-town practice, where support staff and other "prying eyes" might have access to information that could cause him difficulty in his professional life. On this basis, Paul has elected to use walk-in clinics for his healthcare needs and to avoid what he describes as "the trap of continuity of care" which he reframes as the "continuity of judgement and shaming...". For Paul, the walk-in clinic allows him a degree of anonymity which feels safer and more affirming of his identity and life choices.

Clinical Vignette Analysis

Most healthcare providers would argue that continuity of care is an important aspect of quality of care for patients, especially with respect to primary healthcare. However, the scenario above demonstrates that this is not always true for people who identify as part of the 2SLGBTQ+ community. For many 2SLGBTQ+ people, creating the conditions for relational continuity with a primary healthcare provider is a complicated and potentially risky process. In Paul's case above, due to previous negative experiences with physicians when he was discussing his sexual practices openly, he has chosen to use walk-in clinics instead of a signing up to be a part of the practice of a GP in his local community. Paul is concerned about judgement and shaming from healthcare providers in his small town and he would rather seek services at a walk-in clinic that provides him with some level of anonymity.

Unfortunately, many 2SLGBTQ+ people face discrimination and negative experiences while seeking healthcare and this can lead to avoidance of seeking healthcare at all (or until the health issue is advanced or more urgent). Not having an ongoing relationship with a primary healthcare provider is likely to limit continuity of care and therefore, likely to limit the potential for patient-centered care to take place, while also potentially helping patients avoid the risk of heterosexist assumptions. However, Paul's narrative suggests the potential need to "educate" the doctor about his life experience and is understood as a kind of labour that may not produce the desired outcome of a positive relationship. In this context, the idea of "dominant" or "normative narratives" is highly relevant to the disjuncture between actual patient experience and the goals of patient-centered care, suggesting that continuity is not always helpful and can be deeply paradoxical (Cook and Brunton, 2015; Katon et al., 2010).

This disjuncture between the care delivered and the actual care experienced is due in part to the reliance of narratives on shared meaning making and the nature of meaning as "situated" within the details of a story (La Rose, 2012). However, for healthcare providers who do not share a similar identity, making meaning requires a kind of *epistemological humility* and recognition of *not knowing* as the key to understanding patient stories (Parens, 1995). In this context, being patient-centered requires the practitioner to cultivate comfort with uncertainty, while making a commitment to professional development activities that promote a knowledge of LGBTQ diversity and intersecting identities (Baines, 2017; Veltman and La Rose, 2016). It is important to note that appreciation for difference, diversity, not knowing, critical reflexivity, and epistemic humility by healthcare providers are all fundamental elements of successful 2SLGBTQ+ patient-centered care (see Chapter 13 on Critical Allyship for additional details).

Pause and Reflect on Your Clinical Experiences

- Think about a clinical encounter you had where you treated a patient who identified as having a minority sexual orientation (i.e., the patient did not identify as straight/heterosexual). What was the main reason for the clinical encounter? Reflect on your clinical history taking and think about what types of questions you asked.

- Now think about another clinical encounter that you may have experienced with a similar chief complaint in a heterosexual patient. Were the questions you asked similar in the two scenarios? Did you omit any questions about the patient's history of the presenting illness, medical history, or social history in either case?

Pause and Reflect on Your Clinical Experiences (continued)

- Reflect on whether you made any assumptions about the patient who was not heterosexual that led you to omit any questions that you asked the patient who is heterosexual. Was there a possibility that you could have missed any important diagnoses based on your history taking? Was there a possibility that by not asking some questions, you may have affected the relationship/rapport with your patient in a negative way?

The purpose of this exercise is to challenge assumptions you may have made in history taking and to get you to think about whether the same standard of care is being provided to patients, regardless of their sexual orientation. Given that most physicians and healthcare providers grew up in a heterosexist, cisnormative society, many likely have assumptions and negative beliefs about gender and sexual minorities. It is important to identify these potential biases and assumptions, and to challenge them.

Inclusion Strategies

Strategies to Promote Inclusion of Diverse Sexual Orientations and Gender Identities in Medicine

❖

"Equality means more than passing laws. The struggle is really won in the hearts and minds of the community, where it really counts."
—Barbara Gittings, 1973

❖

Professional Vignette

Dr. Nathan is a GP practicing in a small town in Southern Ontario, Canada. Shortly after she took over the primary practice clinic (which included a full roster of patients) from a retiring family doctor, Dr. Nathan received a call from the local Health Authority asking her to accept a trans-identified patient who was experiencing difficulty receiving appropriate, trans-affirming healthcare and had filed a significant complaint with the Authority. Dr. Nathan had no experience with providing care to trans-identified patients, but as a member of the LGBTQ+ community herself and as an MD who had practiced in rural and remote settings for a significant period of time, she felt confident that she would be able to navigate the process of caring for a patient seeking transition-related care and affirming healthcare in general, and agreed to support this patient by adding her to the already full family practice.

Several weeks later, Dr. Nathan met Dorothy, a trans woman who had been seeking healthcare in her local area for more than 5 years when she joined the clinic. When Dr. Nathan met Dorothy, she was amazed at how well informed she was about her own healthcare needs and the resources and supports that were available to support Dr. Nathan as she cared for Dorothy.

In her first appointment with Dr. Nathan, Dorothy stated that she was seeking hormone therapy and (in the future) support for gender affirming surgeries, but she also had a few other current health concerns such as type 2 diabetes mellitus and high blood pressure. Dr. Nathan listened to Dorothy and paid attention to the issues she raised about how she was treated by other doctors in the past and let Dorothy know that she was open to her feedback and suggestions. Dr. Nathan also took Dorothy's advice about where and how to get resources and supports, following up with educational resources such as those available through Rainbow Health Ontario and the World Professional Association for Transgender Health Standards of Care. Dr. Nathan asked Dorothy if she was open to having Dr. Nathan consult with some other MDs who were experts in trans care, so that she could feel confident that she was doing the best by her patient. Dorothy was open and willing to sign consents and answer questions to help facilitate Dr. Nathan's learning.

As Dr. Nathan stated, "Dorothy came with her own wealth of information, really all I had to do was listen and then follow through with what she told me; it reminded me of my time working in remote communities, where you can't just refer someone to a specialist, because the specialist if 500 miles away. You've got to find other ways to figure it out...."

Professional Vignette Analysis

In the case above, Dr. Nathan was willing to accept the risk of doing something unfamiliar to her by taking on a patient who identified as transgender, even though Dr. Nathan had no previous experience with providing trans-affirming care. Dr. Nathan recognized the importance of taking on a patient who had previous negative experiences within the healthcare system and she was open to truly listening to the patient's experiences. By doing so, she was able to recognize that the patient herself was a tremendous source of information and resources related to trans issues. Dr. Nathan also understood the value of seeking to consult and collaborate with other professionals who had more experience than her in order to ensure that she would be able to provide appropriate trans-affirming care to her new patient.

Pause and Reflect
What do I Bring to this Issue? An Exercise in Self-Reflection
• When a colleague or learner speaks about their partner or spouse using gender neutral language, has that made you feel uncomfortable to ask anything more about them? What was it that made you feel uncomfortable? • What barriers have you created or perpetuated for learners or colleagues to disclose their sexual orientation or their gender identity? • How can you create a more inclusive work-environment for medical trainees and healthcare workers of all sexual orientations and gender identities?

Key Takeaways: Physicians as Change Makers

- Physicians must embrace the opportunity to be change makers and leaders in the inclusion of all people, regardless of their sexual orientation or gender identity.
- By modeling inclusive practices that do not assume anyone's sexual orientation or gender identity in both educational and clinical environments, we can promote a culture that allows for disclosure of sexual orientation and gender identity, without fear of negative impact or career repercussions.

- We must work to eliminate the assumption that views people with minority sexual orientations or gender identities as requiring "fixing" or "correcting".
- Colleagues who identify as having a minority sexual orientation and/or gender identity add value to medical education and healthcare, and can provide valuable input that improves patient care experiences and outcomes.
- When healthcare providers' identities reflect the populations they serve, this is powerful in terms of improving the patient care experience and outcomes.
- As physician change makers, we can also influence the medical admissions system, encouraging the inclusion of sexual orientation, gender identity and gender expression in any statement that welcomes diverse applicants.
- Advocacy for the incorporation of appropriate curriculum related to sexual orientation, gender identity and gender expression in medical schools is essential if we are to develop comfort in caring for people who have a wide variety of sexual orientations, gender identities and gender expressions.
- Advocacy for a more inclusive medical education and training curriculum is also essential in order to bring awareness to the health inequities experienced by people who identify as 2SLGBTQ+.

Conclusion

The need for significant improvements in LGBTQ+ healthcare is clearly demonstrated in research undertaken over the past several decades. This scholarship demonstrates the need for far reaching improvements in health education, research activity and curriculum development focused on the needs of LGBTQ+ peoples (Dubin et al., 2018; Korpaisarn and Safer, 2018; Obedin-Maliver et al., 2011; Varley, 2022). Greater exposure and training regarding issues related to 2SLGBTQ+ health increases provider confidence, competence and comfort in treating individuals who identify as 2SLGBTQ+.

More recent scholarship suggests that LGBTQ+ patients are well aware of negative implications resulting from lack of training and knowledge about their healthcare needs and experiences, with trans-identified patients having the most severe effects and still leading the charge for improvement (Dubin et al., 2018; Korpaisarn and Safer, 2018). As healthcare education on these topics increases for all healthcare providers and as more healthcare providers who identify as 2SLGBTQ+ become increasingly comfortable with challenging heterosexism and cisgenderism within healthcare educational programs and within healthcare environments in general, access to high quality, 2SLGBTQ+-affirmative healthcare will also improve.

On a Parting Note…

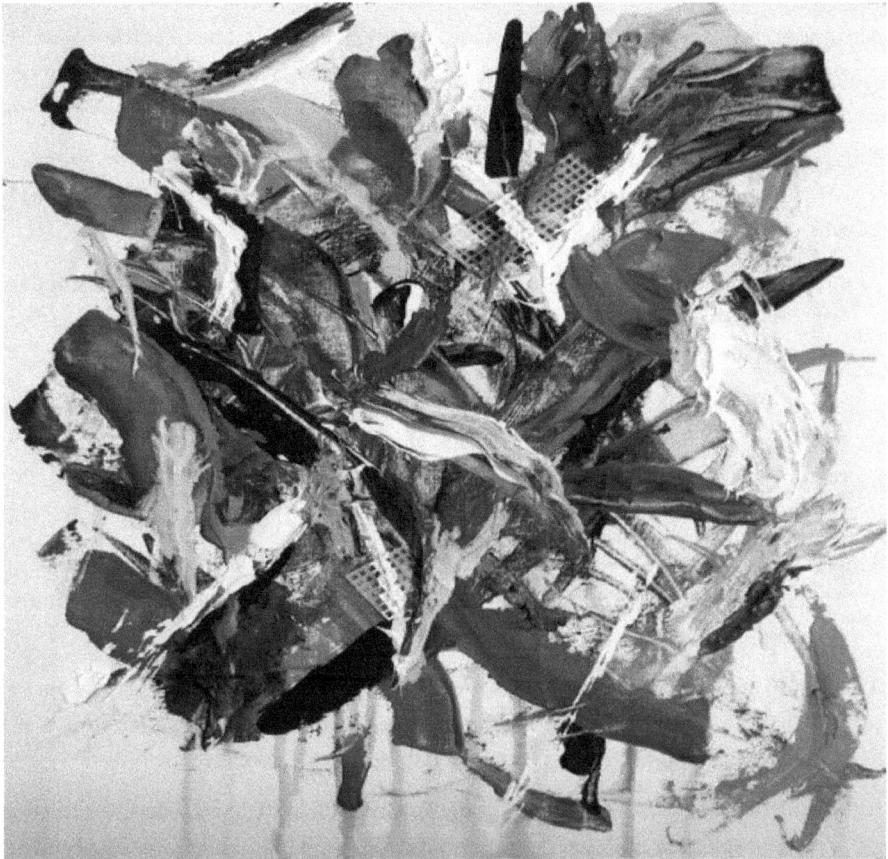

Original artwork by first author, Albina Veltman

References

Alexander, K., Cleland, J., and Nicholson, S. (2017). Let us not neglect the impact of organizational culture on increasing diversity within medical schools. *Perspectives on Medical Education*, 6, pp. 65-67.

Almazan, A.N., and Keuroghlian, A.S. (2021). Association between gender-affirming surgeries and mental health outcomes. *JAMA Surgery*, 156(7), pp. 611-618.

American Psychiatric Association [APA]. (2018). *Position statement on Access to Care for Transgender and Gender Diverse Individuals* [online]. Available from: https://www.psychiatry.org/home/policy-finder

American Psychiatric Association [APA]. (2020). *Position Statement on Issues Related to Sexual Orientation and Gender Minority Status* [online]. Available from: https://www.psychiatry.org/home/policy-finder?k=gender%20minority%20status

American Psychiatric Association [APA]. (1968). *DSM-II Diagnostic and Statistical Manual of Mental Disorders*. 2nd ed. Washington: American Psychiatric Association.

American Psychiatric Association [APA]. (2022). *Diagnostic and statistical manual of mental disorders : DSM-5-TR*. 5th edition, text revision. Washington, DC: American Psychiatric Association Publishing.

American Psychological Association (2015). Guidelines for psychological practice with transgender and gender nonconforming people, *American Psychologist*, 70(9), pp. 832-864.

Baines, D. (2017). *Doing anti-oppressive practice: social justice social work*. 3rd edition. Donna Baines (ed.). Black Point: Fernwood Publishing.

Bauer, G.R., Hammond, R., Travers, R., Kaay, M., Hohenadel, K.M. and Boyce, M. (2009). "I don't think this is theoretical; this is our lives": how erasure impacts health care for transgender people. *Journal of the Association of nurses in AIDS care*, 20(5), pp.348-361.

Bauer, G.R., Scheim, A.I., Deutsch, M.B. and Massarella, C. (2014). Reported emergency department avoidance, use, and experiences of transgender persons in Ontario, Canada: results from a respondent-driven sampling survey. *Annals of emergency medicine*, 63(6), pp.713-720.

Bayer, R. (1981). *Homosexuality and American psychiatry: the politics of diagnosis*. New York: Basic Books.

Branstrom, R. and Pachankis, J.E. (2019). Reduction in mental health treatment utilization among transgender individuals after gender-affirming surgeries: a total population study, *European journal of public health*, 29(4), pp. 727-734.

Burke, S.E., Dovidio, J.F., Przedworski, J.M., et al. (2015). Do contact and empathy mitigate bias against gay and lesbian people among heterosexual first-year medical students? A report from the Medical Student CHANGE Study, *Academic Medicine*, 90, pp. 645–651.

Butler, K., Yak, A., and Veltman, A. (2019). "Progress in medicine is slower to happen": qualitative insights into how trans and gender nonconforming medical students navigate cisnormative medical cultures at Canadian training programs, *Academic medicine*, 94(11), pp. 1757-1765.

Chan, B., Skocylas, R., Safer, J.D. (2016). Gaps in transgender medicine content identified among Canadian medical school curricula, *Transgender health*, 1(1), pp. 142-50.

Canadian Medical Protective Association. (2015). *Treating transgender individuals* [online]. Available from: https://www.cmpa-acpm.ca/en/advice-publications/browse-articles/2015/treating-transgendered-individuals

Coleman, E., Radix, A.E., Bouman, W.P., Brown, G.R., De Vries, A.L.C., Deutsch, M.B., Ettner, R., Fraser, L., Goodman, M., Green, J. and Hancock, A.B. (2022). Standards of care for the health of transgender and gender diverse people, version 8. *International journal of transgender health*, 23(sup1), pp.S1-S259.

Cook, C. and Brunton, M. (2015). Pastoral power and gynaecological examinations: a Foucauldian critique of clinician accounts of patient-centred consent. *Sociology of health and illness*, 37(4), pp. 545-560.

Coutin, A., Wright, S., Li, C. and Fung, R. (2018). Missed opportunities: are residents prepared to care for transgender patients? A study of family medicine, psychiatry, endocrinology, and urology residents, *Canadian medical education journal*, 9(3), e41–e55.

Drescher, J., and Merlino, J.P. (editors). (2007). *American psychiatry and homosexuality: an oral history*. New York: Harrington Park Press.

Dubin, S.N., Nolan, I.T., Streed, C.G., Greene, R.E., Radix, A.E., and Morrison, S.D. (2018). Transgender health care: improving medical students' and residents' training and awareness, *Advances in medical education and practice*, 9 pp. 377-391.

Dyrbye, L.N., Thomas, M.R., and Shanafelt, T.D. (2005). Medical student distress: Causes, consequences, and proposed solutions. *Mayo Clinic proceedings*, 80(12) pp. 1613–1622.

Giffort, D.M., and Underman, K. (2016). The relationship between medical education and trans health disparities: A call to research. *Sociology compass*, 10(11), pp. 999–1013.

Global Action for Trans Equality (2020). *Joint statement on ICD-11 process for trans & gender diverse people* [online]. Available from: https://gate.ngo/icd-11-trans-process/

Grant, J.M., Mottet, L.A., Tanis, J., et al. (2011). *Injustice at every turn: A report of the National Transgender Discrimination Survey* [online]. Available from: https://transequality.org/sites/default/files/docs/resources/NTDS_Report.pdf.

Grbic, D. and Sondheimer, H. (2014). Personal well-being among medical students: Findings from an AAMC pilot survey. *Analysis in brief Association of American Medical Colleges*, 14(4), pp. 1-2.

Greathouse, M., Brckalorenz, A., Hoban, M., Huesman, R., Rankin, S., Stolzenberg, E.B. (2018). *Queer-Spectrum and Trans-Spectrum Student Experiences in American Higher Education: The Analyses of National Survey Findings* [online]. Available from: https://www.academia.edu/37328173/Queer-Spectrum_and_Trans-Spectrum_Student_Experiences_in_American_Higher_Education

Hafeez, H., Zeshan, M., Tahir, M.A., Jahan, N., and Naveed, S. (2017). Health care disparities among lesbian, gay, bisexual, and transgender youth: A literature review. *Cureus journal of medical science*, 9(4), pp. e1184.

Hana, T., Butler, K., Young, T., et al. (2021). Transgender health in medical education, *Bulletin of the World Health Organization*, 99(4), pp. 296-303.

Hatzenbuehler, M.L., Pachankis, J.E. (2016). Stigma and minority stress as social determinants of health among lesbian, gay, bisexual, and transgender youth. *Pediatric clinics of North America*, 63(6), pp. 985- 997.

Hatzenbuehler, M.L. (2009). How does sexual minority stigma "get under the skin"? A psychological mediation framework, *Psychological bulletin journal*, 135(5), pp. 707–730.

Hollenbach, A.D., Eckstrand, K.L. and Dreger, A.D. eds., (2014). *Implementing curricular and institutional climate changes to improve health care for individuals who are LGBT, gender nonconforming, or born with DSD: a resource for medical educators.* Association of American Medical Colleges.

Howard, S., Saewyc, E.M., Cameron, C., et al. (2021). Best Practice Expert Panel, Registered Nurses' Association of Ontario. (2021). Promoting 2SLGBTQI+ Health Equity: Best Practice Guidelines. Toronto, ON [online].

Available from: https://rnao.ca/sites/rnao-ca/files/bpg/2SLGBTQI_BPG_ June_2021.pdf

James, S.E., Herman, J.L., Rankin, S., Keisling, M., Mottet, L., and Anafi, M. (2016). *The report of the 2015 U.S. transgender Survey* [online]. Available from: https://transequality.org/sites/default/files/docs/usts/USTS-Full-Report-Dec17.pdf

Katon, W. J., Lin, E. H., Von Korff, M., Ciechanowski, P., Ludman, E. J., Young, B., and McCulloch, D. (2010). Collaborative care for patients with depression and chronic illnesses. *New England journal of medicine*, 363(27), pp. 2611-2620.

Kidd, S.A., Veltman, A., Gately, C., et al. (2011). Lesbian, gay, and transgender persons with severe mental illness: negotiating wellness in the context of multiple sources of stigma. *American journal of psychiatric rehabilitation*, 14(1), pp. 13–39.

Korpaisarn, S., and Safer, J. D. (2018). Gaps in transgender medical education among healthcare providers: A major barrier to care for transgender persons, *Reviews in endocrine and metabolic disorders*, 19(3), pp. 271-275.

La Rose, T. (2012). Digital media stories through multimodal analysis: A case study of Erahoneybee's song about a child welfare agency, *Journal of technology in the human services*, 30(3-4), pp. 299-311.

MacKinnon, K.R., Tarasoff, L.A., and Kia, H. (2016). Predisposing, reinforcing, and enabling factors of trans-positive clinical behavior change: A summary of the literature. *International journal of transgenderism*, 17(2), pp. 83–92.

Mahowald, L., Gruberg, S., and Halpin, J. (2020). *The State of the LGBTQ Community in 2020: A National Public Opinion Study, Center for American progress* [online]. Available from: https://cf.americanprogress.org/wp-content/uploads/2020/10/ LGBTQpoll-report.pdf?_ga=2.132130252.394860255.1641916454-1963279976. 1641916454.

Mansh, M., Garcia, G., and Lunn, M.R. (2015). From patients to providers: Changing the culture in medicine toward sexual and gender minorities, *Academic medicine*, 90(5), pp. 574–580.

McPhail, D., Rountree-James, M., Whetter, I. (2016). Addressing gaps in physician knowledge regarding transgender health and healthcare through medical education, *Canadian Medical education journal*, 7(2), e70–e78.

Meyer, I.H. (2003). Prejudice, social stress, and mental health in lesbian, gay, and bisexual populations: Conceptual issues and research evidence, *Psychological bulletin journal*, 129(5), pp. 674–697.

Moagi, M.M., van Der Wath, A.E., Jiyane, P.M., et al. (2021). Mental health challenges of lesbian, gay, bisexual and transgender people: An integrated literature review. *Health SA gesondheid – Journal of interdisciplinary health sciences,* 26(9), a1487.

Mongelli, F., Perron, D., Balducci, J., et al. (2019). Minority stress and mental health among LGBT populations: An update on the evidence, *Minerva psychiatry,* 60(1), pp. 27-50.

Morrison, S.D., Dy, G.W., Chong, H.J., et al. (2017). Transgender-related education in plastic surgery and urology residency programs, *Journal of graduate medical education,* 9, pp. 178–183.

Nama, N., Macpherson, P., Sampson, M., and McMillan, H.J. (2017). Medical students' perception of lesbian, gay, bisexual, and transgender (LGBT) discrimination in their learning environment and their self-reported comfort level for caring for LGBT patients: a survey study, *Medical education online,* 22, 1368850.

Niu, N.N., Syed, Z.A., Krupat, E., Crutcher, B.N., Pelletier, S.R., and Shields, H.M. (2012). The impact of cross-cultural interactions on medical students' preparedness to care for diverse patients, *Academic medicine,* 87, pp. 1530–1534.

Obedin-Maliver, J., Goldsmith, E.S., Stewart, L., et al. (2011). Lesbian, gay, bisexual and transgender-related content in undergraduate medical education, *Journal of the American Medical Association,* 306(6), pp. 971-977.

Parens, E. (1995). The pluralist constellation, *Cambridge quarterly healthcare ethics,* 4(2), pp. 197-206.

Peter, T., Campbell, C.P., & Taylor, C. (2021). Still in every class in every school: Final report on the second climate survey on homophobia, biphobia, and transphobia in Canadian schools. Toronto, ON: Egale Canada Human Rights Trust [online]. Available from: https://egale.ca/awareness/still-in-every-class/

Price, M.N., and Green, A.E. (2021). Association of gender identity acceptance with fewer suicide attempts among transgender and nonbinary youth, *Transgender health,* 8(1), pp. 56-63.

Przedworski, J.M., Dovidio, J.F., Hardeman, R.R., et al. (2015). A comparison of the mental health and well-being of sexual minority and heterosexual first-year medical students: a report from the Medical Student CHANGE Study, *Academic medicine,* 90(5), pp. 652–659.

Reisner, S.L., Vetters, R., Leclerc, M., Wolfrum, S., Shumer, D., and Mimiaga, M.J. (2015). Mental health of transgender youth in care at an adolescent urban community health center: A matched retrospective cohort study', *Journal of adolescent health*, 56(3), pp. 274-279.

Rowe, D., Ng, Y.C., O'Keefe, L., et al. (2017). 'Providers' attitudes and knowledge of lesbian, gay, bisexual, and transgender health, *Federal practitioner*, 34(11), pp. 28-34.

Russell, S.T., Pollitt, A.M., Li, G., and Grossman, A.H. (2018). Chosen name use is linked to reduced depressive symptoms, suicidal ideation, and suicidal behaviour among transgender youth, *Journal of adolescent health*, 63(4), pp. 503-505.

Ryan, C., Russell, S.T., Huebner, D., et al. (2010). Family acceptance in adolescence and the health of LGBT young adults, *Journal of child and adolescent psychiatric nursing*, 23(4), pp. 205–213.

Saewyc, E., Poon, C., Wang, N., et al. (2007). *Not yet equal: the health of lesbian, gay, & bisexual youth in BC* [online]. Available from: www.mcs.bc.ca/pdf/ not_yet_equal_web.pdf

Sanchez, N.F., Rabatin, J., Sanchez, J.P., Hubbard, S., and Kalet, A. (2006). Medical students' ability to care for lesbian, gay, bisexual, and transgendered patients, *Family medicine*, 38(1), pp. 21–27.

Sequeira, G.M., Chakraborti, C., and Panunti, B.A. (2012). Integrating lesbian, gay, bisexual, and transgender (LGBT) content into undergraduate medical school curricula: A qualitative study, *Ochsner journal*, 12(4), pp. 379–382.

Smith, R.W., Altman, J.K., Meeks, S., et al. (2019). Mental health care for LGBT older adults in long-term care settings: Competency, training, and barriers for mental health providers, *Clinical gerontologist*, 42(2), pp. 198-203.

Steele, L.S., Daley, A., et al. (2017). LGBT identity, untreated depression, and unmet need for mental health services by sexual minority women and trans-identified people, *Journal of women's health*, 26(2), pp. 116-127.

Taylor, A.B., Chan, A., Hall, S.L., Saewyc, E.M., and the Canadian Trans & Non-binary Youth Health Survey Research Group. (2020). *Being Safe, Being Me 2019: Results of the Canadian Trans and Non-binary Youth Health Survey* [online]. Available from: https://www.saravyc.ubc.ca/2020/03/18/being-safe-being-me-2019/

The 519 Church Street Community Centre. (2020). The 519 Glossary 2020 [online]. Available from: https://www.the519.org/educationtraining/glossary

The Centre. (2006). *LGTB health matters: an education & training resource for health and social service sectors* [online]. Available from: http://www.sexualhealth centresaskatoon.ca/pdfs/p_lgbt.pdf

The Trans PULSE Canada Team. (2020). *Health and health care access for trans and non-binary people in Canada* [online]. Available from: https://transpulsecanada.ca/research-type/reports/

Tordoff, D.M., Wanta, J.W., Collin, A., Stepney, C., Inwards-Breland, D.J., and Ahrens, K. (2022). Mental health outcomes in transgender and nonbinary youths receiving gender-affirming care, *Journal of the American Medical Association Network Open*, 5(2), e220978.

Travers, R., Bauer, G., Pyne, J., et al. (2012). Impacts of strong parental support for trans youth: A report prepared for Children's Aid Society of Toronto and Delisle Youth Services [online]. Available from: https://transpulseproject.ca/wp-content/uploads/2021/10/Impacts-of-Strong-Parental-Support-for-Trans-Youth-vFINAL.pdf

Varley, K. (2022). The lack of sexual and gender minority curriculum in U.S. medical schools, *Journal of science policy & governance*, 20(2). doi.org/10.38126/JSPG200209

Veltman, A., and La Rose, T. (2019). LGBTQ mental health: What every clinician needs to know, *Psychiatric times*, 36(12), pp. 21-23.

Veltman, A., and La Rose, T. (2016). Anti-oppressive approach to assessment, in, Hategan, A., Bourgeois, J.A., Seritan, A.L., and Hirsch, C. (eds.) *On-call geriatric psychiatry: a handbook of principles and practice*. New York: Springer Publishing Company, pp. 55-62.

Veltman, A., and La Rose, T. (2018). Marginalized Geriatric Patients, in Hategan, A., Bourgeois, J., Hirsch, C., and Giroux, C. (eds.) *Geriatric psychiatry*. New York: Springer International Publishing, pp. 629-643.

Veltman, A., La Rose, T., and Chaimowitz, G. (in press). Canadian Psychiatric Association Position Paper. Mental Health Care for People Who Identify as Two Spirit, Lesbian, Gay, Bisexual, Transgender, and (or) Queer (2SLGBTQ+), *Canadian Journal of Psychiatry*.

Wahlen, R., Bize, R., Wang, J., Merglen, A., and Ambresin, A-E. (2020). Medical students' knowledge of and attitudes towards LGBT people and their health care needs: Impact of a lecture on LGBT health, *PLoS ONE*, 15(7), e0234743.

Wittgens, C., Fischer, M.M., et al. (2022). Mental health in people with minority sexual orientations: A meta-analysis of population-based studies, *Acta psychiatrica scandinavica*, 145(4), pp. 357–372.

World Health Organization (2019). *HA60 Gender incongruence of adolescence or adulthood*. International classification of diseases,11th revision [IDC-11] [online]. Available from: https://icd.who.int/browse11/l-m/en#/http://id.who.int/icd/entity/90875286

Appendix 6.1: Glossary of Terms

The following terms and definitions may be used differently by different people in different regions and are not standardized. They are compiled from several sources (Howard et al, 2021; The 519 Glossary, 2020; Veltman & La Rose, 2019), with the acknowledgement that they will change over time as the thinking, attitudes and discourses around 2SLGBTQ+ issues continue to evolve.

Term	Definition
Ally	Someone who advocates for and supports members of a community other than their own, reaching across differences to achieve mutual goals.
AFAB/AMAB	Acronyms meaning "assigned female at birth/assigned male at birth".
Asexual	Sometimes called "ace" for short, asexual refers to a complete or partial lack of sexual attraction or lack of interest in sexual activity with others. Asexuality exists on a spectrum where asexual people may experience no, little or conditional sexual attraction.
Biphobia	Irrational fear and dislike of bisexual people. Bisexuals may be stigmatized by heterosexual people as well as by lesbians, gay men and transgender people.
Bisexual	A person who is attracted to and may form emotional, romantic and/or sexual relationships with people with the same and to people with a different gender and/or gender identity to themselves. People who identify as bisexual need not have had equal experience- or equal levels of attraction- with people across genders, nor any experience at all: it is merely attraction and self-identification that determine orientation.
Cisgender	A person who by nature or by choice conforms to gender- and/or sex-based expectations of society (also referred to as gender normative).
Cisgenderism	Assuming every person to be cisgender, therefore marginalizing those who identify as transgender in some form. It is also believing cisgender people to be superior, and holding people to traditional expectations based on gender, or punishing or excluding those who do not conform to traditional gender expectations.
Coming out	Recognizing one's own sexual orientation or gender identity and being open about it with oneself and/or with

Term	Definition
	others. This often occurs in a significant moment as well as throughout one's life, with each person to whom one chooses to come out.
Discrimination	Negative behaviour or actions toward a person or group of people based on prejudicial attitudes and beliefs about the person's or group's characteristics, such as sexual orientation, gender identity or gender expression.
Gay	A person whose primary sexual orientation is to members of the same sex or gender. A person of any gender identity can identify as gay, although many female-identified people who are attracted to other female-identified people prefer the term lesbian.
Gender-affirming surgeries	Surgical procedures by which a person's physical appearance and function of their existing sexual characteristics are altered to resemble that of the sex or gender they are transitioning to.
Gender creative	Sometimes also known as "gender non-conforming" or "gender expansive"; often in reference to children, but not always; Someone who is gender creative is someone who rejects expected gender roles and stereotypes, expresses a gender identity that is different from the one they were assigned at birth or one that cannot be (or refuses to be) defined within the male/female binary.
Gender expression	The way in which a person expresses their gender identity through clothing, behaviour, posture, mannerisms, speech patterns, activities and more.
Gender identity	One's internal and psychological sense of oneself as male, female, both or neither.
Genderism	Sometimes referred to as cisgenderism; The assumption that all people must conform to society's gender norms, and specifically, the binary construct of only two genders, corresponding to the two sexes (female and male). This belief in the binary construct as the most normal and natural and a preferred gender identity does not include or allow for people to be intersex, transgender, or genderqueer.
Gender nonconforming	A person who does not conform to society's expectations of gender expression based on the gender binary or expectations of masculinity and femininity.
Genderqueer	A person who experiences a very fluid sense of their gender identity and who does not want to be constrained by absolute concepts. Instead, they prefer to be open to relocating themselves on the gender continuum.

Term	Definition
Gender variant	A synonym for gender nonconforming, which is preferred to gender variant because variance implies a standard normativity of gender.
Heterosexual	A person whose primary sexual orientation is to people of a different sex or gender than their own. Heterosexual people are often referred to as "straight".
Heterosexism	The assumption that everyone is, or should be, heterosexual, and that heterosexuality is inherently superior to and preferable to all other sexual orientations.
Heterosexual privilege	Benefits derived automatically by being (or being perceived as) heterosexual that are denied to all other non-heterosexual sexual orientations.
Homosexual	A person who has emotional, romantic and/or sexual attraction predominately to a person of the same gender. As this term is historically associated with a medical model of homosexuality, most people would prefer to self-identify as gay, lesbian or queer.
Homophobia	The irrational fear or hatred of, aversion to, and discrimination against homosexuals or homosexual behaviour.
Internalized homophobia	The experience of guilt, shame or self-hatred in reaction to one's own feelings of attraction for a person of the same sex or gender as a result of homophobia and heterosexism.
Interpersonal or external homophobia	Overt expressions of internal biases, such as social avoidance, verbal abuse, derogatory humour and physical violence.
Intersex	A person who has some mixture of female and male genetic and/or physical sex characteristics. Intersex people may have external genitalia that do not closely resemble typical male or female genitalia, the appearance of both female and male genitalia, the genitalia of one gender and the secondary sex characteristics of a different gender or have a chromosomal make-up that is neither XX nor XY. An outdated term formerly used was hermaphrodite. An intersex person may or may not identify as part of the transgender community.
Institutional homophobia or heterosexism	Refers to the many ways that governments, businesses, religious institutions, educational institutions and other organizations set policies and allocate resources that discriminate against people based on sexual orientation.

Term	Definition
Lesbian	A female-identifying individual whose primary sexual orientation is to other female-identifying individuals or who identifies as a member of the lesbian community.
Non-binary	An umbrella term for gender identities that fall outside of the man-woman binary, anywhere along the gender spectrum.
Pansexual	A person who is attracted to other people regardless of gender identity.
Prejudice	An unjustified or incorrect attitude toward an individual or group of people based solely on their membership in a social group, such as the 2SLGBTQ+ community.
Queer	In contemporary usage, queer is an inclusive, unifying, sociopolitical and self- affirming umbrella term encompassing a broad range of sexual and gender expression, including people who identify as gay, lesbian, bisexual, transgender, intersex, genderqueer or any other nonheterosexual sexuality or nonconforming gender identity. Queer is a reclaimed term, which was previously seen as derogatory, but many people (though not all people) within the 2SLGBTQ+ community are comfortable using this term.
Questioning	A self-identification sometimes used by those exploring personal issues of sexual orientation and/or gender identity.
Reparative or conversion therapy	A range of pseudo-scientific treatments that aim to change a person's sexual orientation from non-heterosexual to heterosexual or a person's gender identity from non-cisgender to cisgender.
Sexual behaviour	Refers specifically to sexual actions or what a person does sexually. Sexual behaviour is not necessarily congruent with sexual orientation and/or sexual identity.
Sexual identity	Refers to a person's identification to self (and others) of one's sexual orientation. It is not necessarily congruent with sexual orientation and/or sexual behaviour.
Sexual orientation	Refers to how one thinks of oneself in terms of one's emotional, romantic or sexual attraction, desire or affection for another person.
Transgender or trans	Someone whose gender identity or expression differs from their assigned gender at birth. It is often used as an umbrella term that includes people who identify as Two Spirit, intersex, genderqueer and non-binary.

Term	Definition
Transition	A complicated, multi-step process that can take years as transgender people align their anatomy and (or) their gender expression with their gender identity.
Transphobia	Irrational fear or dislike of transgender people.
Two Spirit	A term used by some North American Indigenous people to describe those people in their cultures whose nature is comprised of both male and female spirits. People who identify as Two Spirit may also identify as gay, lesbian, bisexual, transgender, intersex, or have multiple gender identities.

Chapter 7
See No Evil: The Politics of Appearance

Noam Raiter, MD, Shania Bhopa, MSc, Ana Hategan, MD,
Heather Sylvester, Hons BSc, MD

❖

"To lose confidence in one's body is to lose confidence in oneself."
—Simone de Beauvoir, 1953

❖

Abstract: Appearance moderates the way in which the world regards individuals and can have significant impacts on both opportunities and barriers. This chapter examines the appearance-related appraisals that physicians encounter as physicians are subject to scrutiny by both their patients and their colleagues. Factors such as physician age, personal style preferences, racial features, body size, and gender identity are explored as they are reported to affect patient satisfaction and confidence in their physician. Harmful stereotypes emanating from a physician's presentation may lead to pressure for conformity within the clinical setting that is detrimental to both physician and patient wellbeing.

Keywords: ageism, appearance, body image, diversity, identity, physical appearance

Introduction

The physician workforce in most Western nations is increasingly diverse, and should approximate the diversity of their national populations. However, this in itself is a source of tension in a variety of ways, with physical appearance being one such area. Although the book covers various aspects of diversity, this chapter will focus on overt aspects including age, personal style preferences, racial features, body size, and gender. Humans judge each other within a fraction of a second of meeting (Willis and Todrov, 2006). On encountering a stranger, studies show that within a tenth of a second, impressions are already formed based on the stranger's appearance and, importantly, longer exposures do not significantly alter those impressions (Willis and Todrov, 2006).

Age, clothing, race, size and other aspects of appearance moderate the way in which the world regards individuals, and can have significant impacts on both opportunities and barriers. The unconscious rapid sorting mechanisms and heuristics that underlie responses to people and situations can be detrimental when implicit conclusions that are without merit, are transmitted to interpersonal behaviours and actions.

An individual's appearance does not correspond with intelligence, compassion or professionalism. However, this knowledge can often be overlooked in medicine, where patients and health providers are both subject to assumptions and judgment based on their appearance. Physician appearance may not be the most important aspect of the doctor-patient or colleague-to-colleague relationships but research shows it certainly plays a role. Several studies have emphasized that patients may have significant preference for physicians who possess certain physical traits. This preference is also observed in the way physicians view their colleagues and themselves. Knowing this, it is important to acknowledge the implications that physician self-presentation has on engagement with patients and the cascade of effects it creates. However, it is also vital to enter these discussions with the hope of building a medical field that is inclusive, promotes authentic self-expression and promotes positive body image rather than conformity to the status quo.

This conversation is critical, as the pressure for conformity within the clinical setting can be detrimental to workplace satisfaction and sense of purpose within one's career. Physician wellbeing has direct impacts on patient care; thus it is important for physicians to feel confident, accepted, and authentic in the workplace (West et al., 2018). Furthermore, many of the physical appearance traits that are discriminated against in the medical workforce may also be reflected in many of our patients. Creating a workforce with diverse physical traits also creates a workforce that reflects the diverse patient population and can better support the varied patient population we serve.

This chapter will explore a number of prevalent preconceptions related to appearance, with the goal of addressing the mitigation of bias, discrimination and judgment that stems from appearance.

The Issues

Appearance, body image and authentic self-expression involve several facets including ones' age, stylistic choices, racially or ethnically specific physical characteristics, gender expression, and body shape and size. The following section will discuss the issues at hand in relation to these facets, noting that they are interconnected, and the intersectionality of these facets expose affected physicians to an even greater degree of scrutiny.

Ageism

"How old are you anyways?", a phrase many physicians, both "too young" and "too old", have come to know and expect from their patients. Ageism in the medical field is not a new phenomenon and its roots date back to archaic definitions of professionalism and society's misconceptualizations of age-related capabilities (Levy and Macdonald, 2016). As trends in physician age demographics change and the average age of physicians continues to rise (AAMC, 2020) whilst at the same time generating some relatively young physicians, it is necessary that we bring these topics to the forefront of our daily discussions. In so doing, it is possible to cultivate a medical field that is inclusive and progressive as the breadth of the physician age spectrum allows a spectrum of experiential expertise and intergenerational mentorship in the workforce.

At the root of ageism towards medical professionals is a patient's desire to have a competent physician. The desire to have a physician who is old enough to have gained vast knowledge and life experience, but also young enough to be sharp, up to date on new research, and relatable with the patient's personal experiences. However, much of ageism is based on how old a physician looks rather than on their clinical and professional competence. Traits such as grey hair and wearing glasses may make an individual appear older. On the flip side, physicians may appear to be younger through minimal physical signs of aging, fashion choices, or even the way they talk.

Hair and Clothing

Despite the poor correlation between one's stylistic choices, intelligence and career suitability, patients appear to place much emphasis on what their physician wears, how they style their hair, and other personal appearance choices. In a 2019 study, over half of participants stated that the way their physician dresses is important to them and one third said it directly impacts their satisfaction with patient care (Petrilli et al., 2018). A majority of participants stated that their preferred style of dress was formal attire. Physicians who were dressed in this category of clothing were deemed more knowledgeable, trustworthy, caring, and approachable by their patients. This trend was even more pronounced for older participants.

Although a majority of younger patients still prefer formal dress, they are more open to physicians wearing scrubs or casual dress compared to their older counterparts (Petrilli et al., 2018). Such age-related trends also have been reported in various other studies (Gherardi et al., 2009; Lill and Wilkinson, 2005) and suggest that newer generations are more flexible with what "dressing professionally" means while older generations maintain more traditional views on physician clothing choices. This phenomenon of increased casualization can be observed in many facets of our modern society beyond clothing such as vocabulary, social norms, and more (Parsi and Taub, 2002).

Pause and Reflect

Was there a time you were critical of a colleague's choice of hairstyle or clothing at work?

- What were your judgments? What informs these perceptions? Did you have a discussion with someone else about their opinions of the colleague's appearance?
- Take a moment to analyze the origins and influences of your perception. What aspect of their presentation were you reacting to? Does it have any impact on their professionalism, performance or tone of the space around them?
- Does their appearance constitute a safety concern for peers, learners or patients? How can you reframe the tone of your inner dialogue?

A common theme that was represented across the body of literature was patients' preference for physicians wearing their white coat during encounters (Gherardi et al., 2009; Rehman et al., 2005; Zollinger et al., 2019). The white coat has historically served as a symbol of hierarchical elitism and contributes to medicine's often paternalistic culture (Wear, 1998). It is well known that a patient-physician relationship that promotes patient centered care leads to better health outcomes and patient satisfaction (Gluyas, 2015). Furthermore, there are many well cited hygiene concerns surrounding wearing a white coat in medical practice but even when patients were made aware of this, their preference for the white coat did not reflect a change (So et al., 2015). This suggests that patient preferences for physicians' dress are not solely based on their desire to receive optimal medical care but are also influenced by their beliefs surrounding professionalism and the medical field.

Patient preferences do not end with physicians' clothing. A number of studies examined patient preferences with respect to physician hairstyles in the clinic. A majority of patients prefer their male physicians to have short hair and their female physicians to have their hair pulled back into a pony tail. Uncolored hair was preferred for both genders (Van der Merwe et al., 2016).

This topic is further complicated by the role of gender bias in physician style choices. One study found that when wearing casual dress in clinic, male physicians received more positive ratings than their female colleagues. Even when wearing more formal outfits, female physicians were more likely to be misidentified as other healthcare workers such as nurses and medical technicians (Xun et al., 2018). Another study examined skirt and dress lengths for women physicians, showing that patients have expectations, essentially 'moral' expectations of female physicians (Van der Merwe et al., 2016). As described elsewhere in Chapters 1 and 5, sexism in medicine has had profound impact on female physician career trajectories, safety of the work environment, and wellbeing. Dismantling gender specific standards for professional dress may serve as one small step towards bringing down barriers that have no correlation to the competence of female and gender diverse physicians, and concurrently serve to hold back their career potential.

The literature shows that the clothing a physician wears matters to patients. Although patient perspectives are important, we must also work towards creating a medical field that promotes physician wellness by allowing physicians to wear clothing that they are most comfortable and confident in within the realm of professionally acceptable dressing.

Tattoos and Piercings

Common societal perceptions of professionalism often entail an individual who is conservatively dressed and free of expressive piercings, tattoos, and other accessories. There is a widespread erroneous belief that piercings indicate decreased trustworthiness and competence by both patients and medical colleagues (Newman et al., 2005). In a study analyzing medical faculty perceptions about colleagues with non-traditional facial piercings, 24% of physicians indicated that it would bother them to work in a clinical setting with a male physician or trainee with an ear piercing and 58% by a physician of either gender with a nose piercing (Newman et al., 2005). Eyebrow piercings were felt to be inappropriate by 73% of physician respondents (Newman et al., 2005) although these endorsements have likely decreased over time. Results from a survey conducted in the emergency department indicated that 48% of patients believe it is inappropriate for their physicians to have a nose stud and 52% said the same regarding their physician having a lip piercing (Newman et al., 2005).

In addition to perceptions about piercings and perceived professionalism, physicians with tattoos are often subject to many biased beliefs from colleagues and patients alike (Johnson et al., 2016). In a 2016 study from the USA, participants rated tattooed practitioners with lower confidence when compared with non-tattooed practitioners (Johnson et al., 2016). As long as these biased beliefs continue to permeate the medical system, it creates inaccurate perceptions about patients and physicians who have piercings.

Clinical Vignette

"I'd like to speak to a *real* physician please," the patient said with a straight face as he was looking directly through me. I tried to think of a response but after 8 hours of my emergency medicine shift as a resident physician, I had very little fight left in me. As I walked towards my preceptor for the shift I thought of ways to explain why the patient insisted on talking to him instead. Did I mess up the patient's name? Was it the way I walked in the room? Could he tell I was only just starting my career? I explained that all I did was to introduce myself, but the patient had already made up their mind about me. By taking one look at me he decided I was not a competent or professional physician, or in his words, not a "real physician".

About five minutes later, a new patient chart was dropped in front of me by the nurse. A 22-year-old female with chest pain. I did my best to put aside the troubles of my past patient encounter and head with a clear mind into this new encounter. The patient looked at me and gave me a look that could only be read as relief. "I love your tattoos" she said as she looked directly at one of my several tattoos.

A lily on my inner left forearm. A tattoo that I got in honor of my best friend who passed away by suicide last year as it was her favourite flower. In the months before her passing both she and I grew increasingly frustrated at her limited access to mental health resources. Eventually, she fell through the gaps of our medical system. I got this tattoo not only to remember her but also to remember the type of physician I want to be. To always see patients as individuals, to always advocate for their needs, to come to every encounter with an open mind and compassion. I thanked her for the compliment, and we got to talking about what brought her in today. I gathered all the information and as I walked out of the room, she stopped me, "I am so glad you are my doctor. Seeing your tattoo when you walked in reminded me that you're a human being too and it made me feel more comfortable opening up to you".

Walking towards the charting station, all the pieces of the puzzle began clicking together. Unlike most days in the emergency room, today I wasn't wearing a long sleeve shirt under my scrubs. As such, tattoos usually hidden on my forearms were now exposed. So, perhaps this the reason that first patient refused to talk to me? Is this why he didn't see me as a "real doctor"? Nonetheless, I then reminded myself, this was also the reason I was able to best connect with and therefore best treat my second patient. How many more patients would benefit from having more diversity in their physicians? Physicians with tattoos like theirs. Or piercings. Or colored hair. Or outfit choices that strayed away from blue scrubs or a white button-down shirt with black trousers. Physicians who weren't afraid to own their individuality.

Clinical Vignette Analysis

This vignette highlights the unfortunate discrimination faced by physicians with expressions of personal style that strays from what is perhaps the status quo in the medical field. It also highlights how important it is to have representation of individuals with diverse physical appearances as an inclusive health workforce shapes the patient care experience. Most physicians can think of at least one instance where we made a snap judgement about a colleague or patient based on their appearance. This should be tempered by a time when seeing someone who looked like us allowed us to feel seen and welcome in a new space or community. Rewiring generations of biased beliefs and stigmatization does not evolve overnight, but it can start with increased representation and a decision that as a medical community we will welcome any and all individuals so that hopefully over time, our patients will also follow suit.

Race, Religion, and Cultural Practices

Physician's race or religion can play a role in career progression and their patient-physician satisfaction ratings. Although the healthcare setting should be a safe space, like society, the medical field also demonstrates discrimination towards minority groups, and this can affect physicians' ability to dress in a way that feels most authentic to their heritage. Although race and religion encompass much more than physical appearance, things such as cultural dress or hair styles are a large part of how individuals may outwardly express their beliefs and affiliations.

There is much research on how physicians' religious and cultural beliefs affect their practices, however research on the experiences of physicians in relation to their religion is relatively sparse. This raises questions in terms of the basis for some institutions' policies that limit religious and ethnocultural wear when it is not clearly tied to infection control or physical safety. Continued work on religious and cultural bias constitutes a critical component to the broader EDI dialogue in the medical microcosm.

Gender and Sexual Identity Expression

Until less than 50 years ago, homosexuality was considered a pathologic disorder by the *Diagnostic* and Statistical Manual of Mental Disorders (Ng, 2010). Despite the critical progressive strides that have been made towards gender equality, gender inequity and societal biases still remain towards those from gender and sexual minorities. It is well known that the sexual preferences and gender identities of physicians influence colleague-to-colleague and doctor-to-patient interactions and relationships. Although gender and sexual orientation go deeper than one's physical appearance, this is what most people are judged on at first glance. Variables that may affect perception of one's sexual or gender orientation include fashion choices, body piercings, hair colouring and more (Madrigal et al., 2021).

In one North American study, approximately one in ten patients responded that they would refuse to see a gay, lesbian or bisexual physician, stating that their physician may be incompetent or that they would feel uncomfortable (Druzin et al., 1998). Knowing this, and often having experienced such discrimination personally, physicians and medical trainees from sexual and gender minority groups may be hesitant to express their true identity through their outward appearance. A study in 2021 found that 67% of medical students report concerns that disclosure of their sexual identity would affect their future career and relationships with their peers (Madrigal et al., 2021). Fostering a culture in medicine that teaches trainees and early career physicians to fear authentic self-expression limits inclusion for both physicians and patients.

Pause and Reflect

Questions to consider as a trainee, practicing physician, or clinical ally:

- Reflect on a recent encounter in which the gender or sexual orientation of a colleague appeared to or explicitly influenced the encounter.
- Were there any elements of social exclusion? How did this emanate in the encounter?
- In considering your clinical setting, what inclusive practices exist for gender and sexual minorities? What daily habits can be adopted to further promote an accepting and progressive clinical culture?
- In what ways can we advance medical education and training in order to progress from awareness to anti-oppressive practices in relation to sexual and gender minority groups?

Weight, Height, and Body Type

Weight bias is an unfortunately prevalent phenomenon in our society, with the perception that one's body type indicates their health behaviours and their value to society. Weight bias is deeply entrenched in many parts of modern society and as such affects the perception of physicians based on their weight and body type. This is reflected in the literature which indicates that physicians who are perceived to be overweight or obese are vulnerable to biased attitudes from patients and are viewed to have decreased credibility in their medical opinions (Puhl et al., 2013). Such assumptions are likely grounded in the contemporary views of what "healthy" is and the expectation that health providers must exemplify such standards.

This issue not only impacts how patients see their physicians but also how physicians view themselves. A recent study found that physicians with a body mass index (BMI) in the "normal-weight" range have greater confidence in their ability to provide nutrition and exercise counseling to their patients compared to physicians with higher BMI who believe that patients would be less likely to trust lifestyle advice from them (Puhl et al., 2013). Importantly, two recent studies indicated that weight bias among medical professionals dates back to their undergraduate years (Lawrence et al., 2021). Body type and body composition often do not constitute an indicator of overall health; thus it is important to acknowledge the multifaceted nature of health.

Similar to physician's weight, their height can also impact the way they are perceived. Height is particularly relevant in the workplace where issues of persuasion and power come into play (Judge and Cable, 2004). When considering the correlation between height, self-esteem, and performance it is appears that height may be seen as a proxy for one's competence as a physician (Judge and Cable, 2004). Further research is required regarding this topic, however, many physicians from both ends of the height spectrum can share anecdotal experiences where this physical trait was used to define their competence and personal traits. Individuals who are shorter in height may require assistive tools such as a stool to support them when leaning over the operating table. Such simple needs may inadvertently translate to diminished power and authority in the workplace.

Professional Vignette

I arrived at work on a Tuesday like any other. I greeted the other members of my team at the family medicine practice. Our practitioner team consists of four physicians, one physician's assistant and two nurses. I entered the exam room to see my first patient of the day, a 56-year-old male with hypercholesterolemia and non-alcoholic fatty liver disease. I came in ready to pull up his risk scores, educate him on the importance of improving his metabolic health and hopefully get him leaving with a new statin prescription and some lifestyle resources. He was the same age as me and had 2 daughters just like I did. Unfortunately, the conversation did not go to plan. He thanked me for explaining his recent blood work results but told me he would deal with matters himself and walked out of the room. These encounters always stick with you. The ones where you feel like you did everything "right" but yet there was a divide between you and the patient that you just cannot seem to breakthrough.

A few hours later, I finally found a minute to sit down to eat my lunch. I was catching up on the news when I overheard the nurses and one of the other physicians talking in the hallway. "Did you see the patient storm out this morning?" one said. Another voice responded, "Well, do you blame them? I wouldn't be taking lifestyle or diet advice from Dr. Marshall either". The third voice piped in, "I know. Have you seen the size of the lunch they are eating today? Who is checking their bloodwork? Where is their diet plan?" I felt a sharp stab in my chest and dropped my fork. If only they knew what was going on, on the other side.

Professional Vignette Analysis

Based on the experiences described in this vignette, the physician experienced weight-based discrimination and stigmatization from his colleagues (and perhaps from his patient, too). This vignette finishes off with the physician reflecting on the aspects of their life that their colleagues do not have insight into. Perhaps they do not know that he has struggled with weight his entire life. That despite every diet and exercise program he has tried, his genetics just do not allow him to lose that extra weight. Or that he was diagnosed with an endocrinologic disorder that affects his weight. Or that he has also been struggling with a binge-restrict cycle of disordered eating.

Further, if this physician was hoping to lose weight, how does overhearing other healthcare professionals talk about their situation affect their motivation to seek care themselves? If colleagues that they know and trust hold such discriminatory judgments about them, what will their own physician think of them?

Such stigmatizing beliefs about body weight and habitus reduce health into a unidimensional concept. In reality, a healthy individual may come in different shapes and sizes, and a wide variety of background experiences may shape what living a "healthy lifestyle" means to each person.

Importantly, we must also ensure that we do not discredit the extensive educational training received by physicians by making snap judgements about their ability to provide care based on their appearance.

The Opportunity

Although seemingly innocuous, the politics related to appearance are but one of many pressure points for medical professionals in terms of impractical patient expectations that potentially contribute to the burnout pipeline. As such, a culture that allows for individuality in physician dress and dissolves traditional standards of professionalism may foster a healthier medical culture in that it reduces one element of the toxic culture of stereotypes. Although research on specific interventions is limited, this section will highlight existing work as well as pose ideas for further opportunities. We continue to see the incoming cohort of physicians promoting inclusivity in dialogue, face-to-face interactions and in clinical settings. The opportunity to continue exchanging information and sharing one's perspective can promote enhanced inclusivity in the workplace.

❖

"To be yourself in a world that is constantly trying to make you something else is the greatest accomplishment."
—Ralph Waldo Emerson, nd

❖

Ageism

The body of literature suggests that neither younger nor older physicians are more competent than the other and each group has unique skill sets that should not be undermined. As such it is important to tackle age-related stereotypes and biases to ensure dignity and respect is maintained regardless of age. This is particularly important in light of the evolving physician workforce. In fact, this evolving age demographic of the physician workforce may facilitate the shift in common but inaccurate perceptions and ideologies that continue to be perpetuated by physicians, other healthcare providers and patients alike.

Stylistic choices

The stylistic choices of physicians such as clothing and hairstyles evidently have an impact on their patient and peer relationships. The shift to wearing casual clothing amongst newer physicians relative to their older counterparts provides an opportunity to discuss the importance of a shift in perceptions about physician professionalism and competency. Stepping away from paternalistic choices such as the white coat may foster more patient-centered relationships by removing one component of the power dynamics in the medical setting. In addition, allowing physicians to express themselves through their hairstyle and clothing choices may offer clinicians a better sense of inclusion, purpose, and authenticity in the workplace. Importantly, creating a workforce with diverse physical appearance can allow patients with similar stylistic choices to feel comfortable in the clinical setting, thus reinforcing the importance of physicians leading by example and embracing their authentic selves.

A 2017 study found that patient preferences were impacted by what they see their own physician wearing regularly (Van De Car e. al., 2017). For example, patients with physicians who regularly wore scrubs in their clinic were more accepting of scrubs as appropriate professional wear. This finding highlights that physicians have an opportunity to largely impact this conversation and change patients' perspectives to ensure a more open-minded approach to clothing choices in the medical field. This is particularly relevant with respect to the dialogue on ethnocultural dress.

Tattoos and piercings

Given that one's outward appearance has little bearing on intelligence, compassion, and competence as a physician, it may be time to reexamine this expectation of conformity regarding the role of piercings and tattoos in the professional setting. Engaging in discussion regarding the way we understand historical social taboos such as tattoos and untraditional piercings presents an important element of appearance-based judgements of physicians (Stirn, 2003).

Creating a more inclusive environment will attract a broader range of physicians that can be reflective of the patient population that they serve. This can increase patient engagement and trust through relatability. As discussed above, creating a workplace that allows for authentic expression can improve physician wellbeing and ultimately improve career satisfaction.

Race, religion, and cultural practices

As discussed earlier, physical identifying characteristics that may indicate a physician's race, religion or culture are often subject to bias and discriminatory actions. This raises questions regarding some institutions' policies that limit religious and ethnocultural wear when it is not clearly tied to infection control or physical safety. For example, policies surrounding head coverings in operating rooms or the availability of only short sleeved scrub tops in hospitals may prevent physicians from entering fields that prescribe these specifications or prevent physicians who have already entered these fields from dressing in a way that aligns with their beliefs (Malik et al., 2019).

While maintaining the standards of sterility supersedes personal choices in terms of appearance, we must still ensure that we create an environment that is inclusive to all individuals. Promoting a culture that is inclusive to physicians of all backgrounds will not only positively contribute to physician wellness but also to patient care for those who also identify with similar backgrounds and may otherwise feel stigmatized for their choice of dress (Jetty et al., 2021).

Gender and Sexual Identity Expression

Given the nuances associated with disclosures of sexual orientation by healthcare professionals, it is important to review the impact of discrimination on those within the 2SLGBTQ+ community in clinical and nonclinical settings (Ng, 2010). The Minority Stress Model (MSM) is a theory that elucidates how stress can negatively affect self-perception and health as a result of discriminatory workplace experiences of gender or sexual minority identities (Baams et al., 2015).

The Minority Stress Model shows that when minority individuals experience sustained prejudice, it can cause stress responses of the physiological and psychological variety that accrue over time to cause poor mental and physical health. For gender and sexual minorities and other minority groups, there can be cascading effects on overall self-esteem, self-perception, self-efficacy and body image. This has impacts on wellbeing, increases burnout risk, and ultimately has an adverse impact on patient care.

It is well known that physicians representing the 2SLGBTQ+ community serve an important role as advocates for 2SLGBTQ+ health care issues (Eliason et al., 2011), added to which medicine must strive to resemble the population it serves if we are to remain effective healthcare providers. As such, the costs of non-disclosure must be considered, including the loss of personal integrity as well as the emotional effects of "passing" and "pronoun switching". It is important to consider how to break down the existing barriers in order to promote the wellbeing of both physicians and patients.

Body Weight and Height

The stereotypes associated with physician weight and height can have detrimental effects for both physicians and their patients. Stigma related to a physician's habitus, specifically their weight, poses negative consequences for the health of both patients and physicians. Fearing discrimination and judgement may cause physicians to be reluctant to access necessary medical care and embark on healthy lifestyle changes if such is actually indicated, as it is known that larger body types do not always indicate a state of poor health (Nyblade et al., 2019).

Distinguishing between the physical appearance of physicians and their perceived health status in relation to their ability to provide competent medical care is also essential as body habitus should not be correlated with career progression, and discrimination in relation to body habitus bears a psychological toll (Carr and Friedman, 2005).

The opportunities for achieving equity with respect to body weight and height chiefly involve the use of education, anti-discriminatory policy and ongoing dialogue to inspire a cultural shift. Over the years we have seen shifts in the language used to describe physical appearance, with gradual but forward momentum in the use of inclusive language. The healthcare and academic teaching environment are the right place to spearhead seismic shifts in the gaze cast at bodies, the language used to describe habitus, and the perceptions tied to bodies.

The gap in disentangling competence, merit and expectations from habitus suggest that it is essential to examine the underlying resistance to change. The opportunities to continue to shift the sociocultural expectations and perceptions about body habitus should share a common goal- to enhance inclusivity in the healthcare environment.

Although many healthcare institutions have made strides, there is still a gap in clinical skills training on inclusive language and unconscious bias for physicians and learners. Diversifying the academic and clinical education workspace, empowering physicians and their interprofessional colleagues to foster inclusive environments and promoting a positive workspace will improve physician wellbeing and patient experience concurrently. Thus, it makes sense to commit to this change. Similar to the topic of cultural dress, reducing discrimination related to body habitus can begin at the policy and administrative level transcending through the institution and laterally across the academic curriculum as well.

Inclusion Strategies

As the previous section has outlined, the impacts of bias and discrimination based on physician appearance can have wide reaching and long-lasting effects on the physician-patient relationship, interprofessional interactions, physician career prospects, physician wellness, and both patient care experiences and patient outcomes. The facets of appearance discussed including age, clothing, jewelry, race, gender, weight and more all speak to an overarching opportunity: to diminish barriers for career entry and progression for affected physicians and trainees, thus creating a diverse workforce that in turn promotes equity and inclusion in the care of patients of all backgrounds. Some general and specific inclusion strategies to mitigate appearance-related bias and discrimination are presented in Table 7.1 and Table 7.2.

Table 7.1 *General inclusion strategies to decrease appearance-related bias and discrimination*

General Inclusion Strategies
• Explore, identify and remove institutional barriers that limit career entry and progression in relation to appearance-related bias • Intentional commitment and action on increasing representation in relation to intersectionality • Utilize onboarding and recurring education and training activities to enhance interprofessional knowledge and skill in equity-informed care practices. Tying inclusive practices and accountability to staff advancement poses an opportunity to ingrain diversity as a source of growth in the academic and clinical workspace

Table 7.2 *Specific inclusion strategies to mitigate appearance-related bias and discrimination*

Specific Inclusion Strategies	
Ageism	Increase bi-directional mentorship in order to allow both younger and older physicians to foster each other's growth and indirectly mitigate bias and discrimination towards interdisciplinary colleagues and patients.
Stylistic Choices (e.g., clothing, hair, piercings, tattoos)	Reassess workplace and clinical area specific dress code policies to ensure they do not inadvertently discriminate based on appearance and that standards solely relate to safety.
Race, Religion, and Culture	Promote inclusive guidelines that maintain safety and sterility while also allowing for expression of one's race, religion, or culture. Suggestions include a wider variety of options for hospital scrubs that allow for individual modesty choices and equivalent head coverings that suit various religious preferences.
Height, Weight, and Body Size	Create more physically inclusive work environments by providing ergonomic accommodations that cover the height, weight, ability and shape spectrum of the workforce.
Gender Expression	Increase gender diversity in the medical field and decrease discrimination towards 2SLGBTQ+ individuals through policy and action.

Key Takeaways

- Physicians are subject to bias and discrimination based on their physical appearance.
- Lack of inclusion based on physical appearance is prevalent and impactful in that it adversely affects the wellbeing and satisfaction of patients and physicians alike.
- Factors such as age, clothing, hair, tattoos, piercings, racialized features, weight, and height affect patient's opinions of their physicians.
- Physicians at both ends of the age spectrum are subject to bias and discrimination that is often without merit as studies show equally positive patient outcomes for both younger and older physicians.
- Patients, physician peers, and other healthcare workers show negative responses towards physicians with tattoos and piercings.
- Patients show bias to female physicians with unconfined hair and casually dressed physicians, however there is no correlation to clinical skill or patient outcome although it affects patient trust, communication and willingness to receive care.
- Physicians from racial, cultural, and ethnic minorities face additional barriers when their ethnoracial, cultural and religious affiliations are visible. Individual bias and systemic factors may limit physicians' ability to dress in a way that aligns with their values and preferences.
- Physicians from sexual and gender minority groups face significant bias within the clinic setting. This impacts interactions with colleagues, patient interactions and interferes with the ability to work inclusively.
- The medical microcosm can present a challenging workspace and invalidating environment in that some physicians are forced to mute or disguise visible aspects of their core identity.
- Bias stemming from appearance is widespread in medicine and creates unsafe spaces for both physicians and patients alike, however there are many opportunities to incorporate inclusion strategies such as those illustrated in the Tables 7.1 and 7.2.
- Key inclusion strategies range from general principles at the institutional level to specific initiatives at the clinical level, both of

which require intention and commitment across all levels of the medical microcosm.

Conclusion

It is evident that several components of physician presentation such as age, clothing, ethnicity, size, and gender can impart bias in how a physician is perceived by their peers and their patients. Not only is it important to create a culture in medicine that is accepting of a diverse population of physicians in order to support physician wellbeing, but it is also critically important to do so in order to promote wellbeing for patients of all backgrounds.

On a Parting Note...

A Letter to My Daughter by Heather Sylvester, MD

Dear Alexandra,

When we were at the coffee shop and I asked you what interested you about LBGTQ2S Medicine and Transgender Medicine in particular, you said, "Mom I'm bisexual." It was at that moment that my love for you achingly intensified. What I mean is that your openness to be who you are and the drive in you to allow others to do the same while speaking out against the opposite resonates deeply with me and touches me to the core.

As a physician, who has been in practice for almost 40 years, I lived through prejudice against women as a medical trainee. When the staff physician, on his weekly rounds, asked me in front of 4 other male medical trainees, "What do you think is the average size of the adult male testicle?" The male physicians on the team snickered as I was sent to examine the "hepatic encephalopathy in Rm 225" and come back with "the correct answer". Many of my female classmates can recount their own experiences with misogyny not dissimilar to my own. My coping strategy was simply to keep my head down and comply, not wanting to disrespect the hidden curriculum in order to find my way to graduation day.

But you! You and your newly minted physician colleagues are speaking up and out and showing what it is to be living open and at home with your own diverse and unique natures. Whether it be, as a first-year medical student, you calling out a prejudiced staff-person, refusing to flip up your nasal septal piercing in the family medicine clinic or wearing your little rainbow pin on your name tag. I know this is not an angry, fist pumping message but rather a message that your mind and heart are open to receive people as they are, where they are and as who they are. I've seen this countless times as you follow your own path to becoming a family physician. Maybe the face of medicine is changing....

Much love,

Mom

Acknowledgement: The authors offer their special thanks to Alexandra Sylvester, Hons BSc, MD, PGY1 Resident in Family Practice, Dalhousie University.

References

AAMC. (2020). *Physician Specialty Data Report Executive Summary* [online]. Available from: https://www.aamc.org/data-reports/data/2020-physician-specialty-data-report-executive-summary

Baams, L., Grossman, A.H., & Russell, S.T. (2015). Minority stress and mechanisms of risk for depression and suicidal ideation among lesbian, gay, and bisexual youth. *Developmental Psychology*, 51(5), pp. 688–696. https://doi.org/10.1037/a0038994.

Carr, D. and Friedman, M.A. (2005) "Is obesity stigmatizing? body weight, perceived discrimination, and psychological well-being in the United States," *Journal of Health and Social Behavior*, 46(3), pp. 244–259. Available at: https://doi.org/10.1177/002214650504600303.

De Beauvoir. S. (1953): "To lose confidence in one's body is to lose confidence in oneself.".

Druzin, P., Shrier, I., Yacowar, M., & Rossignol, M. (1998). Discrimination against gay, lesbian and bisexual family physicians by patients. *CMAJ : Canadian Medical Association Journal*, 158(5), pp. 593–597.

Eliason, M.J., Dibble, S.L., & Robertson, P.A. (2011). Lesbian, gay, bisexual, and transgender (LGBT) physicians' experiences in the workplace. *Journal of Homosexuality*, 58(10), pp. 1355–1371. https://doi.org/10.1080/00918369.2011.614902.

Emerson, R. W. (2014). Ralph Waldo Emerson Essays: "To be yourself in a world that is constantly trying to make you something else is the greatest accomplishment.".

Gherardi, G., Cameron, J., West, A., et al. (2009). Are we dressed to impress? A descriptive survey assessing patients' preference of doctors' attire in the hospital setting," *Clinical Medicine*, 9(6), pp. 519–524. https://doi.org/10.7861/clinmedicine.9-6-519.

Gluyas, H. (2015). Patient-centred care: Improving healthcare outcomes. *Nursing Standard*, 30(4), pp. 50–59. https://doi.org/10.7748/ns.30.4.50.e10186.

Gomez, L.E. & Bernet, P. (2019). Diversity improves performance and outcomes. *Journal of the National Medical Association*, 111(4), pp. 383–392. doi.org/10.1016/j.jnma.2019.01.006.

Jetty, A., Jabbarpour, Y., Pollack, J., et al. (2022). Patient-physician racial concordance associated with improved healthcare use and lower healthcare expenditures in minority populations. *Journal of racial and ethnic health disparities*, 9(1), pp. 68–81. doi.org/10.1007/s40615-020-00930-4.

Johnson, S.C., Doi, M.L., & Yamamoto, L.G. (2016). Adverse effects of tattoos and piercing on parent/patient confidence in health care providers. *Clinical Pediatrics*, 55(10), pp. 915–920. https://doi.org/10.1177/0009922815616889.

Judge, T. A., Cable, D. M. (2004). The effect of physical height on workplace success and income: Preliminary test of a theoretical model. *Journal of Applied Psychology*, 89(3), pp. 428-441. https://doi:10.1037/0021-9010.89.3.428

Lawrence, B. J., Kerr, D., Pollard, C. M., *et al.* (2021). Weight bias among health care professionals: A systematic review and meta-analysis. *Obesity*, 29(11), pp. 1802–1812. https://doi.org/10.1002/oby.23266.

Levy, S. R., Macdonald, J. L. (2016). Progress on understanding ageism. *Journal of Social Issues*, 72(1), pp. 5–25. https://doi.org/10.1111/josi.12153.

Lill, M. M., Wilkinson, T. J. (2005). Judging a book by its cover: Descriptive survey of patients' preferences for doctors' appearance and mode of address. *BMJ*, 331(7531), pp. 1524–1527. https://doi.org/10.1136/bmj.331.7531.1524.

Madrigal, J., Rudasill, S., Tran, Z., Bergman, J., & Benharash, P. (2021). Sexual and gender minority identity in Undergraduate Medical Education: Impact on experience and career trajectory. *PLOS ONE*, 16(11), e0260387. https://doi.org/10.1371/journal.pone.0260387.

Malik, A., Qureshi, H., Abdul-Razakq, *et al.* (2019). *'I decided not to go into surgery due to dress code'*: A cross-sectional study within the UK investigating experiences of female Muslim medical health professionals on bare below the elbows (BBE) policy and wearing headscarves (hijabs) in theatre. *BMJ Open*, 9(3), e019954. https://doi.org/10.1136/bmjopen-2017-019954.

Newman, A. W., Wright, S. W., Wrenn, K. D., & Bernard, A. (2005). Should physicians have facial piercings? *Journal of General Internal Medicine*, 20(3), pp. 213–218. https://doi.org/10.1111/j.1525-1497.2005.40172.x.

Ng, H. (2010). Should a gay physician in a small community disclose his sexual orientation? *The Virtual Mentor*: VM, 12(8), pp. 613–617. https://doi.org/10.1001/virtualmentor.2010.12.8.ccas2-1008.

Nyblade, L, Stockton, M. A., Giger, K., *et al.* (2019). Stigma in health facilities: Why it matters and how we can change it. *BMC Medicine*, 17(1). https://doi:10.1186/s12916-019-1256-2

Parsi, K. & Taub, S. (2002). The trend toward casual dress and address in the medical profession. *The Virtual Mentor*: VM, 4(5). https://doi.org/10.1001/virtualmentor. 2002.4.5.ebyt1-0205.

Petrilli, C. M., Saint, S., Jennings, J., *et al.* (2018). Understanding patient preference for physician attire: A cross-sectional observational study of 10 academic medical centres in the USA. *BMJ Open*, 8(5), e021239. https://doi.org/ 10.1136/bmjopen-2017-021239.

Puhl, R.M.,Gold J.A., Luedicke, J. et al. (2013). The effect of physicians' body weight on patient attitudes: Implications for physician selection, trust and adherence to medical advice. *International Journal of Obesity*, 37(11), pp. 1415–1421. https://doi.org/10.1038/ijo.2013.33.

Rehman, S.U., Nietert, P. J., Cope, D. W., & Kilpatrick, A. O. (2005). What to wear today? Effect of doctor's attire on the trust and confidence of patients. *The American Journal of Medicine*, 118(11), pp. 1279–1286. https://doi.org/10.1016/ j.amjmed.2005.04.026.

So, E. C. T., Fung, F. H. F., Yeung, J. K. H., et al. (2013). Patient perception of physician attire before and after disclosure of the risks of microbial contamination. *International Journal of Medical Students*, 1(3), pp. 109–114. https://doi.org/10.5195/ijms.2013.216.

Stirn, A. (2003). Body piercing: Medical consequences and psychological motivations. *The Lancet*, 361(9364), pp. 1205–1215. https://doi.org/10.1016/s0140-6736(03)12955-8.

Tsugawa, Y., Newhouse, J. P, Zaslavsky, A. M., Blumenthal, D. M., Jena, A. B. (2017). Physician age and outcomes in elderly patients in hospital in the US: observational study. *BMJ*, 357, j1797. https://doi:10.1136/bmj.j1797.

Willis, J., Todorov, A. (2006). First impressions. *Psychological Science*, 17(7), pp. 592–598. https://doi.org/10.1111/j.1467-9280.2006.01750.x.

Van De Car, W., Starostanko, A., & Wendling, A. (2017). Rural patient preference for physician attire. *PRiMER*, 1. https://doi.org/10.22454/primer.2017.1.3.

Van der Merwe, J.W., Rugunanan, M., Ras, J., Röscher, E-M., Henderson, B.D. & Joubert, G. (2016). Patient preferences regarding the dress code, conduct and resources used by doctors during consultations in the public healthcare sector in Bloemfontein, Free State. *South African Family Practice*, 58(3), pp. 94–99. https://doi.org/10.1080/20786190.2016.1187865.

Wear, D. (1998). On White Coats and professional development: The formal and the hidden curricula. *Annals of Internal Medicine*, 129(9), p. 734. https://doi.org/10.7326/0003-4819-129-9-199811010-00010.

West, C. P., Dyrbye, L. N., & Shanafelt, T. D. (2018). Physician burnout: Contributors, consequences and solutions. Journal of Internal Medicine, 283(6), pp. 516-529. https://doi:10.1111/joim.12752

Xun, H., Chen, J., Sun, A. H., *et al.* (2021). Public perceptions of physician attire and professionalism in the US. *JAMA Network Open*, 4(7), e2117779. https://doi.org/10.1001/jamanetworkopen.2021.17779.

Zollinger, M., Houchens, N., Chopra, V., *et al.* (2019). Understanding patient preference for physician attire in ambulatory clinics: A cross-sectional observational study. *BMJ Open*, 9(5), e026009. https://doi.org/10.1136/bmjopen-2018-026009.

Chapter 8
Hear No Evil: The Violence of Silence

Smrita Grewal, MD, Tara Burra, MD

❖

"In the end, we will remember not the words of our enemies, but the silence of our friends."
—Martin Luther King Jr, 1967

❖

Abstract: This chapter explores the issue of silence on racist, discriminatory, and oppressive practices in medicine. Microaggressions in medicine and their harmful consequences are examined, and examples of their occurrence in medical training and clinical practice are provided. The chapter highlights the pressing need to break the silence surrounding power dynamics, privilege, and oppression. Additionally, the authors explore the role of silence in perpetuating stereotypes and implicit bias through personal self-reflection, including examining the model minority stereotype. Recommendations are presented by way of self-reflection exercises that address internalized biases, experiences of privilege and experiences of oppression in healthcare settings.

Keywords: implicit bias, microaggressions, microinterventions, model minority stereotype, patient safety movement, psychological safety, transformative learning theory

Introduction: A brief history of silence in medicine

There has been a long history of silence with respect to oppressive practices in the field of medicine. Silence in the face of racist, discriminatory, and repressive policies has caused profound harm, with enduring effects in many communities. Forced sterilizations of women associated with eugenic and racist policies, physician participation in the Holocaust, the Tuskegee public health "experiments" on Black Americans, and studies of nutritional deprivation of Indigenous children forcibly separated from their parents to attend residential institutions (ostensibly called "schools") provide but a few examples from the twentieth century.

Multiple factors have contributed to the problem of silence. Medicine has historically had a dehumanizing and hierarchical educational system with limited diversity amongst learners and faculty (Craig et al., 2018). Limited representation of minority groups narrows the range of perspectives that can be shared. The intra and inter-professional hierarchies within medicine also perpetuate silence by inhibiting the voices of those without power. In addition, curricula have emphasized the biomedical sciences, with insufficient integration of knowledge from the social sciences and humanities.

Knowledge from the social sciences and humanities is necessary for a depth of understanding of social constructs such as race and social processes such as racism (Sharma and Kuper, 2016). Further, the emphasis in medical training on demonstrating one's knowledge through diagnostic problem-solving and treatment planning contributes to a medical culture in which there is comfort with certainty. Conversely, uncertainty is associated with considerable psychological discomfort. As Sharda (2020) suggests, "we must know the answer, the diagnosis, the treatment. Not knowing is considered failing, and failing is not tolerated." The hierarchical workplace culture tends to reinforce perfectionism: working faster, harder, and longer, to avoid failure and to please one's superiors.

Avoidance of discomfort perpetuates our profession's silence: dialogue about racism and discrimination is inherently complex, imbued with uncertainty, and uncomfortable. As noted by Sharma and Kuper (2016), talking about race entails the potentially painful process of discarding claims of cultural and racial neutrality. Unfortunately, silent complicity in the face of racist acts within medical care continues, affecting both providers and the communities served. Narratives from both physicians and patients who are ethnic minorities within the healthcare environment are rife with descriptions of ongoing racism (Dhara, 2020, Mahabir et al.,

2021 Sharda, 2020), which runs the gamut from implicit bias and stereotyping to microaggressions to clear acts of discrimination.

The Issues

Microaggressions

The term *microaggression* was coined in 1970 by Chester Pierce, an African American psychiatrist at Harvard University, to describe common, often daily, experiences of African Americans (Pierce, 1970). Subsequent research has shown that many other racial and ethnic groups in Canada and the United States also experience microaggressions, including, but not limited to, Indigenous peoples, Asians, South Asians, Latinxs, and Arabs (Williams, 2020.) Pierce and colleagues (1978) describe microaggressions as "subtle, stunning, often automatic, and non-verbal exchanges which are 'put downs'" (p.66). Sue and colleagues (2007) provide the following definition: "racial microaggressions are brief and commonplace daily verbal, behavioral, and environmental indignities, whether intentional or unintentional, that communicate hostile, derogatory or negative racial slights and insults to the target person or group" (p. 273). They describe nine themes that emerge from interactions in which microaggressions are apparent. Based on these themes by Sue and colleagues (2007), in Figure 8.1, we have provided examples of each theme that we have directly or indirectly observed in our medical training and clinical practice.

Alien in own land
corresponding to an assumption that a person of colour is not a true [North] American

• e.g., "Where are you from?"or [after viewing our degrees] "Where's your name from? "Your name sounds Indian, but you don't look Indian"

Ascription of intelligence
in which assumptions about superior or inferior intelligence are assigned on the basis of race

• e.g., a patient ascribes attending physician status to a white male medical student rather than a female or minoritized team member

Colour blindness
the failure to acknowledge race ignores the existence of structural and systemic racism, negates the lived experiences of people of colour, and serves to perpetuate racism. Difference needs to be acknowledged without reinforcing racial hierarchies

• e.g., the idea that health care is delivered based on guidelines that are applied to everyone in the same way, regardless of race

Criminality/ assumption of criminal status
people of colour are assumed to be dangerous, engaged in criminal behaviour or in some way deviant because of their race

• e.g., elevated rates of use of seclusion and restraint for Black and Indigenous patients compared to White patients, elevated rates of liberty deprivation for racialized psychiatric patients such as with the increased use of community treatment orders for BIPOC* patients

Figure 8.1. *Themes of Microaggressions with Examples from Medical Training and Practice (themes based on Sue et al., 2007). (cont. on next page)*

* BIPOC: Black, Indigenous, People of Colour

| Denial of individual racism | statements made by a person that assert they do not hold any racist beliefs or exhibit any racist behaviours |

• e.g., "Why do I need to attend equity, diversity and inclusion training?...I'm not racist"

| Myth of meritocracy | assertions are made that race does not impact success or access to opportunities |

• e.g., "Everyone can succeed in medicine, if they work hard enough" "Why is affirmative action needed?"

| Pathologizing cultural values/ communication styles | an assumption there is a single ideal way to communicate and/or express one's values |

• e.g., describing emotional expression in minority groups as histrionic or dysregulated or attributing quietness as disinterest without clarifying the person's rationale for remaining quiet when this behaviour may represent an intentional code switch for a BIPOC person to preserve a sense of safety due to past adverse experiences associated with speaking up (see chapter 9 for further elaboration)

| Second-class citizen | circumstances in which a White person is given preferential treatment as a consumer over a person of colour |

• e.g., a White male patient is offered expedited access to a specialist consultation after his White male family physician advocated for him to be seen more quickly.

| Environmental | aspects of the built environment that reflect which groups are privileged in that space |

• e.g., there are religious spaces in some publicly funded hospitals that focus on Christian practices, with fewer established spaces for other faiths (e.g., Judaism or Islam) or Indigenous cultural practices such as smudging

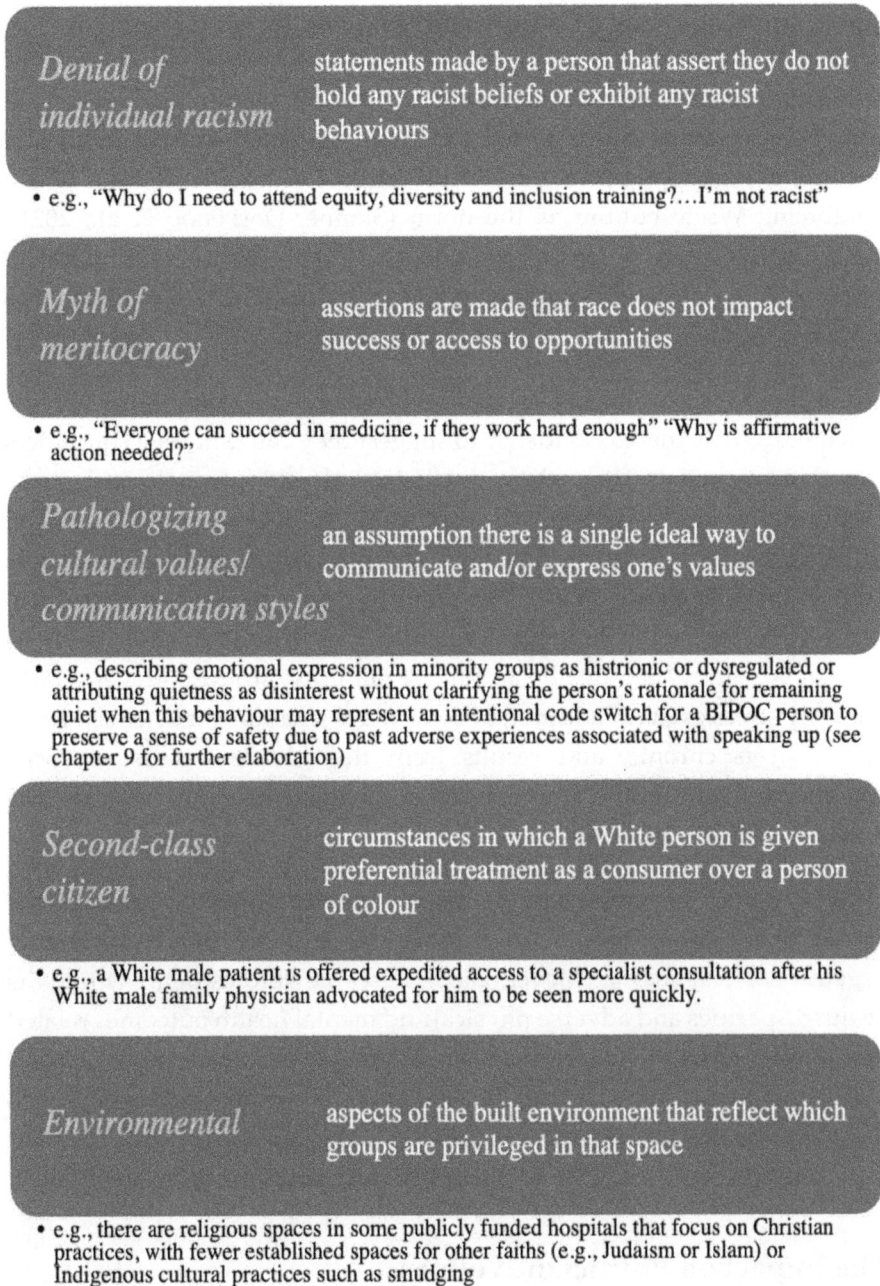

Figure 8.1. *Themes of Microaggressions with Examples from Medical Training and Practice (themes based on Sue et al., 2007).*

* BIPOC: Black, Indigenous, People of Colour

The Consequences of Microaggressions in Medicine

Microaggressions perpetuate systemic racism by reinforcing stereotypes and prejudices that result in the othering (e.g., alien in own land) and devaluing (e.g., assumption of criminal status) of people of color whilst reinforcing White culture as the norm (Skinner-Dorkenoo et al., 2021). Additionally, some microaggressions serve to obscure and maintain systemic racism by promoting ideas such as false color blindness and the myth of meritocracy (Skinner-Dorkenoo et al., 2021).

While the adverse impacts of microaggressions are contested by some (Lilenfeld, 2017), there is evidence to suggest they cause harm to providers and patients alike. They elicit psychological and physiological stress responses; lead to feelings of confusion, exclusion, anger, anxiety, helplessness, fatigue, frustration, and fear; and contribute to chronic stress (Meyer, 2003; Williams, 2020). The minority stress model is a conceptual framework for understanding the harm that discrimination, such as microaggressions, has on the health of minority groups (Meyer, 2003). Minority stress exists in addition to the general stressors experienced by all people; it is chronic, and results from the adverse effects of social conditions, institutions and structures characterized by stigma and prejudice (Meyer, 2003).

Minority stress encompasses the impact of discriminatory events, the vigilance or anticipation of discrimination, and the internalization of negative societal stigma (Meyer, 2003). Research studies demonstrate the health disparities and adverse physical and mental health outcomes related to minority stress (Flentje et al., 2020). Microaggressions present a barrier to treatment with some patients ceasing or never seeking treatment due to the commission of microaggressions by clinicians (Williams, 2020) or expectation of same as captured by the minority stress model (Meyer, 2003).

The Impact on Physician Wellness

Conversely, doctors from ethnic minorities shoulder the burden of microaggressions from both colleagues and patients; yet with the latter, they may feel ethically bound to continue to provide care to the patient-aggressor. Regulators have been slow to address this; for example, in Canada this topic was not broached by the College of Physicians and Surgeons of Ontario until as late as 2021 (CPSO, 2021). Similarly, the Royal College of Physicians and Surgeons of Canada (RCPSC) did not begin to weigh in on this issue until 2020 (RCPSC, 2020). The provider's experience of discrimination can lead to a "freeze effect" which leads to silence in response to microaggression (Sue et al., 2019).

Racial stereotypes and microaggressions persist within the field of medicine, consistent with society more broadly. Medicine mirrors society, yet the privilege of our education and knowledge of the human condition should compel us to refute the racial typecasting we know to be harmful. As practitioners, we are immersed in a milieu of continued silence which is, at once, astounding and unsurprising. Yet, there are increasingly more and more voices, which taken together, provide a chorus for change: the desire to shift to structural competence in medicine. We know that our chief accountability is responsible healthcare, and we are in a privileged position to usher in change.

Professional Vignette

By Smrita Grewal

My parents immigrated to Canada through the points-based system for their work as teachers and later as school principals. With two young children and no money, finding work took precedence over equating their teaching degrees to Canadian standards. Soon after we arrived, my father found a job as a security guard and my mother as a cashier at a fast-food chain. They enrolled at community college and did night classes when time and money allowed. I remember them being puzzled when the local elementary school suggested my sister and I repeat a grade. The school later informed them that it would not be necessary because they had since realized we spoke English well.

At age 6, I returned from school to find my father unpacking a newly purchased volume of the children's Britannica Encyclopedia that would take him a year to pay off. The red books were fixtures on our shelves for years, symbolizing their faith that education would mean freedom.

> My mother tried to enroll me in ballet classes after seeing an advertisement at the supermarket. Although I did not understand it and could not name it at the time, I felt ashamed hearing the instructor tell my mother I did not have "the right look" for ballet.
>
> As a medical student, I think of the moment when I was silent in response to an attending physician telling me I must be a foreign student because anyone trained in Canada would know the answer to the question asked. In response to countless experiences of being mocked for my name, having it be repetitively mispronounced or avoided altogether, I began to dread hearing it and pre-emptively would apologize for it.

Professional Vignette Analysis

This professional vignette begins a personal reflection and exploration of my racial identity, positions of privilege and oppression, and internalized biases. Thinking of these experiences, I see how much my parent's wanted acceptance and belonging for us. Our survival as a family, security and legitimacy felt tied to our ability to avoid conflict with dominant social groups, keep our heads down, and work hard. On the other hand, our subjectivity and cultural identity became associated with fear and shame due to our experiences of racial discrimination. We inadvertently internalized the model minority stereotype and submerged our cultural identity. As Cathy Park Hong writes in the book "Minor Feelings", "We keep our heads down and work hard, believing that our diligence will reward us with our dignity, but our diligence will only make us disappear. By not speaking up, we perpetuate the myth that our shame is caused by our repressive culture and the country we fled."

The Model Minority

The cumulative weight of microaggressions stemming from stereotypes such as the model minority exerts a toll on health and overall wellbeing (Walton and Truong, 2022). The model minority stereotype commonly refers to Asian communities in North America as successful and upwardly mobile due to strong family ties and being hard-working, intelligent, persevering, docile, and quiet (Wu et al., 2014). As outlined in Vo's (2019) dissertation, the term "model minority" was first used by sociologist William Peterson in a 1966 New York Times article. Peterson promoted the narrative that Japanese Americans had overcome racial discrimination through hard work and family values as opposed to other racial groups (Vo, 2019). This portrayal of Japanese Americans as a racial minority "model" was presented in opposition to the Civil Rights Movement to silence African Americans. The press "presented Asian Americans as an example of how a minority group can overcome discrimination through perseverance and hard work alone," minimizing the traumatic impact of exclusionary racist policies on Asian Americans while ignoring the institutional racism, segregation and systemic oppression African Americans face (Padgett et al., 2020).

Despite criticism and resistance, the model minority stereotype persists today and continues to silence the voices of racialized minorities and reduces the diversity, intersectionalities, and inequities among Asian minority groups into one homogenous group or monolith (Yu, 2006). According to Vo (2019), the term "Asian" is "inherently problematic because it denotes homogeneity and disguises the variability and differences within and across different Asian ethnic groups". By creating a racial hierarchy, the model minority myth pits racialized and marginalized minorities against one another, both implicitly and explicitly (Yu, 2006). Moreover, the model minority stereotype coexists simultaneously with Asian minority groups portrayed as "perpetual foreigners" or denigrated as threatening (Yao et al., 2021). The anti-Asian racism and violence during the COVID-19 pandemic illustrate these stereotypes' co-existence (Yao et al., 2021).

Clinical Vignette

On a busy late afternoon in the emergency department of a general hospital, I recently had the opportunity to observe microaggressions, and ashamedly, silence in action. A middle-aged woman of colour arrived via ambulance and joined the long queue to speak with the triage nurse. Her stretcher was parked close by to where I was standing in the queue. She spoke tersely with the paramedic, saying, "don't touch me!" as he moved his arms near her torso and adjusted the blankets that were partially covering her. Her frustration was palpable. He then moved away, and she remained on the stretcher, adjusting the blankets herself, without incident.

Several minutes later, she got off the stretcher and went to the single-occupancy bathroom adjacent to the waiting area. Some time passed, and a White patient approached the bathroom and found it locked. The White patient did not approach the nursing desk for assistance. Subsequently, a White nurse knocked on the bathroom door, spontaneously assisting the patient who was waiting. "Time's up," she yelled through the door at the woman of colour. "Other people need to use the bathroom!" In response, the woman occupying the bathroom yelled something I could not hear clearly. The nurse waited briefly outside the bathroom door and then spoke to one of the security guards, another woman of colour, and stated loudly, "You need to get her out of the bathroom...other people need to use it." And then the nurse added, "you should call for backup, you're going to need it." The security guard nodded. She knocked on the door of the bathroom. The security guard did not call for backup. She yelled through the door "Hello, it's time to leave the bathroom." The woman within again yelled back and a few moments later, she opened the door, left the bathroom and returned to the stretcher. And what role did I play? I was a bystander who watched the entire scenario unfold, regrettably without saying a word.

Clinical Vignette Analysis

This clinical vignette illustrates two of the microaggressions described in Figure 8.1, namely, the second-class citizen and the assumption of criminality. We will examine the microaggressions that are apparent in this scenario, in turn.

Without knowing the intentions of the nurse involved in this scenario, her actions might be deemed by some observers to be an exemplar of patient-centered advocacy for the White patient who was trying to access the bathroom. That is, the nurse proactively requested for the bathroom to be vacated, without the White patient even asking for this assistance. However, her actions can be equally construed as a second-class citizen microaggression against the patient of colour. That is, the White patient's access to the bathroom was given primacy over the continued use of the space by a patient of a different racial background, namely Black, Indigenous and People of Colour (BIPOC) background. The nurse appeared to have concluded the BIPOC patient had exceeded her entitlement to the space, and she was asked to clear the way to provide preferential access for the White patient.

After requesting that the BIPOC patient vacate the bathroom, the nurse stated to the security officer "you should call for backup, you're going to need it." This action was premised on the assumption that her request to vacate the bathroom would likely lead to a physical conflict, necessitating the presence of back-up security personnel. Unfortunately, this is a microaggression that can easily escalate to overt racism within emergency departments or hospital wards, with BIPOC patients disproportionately experiencing seclusion, physical, and chemical restraints, compared to their White counterparts (Smith et al., 2022).

What were the options for a response to break the silence surrounding this situation in the emergency department? While there are suggested models (Paul-Emile et al., 2016; Willams and Rohrbaugh, 2019) and institutional policies for responding to overt racial violence, what are the options for responding to microaggressions? A recent scoping review by Wittkower and colleagues (2022) describes recommended strategies and approaches to train healthcare professionals on how to respond to microaggressions that are perpetrated by patients.

Figure 8.2 summarizes microintervention strategies described by Sue and colleagues (2019) that are applicable to microaggressions perpetrated by patients or fellow healthcare professionals, alike. They define microinterventions as "everyday words or deeds, whether intentional or unintentional, that communicate to targets of microaggressions (a) validation of their experiential reality, (b) value as a person, (c) affirmation of their racial or group identity, (d) support and encouragement, and (e) reassurance that they are not alone" (p. 134). By employing microinterventions, they suggest that those witnessing or experiencing microaggressions can regain a sense of self-efficacy and control, which will enhance psychological wellbeing. Simultaneously, these techniques can disarm and counteract the negative sequelae of microaggressions by posing a direct challenge to the perpetrators.

The Opportunity to Break the Violence of Silence

❖

"The world is a dangerous place to live, not because of the people who are evil, but because of the people who don't do anything about it."
—Albert Einstein, 1953

❖

We Want to Break the Silence, but How?

Given the discomfort inherent in talking about power dynamics, privilege and oppression, what is the path forward to break the silence in medicine? To find our voices, advance dialogue, and instigate change, we posit there is much to be learned from the patient safety movement within healthcare, educational theory, and organizational leadership. Relevant theories and concepts from each of these fields are further discussed.

Beginning three decades ago, numerous studies were published which demonstrated patients were routinely being harmed within modern, complex healthcare systems (Baker et al., 2004, Lleape 1991; Lleape et al., 1994). Following the publication of *To Err is Human* (Kohn et al., 2000), patient safety became an area of scholarship in medicine as part of, and in tandem with, an expanding interest in the quality of healthcare. In a culture that is so uncomfortable with failure, how did the social movement of patient safety take hold within medicine (Lleape, 2021)?

First, patient safety scholars accessed and rigorously analyzed data to provide empirical evidence of the scope of the problem. Efforts were made, that are ongoing, to share narrative accounts from patients and families of the anguish and suffering caused by preventable errors associated with healthcare delivery and to partner with patients and families to improve safety (Bromiley, 2015, National Steering Committee on Patient Safety, 2002).

To build the movement's momentum, its leaders strategically targeted active resistors, both frontline clinicians and organizational leaders, and engaged them through data, patient narratives, and an emphasis on shared values amongst healthcare providers (Mate, 2022). Although more progress is needed, patient safety is a salient example of a sustained social movement that has shifted the culture of healthcare. It serves as a model of harnessing curiosity and courage to address fear, reluctance, and silence.

Physicians' discomfort with *not knowing* contributes to silence and other challenges associated with dialogue about social justice in medicine. Unlike other domains of medical education focused on knowledge and skills, learning about social justice requires the capacity to self-reflect, question assumptions, and engage in new ways of understanding. Transformative learning theory (Baker et al., 2019, Mezirow, 1978) is an adult educational paradigm designed to foster the development of these capabilities. Transformative learning involves becoming critically aware of one's tacit assumptions or expectations and assessing their relevance in understanding one's experience (Mezirow, 2000). Through disorienting experiences, critical reflection, dialogue, and revised interpretation, this educational paradigm aims to modify learners' ways of seeing, being, and doing. In turn, these changes in perspective and action foster the development of learners who become agents of structural and societal change.

Transformative learning is increasingly being adopted in medical education (Baker et al., 2021; Sukhera et al., 2020; Vipler et al., 2021). Given critical reflection and dialogue are integral to the transformative learning paradigm, further dissemination of this approach to medical education will support a new generation of practitioners who are better prepared to break the silence and instigate systemic change. However, educational interventions drawn from transformational learning theory are ideally paired with broader organizational commitments to structural change as individual practitioners are clearly not impervious to the systemic forces that generate inequity. That is, individuals who champion change will be thwarted in sustaining their efforts if the system reinforces the status quo. Bringing about broader systemic changes through education is consonant with the work of scholars such as Freire (1970), Habermas (1984), and hooks,1994), who identified a pivotal role for education in transforming social structures to reduce oppression (Ewert, 1991; Kitchenham, 2008; Sukera et al., 2020).

In recognition of the need for both education and structural change, medical organizations such as the Association of American Medical Colleges (AAMC) and the Royal College of Physicians and Surgeons of Canada (RCPSC), are defining physician competencies in equity, diversity, and inclusion (AAMC, 2022; RCPSC, undated) to inform curricula across the continuum of medical training. Formalized training requirements signal the importance of these competencies and serve as further impetus for organizational change to accomplish and sustain them. While altered training requirements and expectations of physician competencies will contribute to a foundation for structural change, they are unlikely to be sufficient to transform medicine's culture of silence.

We suggest the concept of psychological safety from the organizational leadership literature is a pivotal enabler to support dialogue and action on social justice in medicine. Psychological safety refers to the perceptions of the consequences for taking interpersonal risks, e.g., admitting a mistake, or proposing an innovation, in a particular context such as a healthcare workplace (Edmondson, 1999). Initially proposed in the 1960s, renewed interest in research on psychological safety began in the 1990s and continues (Edmondson and Lei, 2014). Research at the individual, team and organizational level demonstrates that psychological safety facilitates the willingness to contribute ideas and actions toward a shared goal (Edmondson and Lei, 2014).

Psychological safety impacts the ability of teams to learn from failure, which is particularly important to advance work in equity, diversity and inclusion in medicine as we are immersed in systemic failures related to inequity, both historic and ongoing. It also has relevance to leverage the strengths associated with increased workforce diversity: psychological safety moderates the relationship between diversity and team performance as it facilitates more open communication as well as engaged, respectful interactions. As such, psychological safety holds promise to promote organizational learning and collaboration to achieve equity, diversity and inclusion goals in medicine, provided it is paired with leadership vision, support, and prioritized goals.

The patient safety movement, transformative learning theory, explicit physician competencies in social justice, and psychological safety all require dialogue to instigate and sustain change. These dialogues are commonly fraught with tension as individuals are confronted with challenging their own implicit biases and grappling with the ramifications of power, privilege, oppression, and discrimination that pervade all our lives. The discomfort associated with these conversations is necessary: these exchanges create disorienting experiences that prompt critical reflection, further dialogue, and re-evaluation of assumptions that characterize transformative learning. Further, these communications are a process, ideally with many longitudinal opportunities for a group or team to engage in bringing about change. In view of the complexity in facilitating and navigating these discussions, it is likely beneficial for both facilitators and participants to have frameworks to guide their conduct.

Participants in an implicit bias recognition and management curriculum studied by Sukhera and colleagues (2018) described "striving while accepting." That is, the curriculum led to an awareness of a discrepancy between who they strive to be as a health professional and their intrinsic shortcomings associated with their implicit biases (Sukhera et al., 2018). They describe this process of striving while accepting aligns with transformative learning theory (Sukhera et al., 2020): participants strived for a different understanding, while simultaneously acknowledging the limitations imposed by individual biases, which are contextually mediated. Adopting this dialectic to guide discourse amongst healthcare providers about power, privilege and social justice within medicine warrants further study. It holds promise as a framework to guide dialogue and action to advance the equity, diversity and inclusion movement within the medical profession.

The Brave Spaces Framework (Arao and Clemens, 2013) is also pertinent to the goal of addressing silence and avoidance through dialogue and action. This framework was developed to help prepare post-secondary students to navigate the inherent risks associated with social justice dialogues in educational environments. In the Framework, Arao and Clemens (2013) outline five ground rules to guide the creation of educational brave spaces:

1. Controversy with civility: differing and/or conflicting views are expected within a diverse group and the group commits to not only understanding the sources of disagreement, but also working cooperatively toward solutions in pursuit of justice for all people.

2. Own your intentions and impacts: individuals acknowledge the impact of their actions on other people, even if the impact is incongruent with an individual's intention (which may be positive or neutral and still lead to a negative impact).

3. Challenge by choice: individuals will determine for themselves which activities they engage in and to what degree. This ground rule acknowledges that some individuals will be engaged in internal reflection, even if they are not actively engaged in the group's discussion. All participants are encouraged to reflect on which factors influence their decision to challenge themselves to participate in the dialogue.

4. Respect: relating to others in a way that acknowledges their personhood. Participants are encouraged to share what it means to be respectful and which actions demonstrate respect. This exploration is intended to illustrate the cultural and contextual variation in expressions of respectfulness for one another.

5. No attacks: participants agree not to use any form of violence against one another.

Creating a brave space for learning is premised on all participants engaging in the process of setting these expectations for group norms and conduct, which is consistent with the aims of social justice education (Freire, 1970; hooks, 1994), as opposed to facilitators defining them for the group a priori (Arao and Clemens, 2013). Although critiqued for insufficiently acknowledging historical and ongoing inequities (Duchesne et al., 2023; Marquez, 2017; Zheng, 2016), the brave space framework has demonstrated relevance in medical education (Wasserman and Browne, 2021) and, by extension, the continuing professional development of physicians.

Learning and practicing medicine requires the ability to navigate sensitive, emotionally laden, and complicated problems as we care for our patients and ourselves. And yet, we have few models to help us negotiate these complex communication and educational tasks. As the competencies required of physicians continue to evolve, we need to engage with the Brave Space Framework in medicine to not only foster crucial dialogue, but also meet the growing demands for systemic change.

Opportunities to Address Microaggressions

Microinterventions provide a clear means for medical professionals to cease being silent in the face of microaggressions. In Figure 8.2, Sue and colleagues (2019) describe four strategic goals of microinterventions. To distinguish these interventions from generic *comebacks*, the authors carefully describe objectives and the rationale for various microinterventions, including specific tactics that can be employed (Sue et al., 2019 pp. 134-139). First, make the "invisible" visible, by identifying that a microaggression has occurred by undermining the metacommunication, making the metacommunication explicit, challenging stereotypes, broadening the ascribed behaviour to all people, or asking for clarification. Second, disarm the microaggression through the expression of disagreement, setting limits or describing contrasting values. Third, educate the offender by differentiating between intention and impact, appealing to the aggressor's values or principles, pointing out commonality, promoting empathy or describing how the aggressor will benefit from challenging their implicit biases. Fourth, seek external intervention by alerting a leader within the organization, reporting problematic incidents, and seeking out support through one's healthcare providers, peers, support groups or members of one's community.

Microintervention strategies		
Directed Toward Perpetrator Microaggressions	**Directed Toward Institutional Macroaggressions**	**Directed Toward Societal Macroaggressions**
Make the "Invisible" Visible		
• Undermine the meta-communication • Make the meta-communication explicit • Challenge the stereotype • Broaden the ascribed trait to a universal human behavior • Ask for clarification	• Keep a log of inequitable practices as you see them • Run your observations by allies who can corroborate • Solicit feedback from fellow coworkers/students • Monitor trends around recruiting, hiring, retention, promotion	• Create partnerships with academic institutions to analyze data related to disparities in education, health care, employment • Disseminate research on disparity trends to general public and media • Organize peaceful demonstrations
Disarm the Microaggression/Macroaggression		
• Express disagreement • State values and set limits • Describe what is happening • Use an exclamation • Use non-verbal communication • Interrupt and redirect	• Boycott, strike, or protest the institution • Request meetings with intermediary or senior leadership to share perspectives • Exercise right to serve on boards to voice your concerns • Delineate financial repercussions of continued macroaggressions • Notify press or other media outlets	• Protest political leaders who reinforce inequity and division/support those who do not • Revise and veto unjust community policies, practices, and laws • Lobby to your congressmen or senators • Attend televised town hall meetings to voice your concerns
Educate the Offender		
• Point out the commonality • Appeal to the offenders values and principles • Differentiate between intent and impact • Promote empath • Point to how they benefit	• Describe the benefits of workforce diversity • Institute long-term mandated training on cultural sensitivity for all levels • Infuse multicultural principles into organizational mission and values	• Raise children to understand concepts like prejudice, discrimination, and racism. • Challenge silence/lack of response to macroaggression • Identify shared mutual goals among people • Increase community's exposure to positive examples of diverse cultures to offset negative stereotypes and biases
Seek External Intervention		
• Alert Authorities • Report the act • Seek therapy/counseling • Seek support through spirituality/religion/community • Set up a buddy system • Attend support groups	• Report inequitable practices to your union • Create networking/mentoring opportunities for underrepresented employees/students • Maintain an open, supportive, and responsive environment • Call on consultants to conduct external assessments/cultural audits	• Foster cooperation over competition • Foster a sense of community belonging • Create caucuses for allies and targets • Participate in healing circles, vigils, memorials that remind us of the consequences of hate

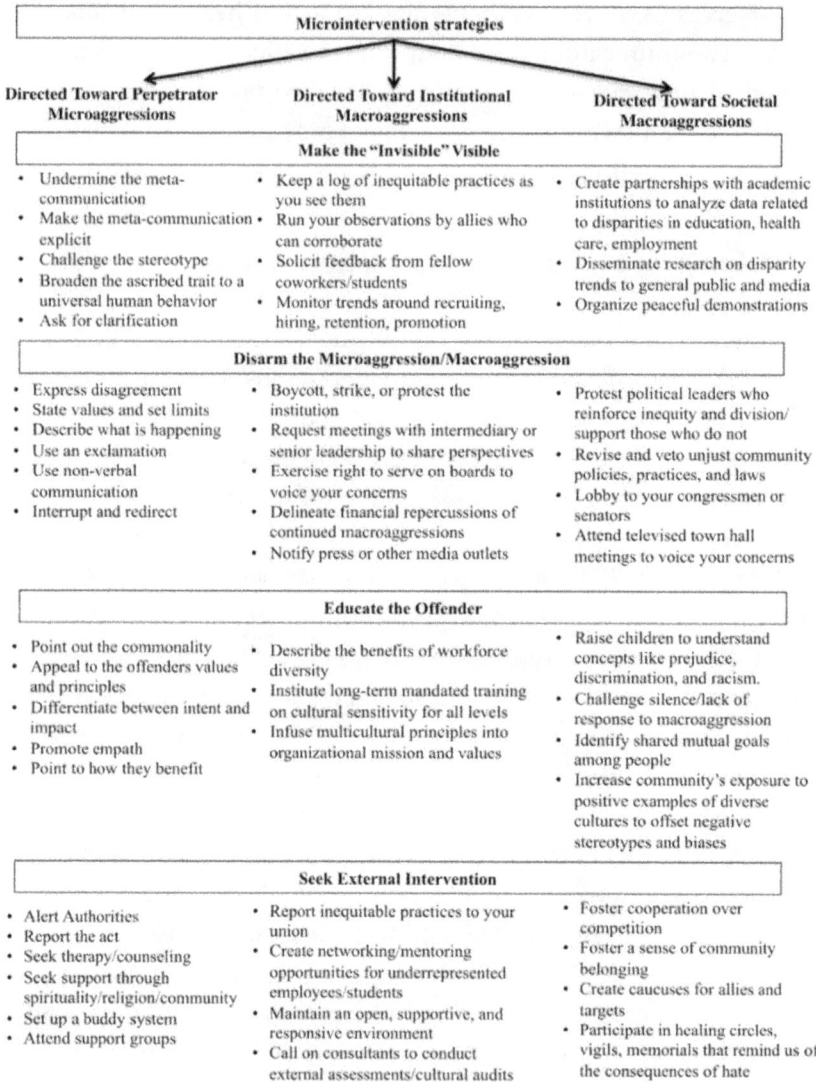

Figure 8.2. *Microintervention Strategies (Reproduced from Sue et al., 2019, p.135 with permission from the corresponding author and the American Psychological Association)*

Equity Building Exercise

Sue and colleagues (2019) suggest that silence, acceptance, passivity and inaction have been the predominant strategies most people have used to cope with microaggressions. They note these ways of managing are ineffective in promoting change. They propose a comprehensive framework that includes specific strategies, microinterventions, that people who are targeted by microaggressions, their allies, and bystanders can employ to bring about change.

Review the paper by Sue et al., (2019) with your colleagues and/or learners you are supervising. Discuss the following:

1. What microaggressions have members of your group experienced or observed in your clinical setting?
2. How are these experiences similar or different from the scenarios described in Table 1 in the paper?
3. For each of the four strategic goals of microinterventions described by Sue and colleagues (2019), below, identify some tactics that could be used to address the observed microaggressions in your setting:
   - make the invisible visible
   - disarm the microaggression
   - educate the perpetrator
   - seek external intervention
4. What do you foresee as the intrapersonal, interpersonal, and/or systemic barriers to implementation of these microintervention strategies in your setting?

Inclusion Strategies

Inclusion Strategies to Address Microaggressions and Internalized Bias

A strong therapeutic alliance forms the foundation of effective clinical care across healthcare settings. Tran et al. (2021) note that "patients mistrust in the therapeutic relationship frequently stems from clinician's stereotype bias and lack of awareness". The following exercise is geared to help facilitate increased self-reflection about individual internalized stereotypes, implicit biases, and experiences of privilege and oppression.

Pause and Reflect

Consider the paper by Mahabir and colleagues, *Experiences of everyday racism in Toronto's health care system: a concept mapping study* (2021). The paper examines individual level effects of current healthcare policies and practices on racial/ethnic groups, with particular attention to racialized groups in a local (Toronto, Canada) healthcare system. Mahabir and colleagues chronicle institutional racism in the healthcare setting and note unequal power social relations. Please review the paper and critically reflect on the following:

    a.   How do your own privileges and oppressions impact your identity and how you interact with other people in your practice environment?

    b.   What implicit biases do you hold?

    c.   How do these biases arise in your interactions with patients? What about with colleagues? What about with the people you report to professionally?

Key Takeaways

- Silence in medicine regarding oppressive practices has caused significant harm to many communities. It is essential to break the silence and have an open dialogue about racism and discrimination in medical care to prevent these harmful practices from continuing.

- Microaggressions perpetuate systemic racism, and addressing microaggressions in the healthcare setting is crucial for creating an equitable and inclusive environment for all patients and professionals. Implementing microinterventions can challenge implicit biases and promote empathy and understanding.

- Healthcare professionals must commit to addressing microaggressions and promoting inclusion in their practice environments to ensure that every patient receives equitable and respectful care.

- Critical self-reflection and addressing individual internalized stereotypes are vital in challenging implicit biases.

- Breaking the silence around power dynamics, privilege, and oppression in medicine requires learning from different fields, including the patient safety movement, educational theory, and organizational leadership.

Conclusion

Silence in response to oppressive practices in medicine, particularly racism and discrimination, perpetuates systemic racism and results in adverse physical and mental health outcomes for both patients and healthcare professionals. Breaking the silence and engaging in open dialogue about the harmful effects of microaggressions and stereotypes, such as the model minority stereotype, is essential to promote inclusivity and equity in healthcare settings.

Implementing microinterventions, critical self-reflection, and addressing individual internalized biases can challenge implicit biases and promote empathy and understanding. However, addressing microaggressions may face elicit intrapersonal, interpersonal, and systemic barriers, and learning from different fields, including patient safety, educational theory, and organizational leadership, is crucial. Psychological safety in conjunction with leadership vision, support, and prioritized goals are instrumental to progress on achieving equity, diversity and inclusion goals.

On a Parting Note...

Silence
Ocean Vuong writes, "sometimes you are erased
before you are given the choice of stating who you are."

We speak English.
I learned to say pre-emptively.

You drove me to that recital, remember?
We stopped for ice cream.
I was angry in the car.
They were making fun of your accent.
I know you said.
Then you asked me if I knew my lines.
I learned my words.
As you learned
To let go of yours.

Audre Lorde writes, "My silences had not protected me.
Your silences will not protect you."
A silence that is imposed
From the outside
Then from the inside

It is not inherent to any identity
It is the coerced surrender of identity

Ta-Nehisi Coates writes, "the moments we spent readying the mask,
or readying ourselves to accept half as much, could not be recovered.
The robbery of time is not measured in lifespans but in moments."

Revelation needs language
Negotiating whether to say something.
Going around the moment.
Silences that do not breathe
Stultifying and arid.

© Smrita Grewal, 2023

References

Arao, B., and Clemens, K. (2013). From safe spaces to brave places: a new way to frame dialogue around diversity and social justice in Landreman, L.M. (ed.) *The Art of Effective Facilitation.* Sterling, VA: ACPA, pp. 135–150.

Association of American Medical Colleges. (2022). Diversity, Equity, and Inclusion Competencies Across the Learning Continuum. *AAMC New and Emerging Areas in Medicine Series.* Washington, DC: AAMC.

Baker, G.R., Norton, P.G., Flintoft, V., Blais, R., Brown, A., Cox, J., et al. (2004). The Canadian adverse events study: the incidence of adverse events among hospital patients in Canada. *Canadian Medical Association Journal,* 170(11), pp. 1678-1686.

Baker, L.R., Wright, S., Mylopoulos, M., Kulasegaram, K., Ng, S. (2019). Aligning and Applying the Paradigms and Practices of Education. *Academic Medicine,* 94(7), p.1060. doi:10.1097/acm.0000000000002693.

Baker, L.R., Phelan, S., Woods, N.N., Boyd, V.A., Rowland, P., Ng, S.L. (2021). Re-envisioning paradigms of education: towards awareness, alignment, and pluralism. *Advances in Health Sciences Education* 26(3), pp. 1045-1058. doi: 10.1007/s10459-021-10036-z.

Bromiley, M. (2015). The husband's story: from tragedy to learning and action. *BMJ Quality and Safety* 24, pp.425–7. doi:10.1136/bmjqs-2015-004129.

Craig, S. R., Scott, R., Blackwood, K. (2018). Orienting to Medicine: Scripting Professionalism, Hierarchy, and Social Difference at the Start of Medical School. *Culture, Medicine, and Psychiatry,* 42(3), pp. 654–683. doi:10.1007/s11013-018-9580-0.

Coates, T.-N. (2015). *Between the World and Me.* Spiegel & Grau.

College of Physicians and Surgeons of Ontario. (2021). Treating patient bias. *Dialogue,* 17(3), pp. 10-21.

Duchesne, E., Caners, K., Rang, L., & Dagnone, D. (2023). Addressing microaggressions with simulation: a novel educational intervention. *CJEM,* 25(4), pp. 299–302. https://doi.org/10.1007/s43678-023-00474-6

Dhara, A. (2020). Our complicit role in systemic racism. *Canadian Family Physician,* 66 (August), pp. 596-7.

Edmondson, A.C. (1999). Psychological safety and learning behavior in work teams. *Administrative Science Quarterly,* 44(2), pp. 350 –83.

Edmondson, A.C., Lei, Z. (2014). Psychological safety: the history, renaissance, and future of an interpersonal construct. *Annual Review of Organizational Psychology and Organizational Behavior*, 1, pp.23-43.

Ewert, J. (1991). Habermas and Education: A comprehensive overview of the influence of Habermas in Educational Literature. *Review of Educational Research*, 61(3), pp.345-378.

Flentje, A., Heck, N.C., Brennan, J.M. and Meyer, I.H. (2020). The relationship between minority stress and biological outcomes: A systematic review. *Journal of Behavioral Medicine*, 43(5), pp.673–694. doi.org/10.1007/s10865-019-00120-6.

Freire, P. (1970). *Pedagogy of the oppressed*. New York, NY: Continuum.

Habermas, J. (1984). *The theory of communicative action: Vol. I. Reason and the rationalization of society*. Boston: Beacon.

hooks, b. (1994). *Teaching to transgress: Education as the practice of freedom*. New York, NY: Routledge.

Kendi, I.X. (2019). *How to be an antiracist*. New York: One World.

Kitchenham, A. (2008). The evolution of John Mezirow's transformative learning theory. *Journal of Transformative Education* 6, pp.104-123.

Kohn, L.T., Corrigan, J., Donaldson, M.S. (2000). *To err is human: building a safer health system*. Washington, D.C: National Academy Press.

Leape, L.L., Brennan, T.A., Laird, N., *et al.* (1991). The nature of adverse events in hospitalized patients. Results of the Harvard medical practice study II. *N Engl J Med* 324, pp.377–84. doi:10.1056/NEJM199102073240605.

Leape, L.L. (1994). Error in medicine. *JAMA* 272, pp. 1851-1857. doi:10.1001/jama.1994.03520230061039.

Leape, L.L. (2021). *Making healthcare safe: the story of the patient safety movement*. Cham, Switzerland: Springer International Publishing.

Li, Y. & Nicholson, H. L. (2021). When "model minorities" become "yellow peril"-Othering and the racialization of Asian Americans in the COVID-19 pandemic. *Social Compass*, 15, p. 2.

Lilenfeld, S.O. (2017). Microaggressions: strong claims, inadequate evidence. *Perspectives on Psychological Science*, 12, pp.138-169.

Lorde, A. (1984). The transformation of silence into language and action. *In Sister Outsider: Essays and Speeches* (pp. 40-44). Crossing Press.

Mahabir, D.F., O'Campo, P., Lofters, A., Shankardass, K., Salmon, C., Muntaner, C. (2021). Experiences of everyday racism in Toronto's health care system: a concept mapping study. *Int J Equity Health* 20, 74. doi.org/10.1186/s12939-021-01410-9.

Marquez, A. (2017). Safe and brave spaces. *Medium* [online]. Available from: https://medium.com/@amarquez628/safe-and-brave-spaces-b9a3b51e107f.

Mate, K. (2022). Addressing pushback on health equity. *Healthcare Executive* 37(1), pp. 44-45.

Meyer, I.H. (2003). Prejudice, social stress, and mental health in lesbian, gay, and bisexual populations: Conceptual issues and research evidence. *Psychological Bulletin*, 129(5), pp. 674–697. doi.org/10.1037/0033-2909.129.5.674.

Mezirow, J. (1978). Perspective transformation. *Adult Education*, 28, pp.100-110.

Mezirow, J. (1997). Transformative learning: Theory to practice. *New Directions for Adult Continuing Education*, 74, pp 5-12.

Mezirow, J. (2000). *Learning as transformation: Critical perspectives on a theory in progress*. San Francisco: Jossey-Bass.

National Steering Committee on Patient Safety. (2002). *Building a Safety System: A National Integrated Strategy for Improving Patient Safety in Canadian Health Care*. Ottawa, ON: Royal College of Physicians and Surgeons of Canada.

Padgett, J. K., Lou, E., Lalonde, R., & Sasaki, J. Y. (2020). Too Asian? The model minority stereotype in a Canadian context. *Asian American Journal of Psychology*, 11(4), 223-232. doi.org/10.1037/aap0000203

Paul-Emile, K., Smith, A.K., Lo, B., Fernandez, A. (2016). Dealing with racist patients. *New England Journal of Medicine* 374(8), pp. 708-711.

Pierce, C. (1970). Offensive mechanisms. In: Barbour, F.B. eds. *The Black Seventies*. Boston, MA: Porter Sargent, pp. 265-82.

Pierce, C., Carew, J., Pierce-Gonzalez, D., Willis, D. (1978). An experiment in racism: TV commercials. In: Pierce C. eds. *Television and* Education. Beverly Hills, CA: Sage, pp. 62-88.

Royal College of Physicians and Surgeons of Canada. (undated). CANMEDS 2025 Theme-specific Expert Working Groups (EWGs) Terms of Reference [online]. Available from: https://www.royalcollege.ca/rcsite/canmeds/canmeds-25/ewg-epanels-e

Royal College of Physicians and Surgeons of Canada. (2020). Statement on Anti-Black Racism [online]. Available from: https://newsroom.royalcollege.ca/statement-on-racism/

Sharda, S. (2020). We need to talk about racism. *BMJ Opinion* [online]. Available from: https://blogs.bmj.com/bmj/2020/03/05/saroo-sharda-we-need-to-talk-about-racism/

Sharma, M., Kuper, A. (2016). The elephant in the room: talking race in medical education. *Advances in Health Sciences Education,* 22(3), pp. 761–764. doi: 10.1007/s10459-016-9732-3.

Skinner-Dorkenoo, A.L., Sarmal, A., Andre, C.J., & Rogbeer, K.G. (2021). How Microaggressions Reinforce and Perpetuate Systemic Racism in the United States. *Journal of Social Issues,* 77(1), 102-119. doi:10.1111/josi.12412.

Smith, C.M., Turner, N.A., Thielman, N.M., et al (2022). Association of Black Race with Physical and Chemical Restraint Use Among Patients Undergoing Emergency Psychiatric Evaluation. *Psychiatric Services,* 73(7), pp. 730-736. Available from: doi:10.1176/appi.ps.202100474

Sue, D.W., Capodilupo, C.M., Torino, G.C., et al (2007). Racial micoaggressions in everyday life implications for clinical practice. *American Psychologist,* 62(4), pp. 271-286.

Sue, D.W., Alsaidi, S., Awad, M.N., et al (2019). Disarming racial microaggressions: microintervention strategies for targets, white allies, and bystanders. *American Psychologist,* 74(1), pp. 128-142.

Sukhera, J., Wodzinski, M., Tenuissen, P.W., et al. (2018). Striving while accepting: exploring the relationship between identity and implicit bias recognition and management. *Academic Medicine,* 93(11 suppl), pp. S82-S88.

Sukhera, J., Watling, C.J., Gonzalez, C.M. (2020). Implicit bias in health professions: from recognition to transformation. *Academic Medicine,* 95(5), pp. 717-723.

Tran, N., Yabes, K., & Miller, A. (2021). How should clinicians help patients navigate "model minority" demands?. *AMA Journal of Ethics,* 23(6). doi:10.1001/amajethics.2021.456.

Walton, J., & Truong, M. (2022). A review of the model minority myth: understanding the social, educational, and health impacts. *Ethnic and Racial Studies,* 46(3), pp. 391-419. doi:10.1080/01419870.2022.2121170.

Vo, Vi. (2019). Interrupting the "Model Minority" Narrative: The Voices of Vietnamese Canadian Youth. University of Western Ontario Electronic Thesis and Dissertation Repository. 6044. https://ir.lib.uwo.ca/etd/6044

Vipler, B., Knehans, A., Rausa, D., Haidet, P., McCall-Hosenfeld, J. (2021). Transformative Learning in Graduate Medical Education: A Scoping Review. *Journal of Graduate Medical Education* 13(6), pp. 801-814. doi: 10.4300/JGME-D-21-00065.1.

Vuong, O. (2019). On Earth We're Briefly Gorgeous. Penguin Press.

Wasserman, J.A., Browne, B.J. (2021). On triggering and being triggered: civil society and building brave spaces in medical education. *Teaching and Learning in Medicine* 33(5), pp. 561-567. doi: 10.1080/10401334.2021.1887740.

Williams, J. C., Rohrbaugh, R.M. (2019). Confronting Racial Violence: Resident, Unit, and Institutional Responses. *Academic Medicine*, 94(8), pp.1084-1088.

Williams, M.T. (2020). Microaggressions: clarification, evidence, and impact. *Perspectives on Psychological Science*, 15(1), pp. 3-26. doi:10.1177/1745691619827499.

Wittkower, L.D., Bryan, J.L., Asghar-Ali, A.A. (2022). A scoping review of recommendations and training to respond to patient microaggressions. *Academic Psychiatry* 46, pp. 627-639.

Wu, E. D. (2014). *The Color of Success: Asian Americans and the Origins of the Model Minority*. Princeton, NJ: Princeton University Press .

Yu, T. (2006). Challenging the politics of the "model minority" stereotype: a case for educational equality. *Equity and Excellence in Education* , 39, pp. 325-333.

Zheng, L. (2016) 'Why your brave space sucks' *The Stanford Daily* [online]. Available from: https://stanforddaily.com/2016/05/15/why-your-brave-space-sucks/.

Chapter 9
Speak No Evil: Lessons in Language and Code-Switching

Olubimpe Ayeni, MD

❖

"In all the years of morbidity and mortality meetings, I have never heard of a patient who died because the doctor had an accent. But I have lost count of the mishaps and deaths from inattention, overconfidence, and plain arrogance. Accents don't hurt patients, attitudes do."
—Ranjana Srivastava, 2018

❖

Abstract: This chapter explores racism and language in medical settings. In an increasingly diverse world, physicians and patients are exposed to different communication norms and styles. These social interactions highlight issues such as perceived competence based on accents, navigating the dualities of identity that arise with code-switching, and the burden of constantly justifying and legitimizing the space that one occupies.

Keywords: *accentism, code-switching, cultural competence, discrimination, language bias*

Introduction: Language and Racism in Medicine

Language is a powerful tool that constantly evolves to reflect sociocultural norms. It is an important part of human connection, expression, and allows us to convey information to others. In medical settings, effective communication has a positive impact on the quality of healthcare just as poor communication can result in bad outcomes. Our world has become a global village, which means that there are many opportunities for interactions between patients and physicians from different linguistic groups. There are nearly 7000 languages spoken globally and the five most spoken are Chinese languages, English, Hindi, Spanish and Arabic; an estimated 650 million speak English as a second language (World Health Organization, 2015).

In this chapter, we will explore the role that language plays in medical settings and how it reflects larger issues such as discrimination and exclusion. For example, certain accents and ways of communicating are perceived to be more desirable than others; these perceptions spill over into the workplace and have an impact on the interactions among physicians, and between physicians and patients. In addition, accentism affects how patients and other physicians perceive the competence of physicians who speak with an accent. Finally, physicians from marginalized communities often straddle the dual roles of communicating one way with more dominant cultures and a different with individuals with whom they share a cultural background. As we move towards inclusivity, it is important to understand the unique challenges that physicians face in their roles as communicators.

Professional Vignette

On the first day of a new clinical rotation, residents from different services meet for the first time in the physician's lounge. While making small talk, one resident asks the other, "Where are you from?"

The resident replies, "I grew up in Toronto."

"No, I mean where are you from *from*?" asks the first resident, emphasizing the second "from" as if to imply that even though her colleague lives in Toronto, she is from elsewhere. She goes on to say, "I mean you're not from around here. I can hear a little something: an accent. Where are you originally from?"

"Oh, I was born in India but moved here as a kid."

"You speak English really well."

Professional **Vignette Analysis**

Physicians who speak with an accent have the added burden of being seen as "others" from the moment they start to speak. While questions and statements about place of origin and accents may seem innocent and may be asked with honest intentions, they can be a distraction and a source of stress. This vignette highlights how this issue comes to light daily for some physicians, even in seemingly benign conversations.

Accents refer to a particular manner of pronunciation and according to the American Speech-Language-Hearing Association, an accent is a phonetic trait from a person's original language that is carried over into a second language (Masztalerz, 2021). Accentism is when non-native accents are stigmatized or discriminated against (Mai and Hoffmann, 2014); they find themselves "judged, marginalised and even penalised for the way their English sounds (Ro, 2021)."

Pause and Reflect: Reactions to English speakers with an accent

Think back to an encounter with a colleague with an accent on which you or someone else present during the encounter commented.

- What was the nature of the comment on the accent?
- If you commented on the accent, what purpose did this serve?
- Were you focusing on the information being presented or on how your colleague speaks? What assumptions were you making about your colleague based on how they speak?
- Have you ever been a silent bystander whilst colleagues or patients commented on a colleague's accent? Have you contributed to negative rhetoric about accents?

The Issues: What are the equity issues associated with language?

Perceived Competence Based on Language

According to Communication Accommodation Theory, people construct and interpret messages based on what they perceive as similarities with the speaker (Lee et al., 2022). There is evidence that non-native accented speakers are discriminated against in different spheres including education, employment, and the media (Roessel et al., 2020). For example, African American English (AAE) speakers have long experienced discrimination because AAE has been associated with incompetence and illiteracy (Pullum, 1999). These linguistic stereotypes extend to medical settings; for instance, when Canadian and Chinese Canadian undergraduates were asked to rate the competence of a doctor with either a standard Canadian accent or a Chinese accent, doctors who speak with a Chinese-Canadian accent were perceived as less competent than doctors who speak with a standard Canadian accent (Chin et al., 2019).

In another study, researchers asked study participants to judge how truthful certain nonsensical statements were, such as "ants don't sleep" when spoken by native and non-native speakers of English (Lev-Ari and Keysar, 2010). They found that people are less likely to trust non-native speakers with foreign accents simply because they are more difficult to understand. In a field like medicine where trust is at the core of building a physician-patient relationship, this type of judgment and bias can be problematic.

Another layer of complexity stems from the fact that certain accents are placed on a pedestal while others are looked down upon. International research reflects these trends. German speakers of English were preferred over West Indian and South Asian English speakers for high-status jobs (Kalin et al., 1980). Similarly, American listeners assigned higher ratings of status (such as competence and intelligence) and personality (such as friendliness and warmth) to English speakers from Western Europe (e.g., France, Germany) but downgraded speakers from South and East Asia (e.g., China, India, Vietnam) (Dragojevic and Goatley-Soan, 2022). The linguistic hierarchy that determines which accents are favored is problematic because of how explicitly racist it is. An accent is accepted as the standard due to the power that a dominant group exerts over marginalized groups.

When performance is judged based on one's accent, it is important to acknowledge that the hierarchy of accents reflects racist views on language (Alim et al., 2020). Since accents are hard wired and challenging to eliminate or switch in adulthood, the speaker with an accent has an unfair disadvantage in social interactions when the accent is devalued. Moreover, those in power have historically dictated acceptable speech patterns. It is important to highlight that linguistic hierarchies exist not because speakers choose to *speak* a certain way, but rather because listeners choose to *listen* in particular ways.

Despite these challenges, efforts at promoting linguistic diversity are crucial in managing a diverse workforce that deals with diverse patient populations. Initiatives such as "accent-reduction" classes which are aimed at foreign-trained physicians must be viewed for the racist connotations that they perpetuate.

❖

It is a peculiar sensation, this double-consciousness, this sense of always looking at one's self through the eyes of others, of measuring one's soul by the tape of a world that looks on in amused contempt and pity.
—W.E.B. DuBois, 1903

❖

Code-Switching in Medical Settings

Code-switching is defined as shifting from the linguistic system of one language or dialect to that of another (Merriam-Webster, 2023). Beyond the strictly linguistic definition, code-switching "involves adjusting one's style of speech, appearance, behavior, and expression in ways that will optimize the comfort of others, in exchange for fair treatment, high-quality service, and employment opportunities" (McCluney et al., 2019).

Adjusting one's way of communicating is an often-benign accommodation that is made to move between the different spheres that an individual must navigate daily. In fact, social norms dictate that one's style of speech, appearance, and behavior should shift to reflect one's ongoing adaptability to different social situations. The issues arise, however, when there is pressure to make these adjustments due to discrimination or a fear of retribution.

To a certain extent, code -witching is a crucial tenet of communication in medical settings. Physicians spend years perfecting their craft and arming themselves with a vast body of knowledge; along with this training comes the adoption of thousands of medical terms and terminology that can reflect one's proficiency in their field. For that knowledge to be translated in clinical practice, physicians must be able to package the information in a way that is palatable to patients. In medical school, students are often taught to simplify their explanations of medical knowledge and to speak at the sixth-grade level to ensure patient comprehension. Code-switching, then, is built into medical communication in the way that physicians package information for their patients; in other words, they speak to patients in a very different way than they would speak to a colleague in the same field.

In elucidating why members of marginalized groups grow so adept at code-switching, their motivations can be explained through examining societal factors. For ethnic minorities, downplaying membership in a stigmatized racial group can elevate social status and the perception of their professionalism. Furthermore, certain behaviors are avoided to distance oneself from stereotypical perceptions that are associated with certain ethnic groups. The challenges arise when downplaying group membership and changing one's behaviour are viewed negatively by members of one's ethnic group (McCluney et al., 2019). The fear of being seen as a "sell out" puts pressure and added psychological baggage on the code-switcher.

 Another reason why minorities code-switch is to show allyship and shared interest with members of dominant groups with hopes of improving upward mobility; people affiliate with people with shared interests or values. Once again, these efforts at fitting in suppressing one's authentic self are exhausting and lead to increased distress (McCluney et al., 2019).

Improving the comfort of patients sometimes comes at an expense to physicians that code-switch in medical settings. For some physicians, code-switching is a pathological response to the racism that they experience as healthcare providers from marginalized groups (Brown, 2021). Some physicians of colour see code-switching as a necessary evil that puts pressure on them to assimilate to a medical culture that is predominately

White and male (Madara, 2021). For these physicians, there is a pressure to conform with the norms of the majority in order to achieve academic success; one must suppress his or her own identity to make others more comfortable. On the other hand, there is pressure on the same individual to make changes to their behaviour to make others (patients and colleagues alike) feel more comfortable. In this duality, code-switching does not feel like a choice, but rather a means to an end in navigating challenging interactions (Brown, 2021). There is a psychological cost on the physician to always be "on" and feel like one cannot truly be themself at the workplace (McCluney et al., 2019).

In contrast to the pressures and negative aspects of code-switching, there are instances where connections can be formed which are beneficial to patients and physicians alike. An example is seen in a scenario that was described by Nathan Wood (2019), then a medical student, where different dialects were used in different clinical settings. What he noticed was that an attending physician spoke African American English when speaking to a patient about personal matters, but the same physician switched to American English when asking or giving medical information. In this scenario, the physician was able to build and establish a rapport by focusing on similarities with the patient; the physician was also able to effectively communicate medical information in a way that the patient could understand and act upon. The perceived benefits to the patient would be improved understanding of health information and increased trust in their health professional, which could in turn lead to enhanced satisfaction and compliance with healthcare recommendations (Wood, 2019).

One potential drawback to switching linguistic styles is if a misread occurs and instead of building a bond, the patient is offended. To minimize this risk, Wood suggests that three conditions should be met when considering switching one's way of communication style. According to Wood, one should have a legitimate claim to or affiliation with the language, dialect, or cultural norm in question. This requires an awareness of self and other to avoid cultural appropriation and strictly performative gestures. In addition, word choice, tone, and body language should all convey clear and honest intentions such a humility and compassion. Finally, code-switching must be done with professionalism; this means excluding vulgar language and offensive slang.

Hybrid Professional and Clinical Vignette

I was seeing a patient for a post-operative visit. She and I are from the same West African ethnic group. We acknowledged each other in English. After that, I reviewed the findings from her surgical procedure. I examined her and reviewed wound care instructions with her. Near the end of the encounter, she asked me if I spoke our non-English language. I said that I did, and she seemed surprised. We then had a spirited conversation where she shared that she was excited about me being the only surgeon that she had met from our ethnic group. We then exchanged stories about our families, where we both changed our tone and mannerisms, and I left the encounter feeling happy about being able to make a connection with her. It happened so naturally that I did not even acknowledge it as unusual at the time.

Hybrid Professional and Clinical Vignette Analysis

Code-switching, as described above, can help to create a safe space and build rapport when communicating in a medical setting. It requires a different form of linguistic mastery that is complementary to the message being presented. It establishes familiarity and is a useful adjunct to enhancing communication and building trust in a doctor-patient relationship.

Communication is critical in our everyday lives and has an impact on our interactions in every industry and sector; the medical field is no exception. Good communication facilitates the exchange of information between physicians as well as between physicians and their patients; it can also assist in coordinating multidisciplinary care, avoiding patient harm, and improving the overall quality of care. The importance of language as a tool when navigating sensitive topics is displayed frequently in medical settings.

More recently, global issues such as the COVID-19 Pandemic and warfare have resulted in the need for international collaboration and humanitarian work for the greater good of society. Physicians are traveling to provide foreign aid and to bolster understaffed workforces. Borders have become porous to the exchange of knowledge and expertise needed to collaborate internationally such as creating vaccines. The need for communicating effectively is even more critical, whether in person or virtually, and discussions about styles of communication are increasingly relevant.

Perceptions of communication and miscommunication often rest on the communication style of the speaker, and less emphasis is placed on the listener in these exchanges. As a result, issues such as accentism and language biases place increased scrutiny on the speaker. In addition, these types of discrimination tend to be based on a set of socially ascribed hierarchies that often place underrepresented groups on a lower level.

When non-native English speakers work as physicians, some of the issues that they face include the pressure to conform linguistically, and questions surrounding their competence based on how they speak. Moreover, these biases can potentially affect how physicians are selected and promoted for positions within the medical field. Biases can potentially demote excellent candidates, not on the strength of their applications but on the basis of misperceptions by their peers. These are just a few of the challenges faced by healthcare providers or medical trainees during their encounters with patients and colleagues.

The Opportunity

What are the opportunities to lead with equity in language and communication?

As we move towards increasingly diverse communities and workplaces, the medical profession must accommodate and reflect this diversity. In the medical literature, the role of language in discussions about diversity and inclusion has received less attention than gender and ethnicity. This trend is changing, however, as more research is being performed about the interplay between language and these other factors. We are increasingly understanding the importance of language in healthcare encounters and recognizing opportunities to lead with equity.

Equity, from a linguistic perspective, necessitates asking questions about whose style of communication is underrepresented and whose is overrepresented. At a minimum, there must be an understanding that all languages and styles of communication are equally worthy. In practice, this means giving people a chance to communicate in ways that they feel comfortable by diminishing the social pressures for them to conform. This will ensure that we are incorporating different world views and seeing them as valuable contributions.

By increasing linguistic diversity through increased representation, there is a potential to enrich physician-to-physician and patient-to-physician interactions. In a clinical trial involving virtual nurses, patients reported "increased satisfaction, trust, liking, preference, perceptions of caring, and willingness to work with the nurses that they personally identified with" (Zhou, 2014). It is well documented that humans tend to accommodate, or adapt, to another person's speaking style to increase perceived similarity (Lee et al., 2022). In theory, then, having a more diverse workforce has the potential for the medical field to reap the benefits of people's real or perceived similarities.

Increased diversity in medicine means we have more opportunities to learn from our peers and eliminate disparities that patients experience. The medical workforce will better represent patients, and this is inarguably a positive shift. As linguistic diversity increases among physicians, we need to acknowledge and respect these differences instead of aiming for assimilation. Physicians are not immune to bias; understanding how our biases may change our perception of our colleagues is a crucial starting point in discussions about linguistic diversity.

Inclusion Strategies

Inclusion Strategies for Language Diversity

Strategies to improve inclusion pertaining to language diversity should take the form of ongoing discussions about reducing exclusion based on language. Minimizing linguistic discrimination in the medical field starts with reviewing medical education and training curricula to assess for knowledge gaps. Outdated curricula will not emphasize the biases that informed medical education in the past.

Discrimination based on language is not considered a social taboo but perhaps it is time to highlight its negative impact. We need to recognize the stress that non-native accented speakers must feel when communicating and work towards focusing on what they are saying as opposed to how they are speaking. This would start with acknowledging that we all have implicit biases which then balloon to shape institutional cultures that perpetrate these biases.

Another way to foster inclusion is to be deliberate in selection, hiring, and promoting staff. If the individuals in charge of selecting and hiring medical trainees come from diverse linguistic backgrounds themselves, there is a higher likelihood that their hiring and promotion practices will in turn create a diverse workforce. Along the same lines, hiring and promotion practices should be as standardized and objective as possible, to reduce and hopefully eliminate biases. It goes without saying that efforts should be made to recruit, support, and retain trainees and physicians from diverse backgrounds.

For physicians who employ code-switching, this cultural fluency should be recognized as a special skill that facilitates inclusivity of the linguistic needs of others. We should examine which biases lead them to accommodate to the linguistic needs of others while finding ways to support them. Strategies for language inclusion do not mean physicians from underrepresented groups should change their way of speaking; we should instead "explore how race and language interplay, and the role of systems that influence the conceptualization and interplay of race and language" (Lee et al., 2022). Table 9.1 outlines some strategies for leaders on improving language inclusion in medical settings.

Table 9.1 *Strategies for leaders on improving language inclusion in medical settings*

1.	Provide interpreter services and consider gender concordance where indicated and feasible.
2.	Recruit, retain, and support minority staff.
3.	Provide multidisciplinary training to increase cultural awareness, knowledge, and skills.
4.	Engage in progressive shifts to cultural humility: Incorporate culture-specific attitudes and values into health promotion materials.
5.	Provide linguistic competency that extends beyond the in person clinical encounter to telephone, virtual, and print communication.

Professional Vignette

During a debriefing session after interviews for fellows in a postgraduate training program, the program directors review their list of applicants. Each director has a chance to provide feedback on their top two candidates from the pool of ten. One at least three occasions, one of the top candidate's accent is brought up. "She interviewed well, but her accent is hard to understand at times. Will that be a problem when she is communicating with patients, staff, and other trainees?" Another staff member speaks up and says, "well, she has more publications than all of us combined, so she clearly knows how to communicate effectively and at a high level. This really should not be a factor that holds her back." A few awkward pauses and stares are exchange, followed by nods. In the end, the consensus is to rank the candidate in question in the top position.

Professional Vignette Analysis

Speaking up and exposing bias is one way to enhance inclusion. Understanding one's privilege is a prime example of this; when placed in a position of power, such as on an admissions panel, it is important to appreciate how decision-making can send a message about the institution's culture. In this vignette, the message that is sent is that the institution will focus on merit over any other factors in their admissions process.

Key Takeaways

- Medicine is becoming increasingly diverse, and language is an often underappreciated contributor to this diversity.
- Linguistic diversity must be understood and appreciated as it intersects with other social variables.
- Increasing diversity in the medical education pipeline means there is potential for a linguistically diverse population of future physicians to hopefully diminish linguistic discrimination and normalize diverse identities.
- Code-switching has both positive and negative aspects, depending on the circumstances, and should be acknowledged as both challenging and rewarding.
- The workplace can create pressures for minorities to code-switch.
- Accentism is common and can create bias with respect to correlations between linguistic patterns, competence and professionalism.
- Accents are part of identity and should not be seen as a factor requiring modification or reduction as accents are a distinct entity from language fluency and communication skills.
- For physicians to be linguistically effective, there must be an understanding of the factors that affect how physicians' communication styles are perceived and incorporated into health encounters.
- Strategies to dismantle linguistic hierarchies in healthcare include providing training to those delivering care to linguistically diverse populations, starting with learners. It is important to identify discriminatory practices that act to perpetuate racist narratives.
- At the individual level, it is essential to be aware of our own linguistic biases and how they shape our worldview, how they shape the workplace culture and how they intersect with the broader mandate of the healthcare institution.
- At the institutional level, educational and clinical spaces should aim to be representative: as linguistically diverse and inclusive as befits the needs of the population served.

Conclusion

Language plays a crucial role in our everyday communication. Good communication between doctors and patients improves outcomes, adherence, and satisfaction. When the spotlight is placed on how doctors use language, interesting challenges and opportunities emerge. Perceptions of how physicians speak need to be judgment-free and cannot create an "us versus them" dichotomy, nor should it allow a space for rhetoric that links linguistic style with competence. It is essential to recognize that there are many other factors at play when language intersects with other sociocultural variables. Focusing on the message while acknowledging the messenger is of vital importance.

Inclusivity in medical settings also involves paying attention to the crucial role that language plays for physicians and patients alike in the equity, diversity and inclusion (EDI) discourse. Language is a critical component of the EDI conversation- with the lights out and inability to distinguish ethno-racial, religious and other markers of sociocultural identity, language burns bright. It can be wielded to include and exclude, to mock and to extol, yet it has no bearing on one's capacity as a physician or on one's entitlement to care as a patient.

On a Parting Note...

Where before some ancestors pulled the veil and passed

to shed the reviled skin on which stones amassed,

I too must now presume to pass by the shedding of my tongue,

as my lingua franca draws opprobrium and denies my intellect.

But when shall it stop? When will my words pass muster and not mockery? When?

Shall I go back from whence I came? Shall you return the treasures plundered to send us all back from where we came and yourself return to the root place from where you came? And thence shall the tongues all speak alike and the Tower of Babel fall once we are each returned from whence we came?

© Mariam Abdurrahman, 2023

References

Alim H.S., Reyes A. and Kroskrity P.V. (2020). The Field of Language and Race: A Linguistic Anthropological Approach to Race, Racism, and Racialization. In Alim, H.S., Reyes, A. and Kroskrity, P.V. (eds.). *The Oxford Handbook of Language and Race* (Online edn: Oxford Academic), pp. 1–21.

Blanchard, A.K. (2021). Code Switch. *New England Journal of Medicine*, 384, pp. e87.

Brach, C. and Fraser, I. (2000). Can cultural competency reduce racial and ethnic health disparities? A review and conceptual model. *Medical Care Research and Review*, 57 (Supplement 1), pp. 181-217.

Brown, IM. (2021). Diversity Matters: Code-Switching as an EM survival tactic. *Emergency Medicine News*, 43(1), p.7.

Cargile, A.C. and Giles, H. (1998). Language attitudes toward varieties of English: An American-Japanese context. *Journal of Applied Communication Research*, 26(3), pp. 338–356.

Chin, L.C., Baquiran, C.L.C., and Nicoladis, E. (2019). A doctor's foreign accent affects perceptions of competence. *Health Communication*, pp. 726-730.

Code-switching. Merriam-Webster. (2023). Available from: https://www.merriam-webster.com/dictionary/code-switching

Dragojevic, M. and Goatley-Soan, S. (2022). Americans' attitudes toward foreign accents: evaluative hierarchies and underlying processes. *Journal of Multilingual and Multicultural Development*, 43 (2), pp. 167-181.

Du Bois, W.E.B. (1903). The Souls of Black Folk. Chicago: A.G. Mc-Clurg.

Flores N. and Rosa J. (2015). Undoing appropriateness: raciolinguistic ideologies and language diversity in education. *Harvard Education Review*, 85(2), pp. 149–171.

Hosoda, M., Stone-Romero, E. F., and Walter, J. N. (2007). Listeners' cognitive and affective reactions to English speakers with standard American English and Asian accents. *Perceptual and Motor Skills*, 104(1), pp. 307–326.

Kalin R., Rayko D.S., and Love N. (1980). The Perception and Evaluation of Job Candidates with Four Different Ethnic Accents. In H. Giles, W.P. Robinson and Smith P.M. (eds.). *Language: Social psychological perspectives*. Oxford: Pergamon, pp. 197-202.

Lee D.N., Hutchens M.J., George T.J., Wilson-Howard D., Cooks E.J., and Krieger J.L. (2022). Do they speak like me? Exploring how perceptions of linguistic difference may influence patient perceptions of healthcare providers. *Medical Education Online,* 27, p1.

Lev-Ari, S. and Keysar, B. (2010). Why don't we believe non-native speakers? The influence of accent on credibility. *Journal of Experimental Social Psychology,* 46 (6), pp. 1093-1096.

Lindemann, S. (2003). Koreans, Chinese or Indians? Attitudes and ideologies about nonnative English speakers in the United States. *Journal of Sociolinguistics,* 7(3), pp. 348–364.

Madara, J. (2021). Reckoning with medicine's history of racism. American Medical Association [online]. Available from: https://www.ama-assn.org/about/leadership/reckoning-medicine-s-history-racism.

Masztalerz, G. (2021). *Accent Modification and Identity: A Phenomenological Study Exploring the Experiences of International Students and Immigrants/Refugees.* BSc thesis. University of Northern Colorado.

Mai, R. and Hoffmann, S. (2014). Accents in business communication: An integrative model and propositions for future research. *Journal of Consumer Psychology,* 24(1), pp. 137–158.

McCluney, C.L., Robotham, K., Lee, S., Smith, R., and Durkee, M. (2019). The costs of code-switching [online]. *Harvard Business Review.* Available from: https://hbr.org/2019/11/the-costs-of-codeswitching

Molina, R. and Kasper, J. (2019). The power of language-concordant care: a call to action for medical schools. *BMC Medical Education,* 19, p. 378. Published online 2019 Nov 6.

Priebe, S. (2016). A social paradigm in psychiatry - themes and perspectives. *Epidemiology and Psychiatric Sciences,* 25(6), pp. 521–527.

Pullum, G.K. (1999). African American vernacular English is not standard English with mistakes. In R.S. Wheeler (ed.). *The workings of language: from prescriptions to perspectives.* Westport: Praeger, pp. 59–66.

Ro, C. (2021). *The pervasive problem of 'linguistic racism'* [online]. Available from: https://www.bbc.com/worklife/article/20210528-the-pervasive-problem-of-linguistic-racism

Roessel, J., Schoel, C., and Stahlberg, D. (2020). Modern notions of accent-ism: findings, conceptualizations, and implications for interventions and research on nonnative accents. *Journal of Language and Social Psychology.* 39(1), pp. 87–111.

Srivastava, R. (2018). Accents don't hurt patients, attitudes do [online] Feb 7, 2018. Available from: https://www.theguardian.com/commentisfree/2018/feb/07/accents-dont-hurt-patients-attitudes-do

Takeshita, J., Wang, S., Loren, A.W., Mitra, N., Shults, J., Shin, D.B. and Sawinski D.L. (2020). Association of racial/ethnic and gender concordance between patients and physicians with patient experience ratings. *JAMA Network Open*, 3(11), e2024583.

World Health Organization. (2015). Bridging the language divide in health. *Bulletin of the World Health Organization* [online]. Available from: https://www.who.int/bulletin/volumes/93/6/15-020615/en/

Wood, N. (2019). Departing from doctor-speak: a perspective on code-switching in the medical setting. *Journal of General Internal Medicine*, 34(3), pp. 464–466.

Zhou, S., Bickmore, T., Paasche-Orlow, M., and Jack, B. (2014). Agent-user concordance and satisfaction with a virtual hospital discharge nurse. *In*: Bickmore T, Marsella S, and Sidner C, (eds.). Intelligent Virtual Agents. vol 8637. Lecture Notes in Computer Science. Cham, Switzerland: Springer: Cham, pp. 528–541.

Chapter 10
Rules of the Race: Stay in Your Lane

Mariam Abdurrahman, MD, Crystal Pinto, MD

❖

With boot to neck and nary a way to grasp breath,
he gasped his last:
"I can't breathe"
—Mariam Abdurrahman, 2023

❖

Abstract: The history of racism in medicine is broad, heterogeneous and can be so deeply entrenched as to be imperceptible. This chapter examines the presence of racism within the organizing fabric of medical institutions and explores the racist underpinnings in medical education that continue to shape the profession today. The impact of medical racism on patients and physicians alike is examined. The chapter explores opportunities for antiracism work within core facets of the field, notably medical education and medical journals as the chief conduit for transmitting information, attitudes and innovations in the field.

Keywords: BIPOC, discrimination, equity-responsive, medical racism, race correction, racial gas lighting, racialized medicine, racism

Introduction

There are increasing calls to acknowledge racism as a public health crisis, as racism is not confined to a social phenomenon but rather a biosocial one that promotes the persisting racial gap in morbidity and mortality (Amutah et al., 2021; Hall and Fields, 2015; Ogedegbe, 2020). While the effects of racism are often insidious and take the form of microaggressions, there are also blatant acts of macroaggression that emphasize the various structural pillars of racism embedded in society. The COVID-19 Pandemic has been particularly instructive in casting a light on these pillars which notably include medicine and healthcare systems, justice, and education.

As George Floyd drew his last breadth on 25 May 2020 (Wikipedia, 2023a), the world watched transfixed as he asphyxiated both physically and metaphorically, for the boot to his neck was indeed the contemporary yoke to his ancestors' necks in the era of slavery. His law enforcement encounter reflected the ongoing nature of Black males and other racialized males' interactions with systematized violence. What were the life antecedents to this fatal incident? How did he arrive at this moment of fatal reckoning? This was not a unique or isolated event, but rather a reenactment of a recurring pattern of racial subjugation. It occurred on the streets, but it could have also taken place in a clinical space and in fact this is the case in various instances, the most recently publicized being Joyce Echaquan's death in a hospital in Quebec, Canada, on 28 September 2020 (Wikipedia, 2023b).

Seminal events like the above remind us that while institutions like medicine are privileged to serve, the privilege has not served racialized patients well, nor is the privilege of a medical license borne equally by physicians. Physicians of minority backgrounds are subject to microaggressions, with racialized physicians experiencing racism both in their patient and interprofessional encounters. The pecking order established by race constitutes a crisis that continues to stifle racialized physicians and medical learners, albeit in a more gradual fashion than George Floyd and Joyce Echaquan's rapid demise.

Racism is "a system of structures, policies, practices, and norms that construct opportunities and assigns values based on one's phenotype" (Jones, 2002). Racism has long been recognized as an underlying cause of health inequity (Amutah et al., 2021; McCord and Freeman, 1990; Ogedegbe, 2020; Williams, 2021). Medicine contributes to the insidious and deleterious effects of racism through the continued misrepresentation of race as biology. As explored in Chapter 1, medicine has a long history of propagating the notion of biological difference between races (Byrd and Clayton, 2001), despite race being a social rather than biological construct as underscored by the Human Genome Project (USDE, 2019). The Project revealed that there is less than 0.1% difference between humans at the DNA level and these differences are not associated with the social categorizations of race.

The conflation of race with biology is deeply ingrained and herein lies the chief challenge to addressing medical racism, racialized medicine and associated equity, diversity and inclusion (EDI) issues in medicine. By definition, the concept of race is itself racist as the "concept of race was developed to stratify and privilege people on the basis of physical appearance and presumed ancestry" (Williams, 2021). Furthermore, racism is itself the chief challenge to advancing research on racism and antiracist approaches (Williams, 2021). Despite recognition of these issues in the medical field and increasing recognition of the impact on health, health equity and wellbeing, there remain significant EDI gaps in medicine. These gaps have been highlighted by current events that continue to reverberate from society into medicine and vice versa.

Events including the widely publicized deaths of George Floyd and Eric Garner at the hands of law enforcement reflect the modern-day chains of slavery that minorities continue to experience in the broader society, whilst the deaths of Brian Sinclair and Joyce Echaquan reflect the deeply embedded systemic racism that continue to permeate medicine today (Allan and Smylie, 2015; Amster, 2022; Wikipedia, 2023ab). In medicine, these emblematic events have triggered deep reckoning about EDI gaps and the role of the field as an oppressor where it should be an advocate, a place of exclusion where it should be inclusive, a space of privilege where it should instead foster equity, and a place of tolerance where it should instead embrace diversity.

Although various micro to macro EDI strategies have been explored, this is yet to be accompanied by meaningful and lasting action likely because it is so difficult to know how and where to begin. The stasis of not knowing can be empowering in the humility of acknowledging that we are mired so deeply as to be near stuck. However, paralysis cannot remain the reason for inaction on this critical front. Nor can we wait for change at the broader societal level given the magnitude of harm associated with racism; in fact, there are calls to address racism as a public health crisis as a result of the health and social harms caused by racism (Paine et al., 2021; Wong et al., 2014). The role of medicine in creating an equity-responsive climate cannot be underscored enough given the spectrum of racial harms that emanate in, or are maintained by medicine, and are deeply buried in clinical practice guidelines, investigations and teaching of the art and science of medicine.

Medicine is a microcosm of society with intricately stratified membership much like the broader society. We know that racial misrepresentation and racial microaggressions derive their power within an inequitable and racially stratified society, ergo the need for systemic solutions that span across medical education and training, clinical practice and medical research.

Professional Vignette

by Crystal Pinto

Before I attended medical school in the most racially diverse city in Canada, I completed my bachelor's degree at the same university. Many of the pre-med classes were held in the same building and in the same rooms in which the medical students attended their lectures. The space was familiar to me, and as I waited outside the room for one of my first classes in medical school to begin, undergraduate students started to pour out of the room. Much like the classes I had been in, the students were reflective of the demographics of the city we lived in – most of them were racialized. After they were gone, the medical students, myself included, filled up the room. The racial demographics were now different, with racialized students very clearly in the minority of a predominantly White-appearing class.

At some point that morning, someone from the Faculty came in to give us one of the orientation speeches that they give at the start of medical school. Somewhere in the middle of the speech, she looked around the room and said, "There are so many things I love about this city, but what brings me the most joy and pride is that I'm standing in front of one of the most diverse medical school classes in the country." The "diversity" of the predominantly White class was read as a point of pride.

Professional Vignette Analysis

Sitting in that room as a non-White medical student, the message I got was that medicine was expected to be predominantly White. The fact that the demographics were so radically shifted from that of the pre-med classes was not noted as a failure. It seemed to me that the inclusion of racialized students was such a radical departure from the norm that any inclusion at all was viewed as a victory for "diversity". Reflecting back on this experience, it was fairly clear to me that my presence in medical school was not something that could be taken for granted. It almost felt like gratitude was expected. This can act as a significant barrier to being able to identify and name the ways in which the institution of medicine contributes to the stressors experienced by racialized minority students.

In my experience, there was often the assumption that the microaggressive behaviours were coming "from a good place." Questions about my accent or my name had to be understood as curiosity. To question or to chafe against people's expectations of me would mean that I might be labelled difficult, and in a system where so much of the evaluation of ability is subjective, that is not a benign risk. I came to think early on in my clerkship training that professionalism was really a measure of how well I could fit into the dominant culture of medicine, and how comfortable I could make the dominant majority around my otherness. This ability to mask my otherness became second nature to me, yet was always something I had to exert effort to maintain.

Pause and Reflect

- Are the racial demographics in your medical school reflective of the communities served by the institution?
- Amongst racialized physicians in your cohort, how many are/were Black or Indigenous?
- What are the expectations of physicians' appearances, grooming, and behaviour, and are these racially coded?
- How does the experience of being "othered" or "alien" impact success and well-being?

The Issues

What are the Issues?

Racism takes various forms, ranging from blatant acts of prejudice (i.e., macroaggressions) to the more insidious form of microaggressions. Sue (2005, p. 108) describes microaggressions as "insidious, damaging, and harmful forms of racism [that] are...everyday, unintentional, and unconscious [and] are perpetrated by ordinary citizens who believe they are doing right". Pierce (1970) originally coined the term in 1970 and notes that the cumulative effect of microaggressions over a lifetime can contribute to increased morbidity and mortality while concurrently crushing confidence. As such, racism is toxic and detracts from the ability to achieve self-actualization for racial minorities as access to opportunities are stratified by the racial pecking order. In medicine, the effects are seen in the pipeline with very low representation of Black and Indigenous students in medical schools, as discussed in Chapter 4. The effect is replicated down the line to medical leadership, clinically and academically, with low representation of racialized physicians in medical leadership roles.

Racial microaggressions are often nebulous, deriving from the metacommunication or hidden messages contained in everyday interactions (Espaillat et al., 2019). The fact that microaggressions are hidden in daily interactions and can be quite subtle widens the gap of racial realities, adding a challenge to attempts to create meaningful dialogue about the issue (Wong et al., 2014). Microaggressions span a spectrum (Table 10.1) and may be intentional, such as with microinsults, or unintentional, such as with microassaults and microinvalidations.

Table 10.1. *Taxonomy of Racial Microaggressions (Sue et al., 2007)*

Category	Definition	Example
Microinsults	Often conscious and explicit racist behaviours (verbal, non-verbal gestures, or environmental cues) that are intended to purposefully hurt a person	Racial denigration, name calling, teasing, avoidant or discriminatory acts

Category	Definition	Example ...*continued*
Microassaults	Often unconscious nonverbal and verbal actions that demean a person's racial heritage	Assumption of criminality due to one's race
Microinvalidations	Often unconscious behaviours (including verbal) that invalidate, negate or minimize the lived realities of racialized persons	Denial or dismissal of racism, ascribed hypersensitivity, "color blindness", regarding racial minorities as foreigners

The unintentional and unconscious elements of microaggression add complexity as most view themselves as decent human beings who believe in equality and strive to do the right thing (Sue et al., 2007; Wong et al., 2014). In the medical setting, this translates to a staunch belief on the part of most physicians that although the system is flawed, they themselves provide care to their patients equitably and harbor no bias towards colleagues of other races. Similarly, physicians may not recognize the relative denominations of privilege within their professional sphere and assume that any differences in status stem from merit.

White male physicians who occupy leadership roles would likely attribute their position to meritocratic achievement, with few acknowledging the head start of privilege, thus engaging in the myth of meritocracy (Sue et al., 2007). This misconception of merit further negates the reality of racialized physicians when their attempts at career advancement are derailed by racism. The challenge in addressing the differential racial realities lies in the subtle and insidious elements of racial microaggressions.

Racial Gaslighting

The subtlety and perhaps the most insidious power of microaggressions is that they not only deny the reality of racialized persons, but they also cause the recipient to question their experience of the event, thus the experience of racial gaslighting. Naming the problem and attempting to engage in constructive dialogue is often suggested as the antidote to many "elephant in the room" situations. However, in this instance constructive release is fraught with the risk of being further invalidated and relegated as being "hypersensitive".

Racialized physicians who also have multiple intersecting minority identities may also find themselves alternating between extremes of being invisible and being hypervisible, a state of perpetual adverse experiences. Young racialized males experience hypervisibility; they may find themselves repeatedly being asked to identify themselves in spite of wearing their identification badges whilst others are asked if they are custodial staff despite visible identifiers that indicate otherwise. Physicians of colour often report encountering surprise, at times outright hostility from patients whilst others describe microaggressions including misidentification by their colleagues (Brown et al., 2021; Rowe et al., 2022; Wheeler et al., 2019). In attempting to name the racism and discuss the experience, their accounts may be questioned and alternate explanations proposed including the suggestion of racial hypersensitivity and the implication that no harm was intended or given.

The invalidation of personal experiences and environmental observations of racism present an added toxic burden that accumulates over a lifetime of recurring exposure, progressively "flattening confidence" (Pierce, 1995 p. 281) and self-efficacy, resulting in a double bind: racialized physicians experience obstacles in their career advancement as a result of systemic discrimination but at the same time the effects of the racism are such that the resultant diminishment of self-esteem and self-efficacy hinder attempts to continue to fight the racial oppression.

In addition to the progressive erosion of confidence, the cumulative effects of microaggression also facilitate the leaky pipeline in medicine and contribute to physician burnout; in fact, the conceptualization of the effects of microaggression share striking similarities to the three domains of burnout (see Figure 10.1a and 10.1b). The pipeline must be nurtured by addressing and preventing downstream leaks at the same time as the pipeline entry is being continuously cultivated to shape successively more equity-responsive generations of learners. The entry level and upstream regions of the pipeline are dually shaped by societal influences and the medical curriculum. Many would balk at the statement that medicine has a longstanding history of racism, and the medical curriculum inculcates racism and misinformation, however these issues are increasingly apparent as subsequently discussed.

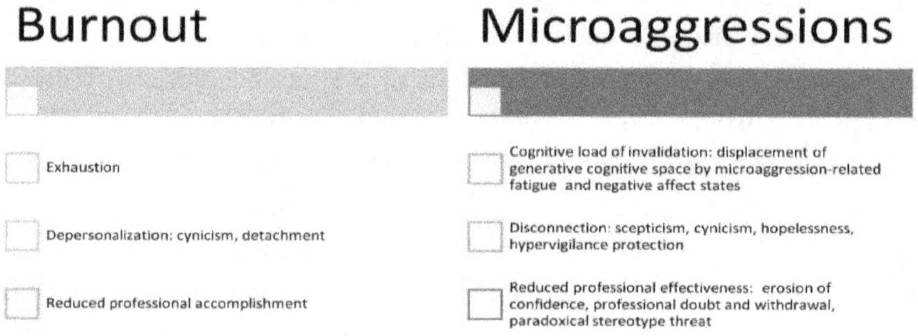

Burnout
Microaggressions
Exhaustion
Cognitive load of invalidation: displacement of generative cognitive space by microaggression-related fatigue and negative affect states
Depersonalization: cynicism, detachment
Disconnection: scepticism, cynicism, hopelessness, hypervigilance protection
Reduced professional accomplishment
Reduced professional effectiveness: erosion of confidence, professional doubt and withdrawal, paradoxical stereotype threat

Figure 10.1a *Conceptual overlap between burnout and the sequelae of microaggressions*

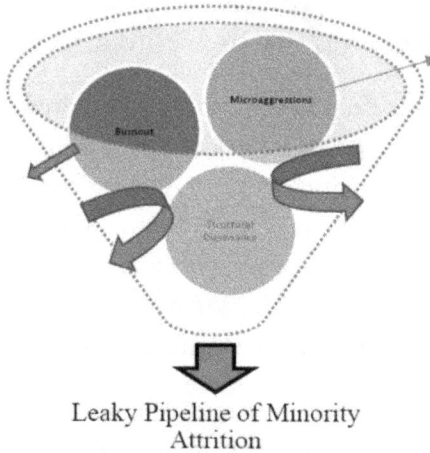

Microaggressions
Burnout
Leaky Pipeline of Minority Attrition

Figure 10.1b. *Interaction between burnout, microaggressive climates and the leaky pipeline*

❖

"The paradox of education is precisely this - that as one begins to become
conscious one begins to examine the society in which he is being educated"
—James Baldwin, 1963

❖

Medical Schools as Training Grounds for Racism

Perhaps unsurprisingly, medical schools' histories with racism have been
as charged as the history of medicine in general. Many medical schools in
Canada banned Black students from enrolling in the early 20th century,
with at least one school continuing until 1965 to enforce the ban, which
remained on its books until 2018 (Henry, 2021.) At the time, the American
Medical Association also wished to exclude Black physicians from its
membership, and was pressuring Canadian Universities to expel Black
students. Black Americans were limited to studying medicine at
Historically Black Colleges and Universities (HBCUs), which lacked the
funding to meet demand. Thus, medical education in North America
remained predominantly White.

Although efforts have been made to increase diversity, these efforts have
not benefited all racialized students equally. A 2012 survey of Canadian
medical schools found that some racial minorities (e.g., Asian students)
were over represented while Black and Indigenous students remain
underrepresented. Given the history of racial oppression, this is not
surprising, nor is the experience of these students once they arrive.
Multiple studies have found that racialized minority students experience
exclusion, and both implicit and explicit forms of racism. This greatly
contributes to their psychological distress, as they try to navigate the degree
of attention to draw to their experience. Some students, especially Black
and Indigenous students often carry the weight of addressing the historic
racism in their programs. Furthermore, they must contend with racial
misrepresentation in the curriculum as the class collectively embarks on the
endeavour of studying misinformation and excelling at their proficiency
with the curriculum material.

Medicine 101: Delivering Racism and Misinformation through the Curriculum

Medicine has a long history of propagating the notion of biological difference between races (Byrd and Clayton, 2001). This occurs in various ways in clinical practice and begins as early as the premedical and preclinical years of medical education. On examining the preclinical curriculum, racial misrepresentation is observed in three broad categories (Amutah et al., 2021; Chadha et al., 2020; Nieblas-Bedolla et al., 2020; Tsai et al., 2016):

- Semantics: imprecise terminology usage in the description of ethnoracial differences and population differences in health
- Epidemiology
  - the presentation of disease prevalence without context
  - pathologization of race through the linkage of increased disease burden with minoritized groups
- Clinical Practice Guidelines: racial categorization or adjustment of diagnostic, screening and treatment variables, e.g., race correction factors in diagnostic equipment

Given that these observations relate to preclinical education, this is quite concerning as a venue for cementing implicit biases and inaccurate understandings of race and biology that medical and premedical students bring with them. In terms of the epidemiology domain, the danger of presenting racial differences in disease burden without context is that it primes learners to attribute these differences solely to racial identity, so that race is in effect a risk factor, yet we know that race does not cause disease although racism does (Amutah, 2021; Deyrup and Graves, 2022).

Once clinical training begins, the previously absorbed biases stand to be reinforced depending on how clinical cases are taught and how the content is presented in reference materials. The racialization of disease is prevalent in textbooks, case-based learning in terms of the heavy reliance on "classic cases", examination questions and the choice of representative patient selected for bedside teaching. For example, a review of examination bank questions showed that *race was incidental to the answer in 7.4% of questions that included a White patient descriptor; in contrast for Indigenous Americans, race was diagnostic 100% of the time* (Ripp and Braun, 2017).

Given the inherent biases embedded in curricular materials, it is important to give attention to these sources in attempting to correct racial misrepresentation and physician bias. Most medical students and residents will readily recite that sickle cell is observed in Black persons whilst cystic fibrosis is observed in White persons, both of which are inaccurate. The adaptation of the curved red blood cell to ward off the *plasmodium* parasite is not racially determined but rather is present in populations at risk for malaria, a fact that is often overlooked in teaching inquiring young minds that are at risk of later perpetuating this incomplete knowledge. In terms of cystic fibrosis, the cognitive bias surrounding the phenotype of a patient may result in overlooking screening for non-White patients presenting with signs and symptoms suggestive of the condition. Similarly, reporting and teaching that asthma rates are elevated in Black children overlooks the fact that the social conditions are the true modifying variable as opposed to a racial predilection for the condition (Amutah et al., 2021; Wright, 2011).

As education and training progress, it quickly becomes second nature to utilize treatment algorithms that include race correction without an understanding of the etiology and justification of correction factors. The controversial kidney correction factor is the most cited example of the adverse implications of a race correction factor that is entirely without scientific merit in terms of creatinine differences across races. By the time trainees are in practice these correction factors are second nature in their work and they in turn transmit this misinformation to their own learners with the confidence of having trained in a reputable medical institution. Surely, we can trust our medical education, right?

The ability to trust in medical institutions is implicit for most learners, thus highlighting the critical role of the institution as a venue for addressing racial misrepresentation and physician bias. The effects of this bias are evident in the differential healthcare access, diagnosis and treatment of minoritized patients relative to the dominant majority (Amutah et al., 2021; Hall and Fields, 2015; Ogedegbe, 2020; Wong et al., 2014). The effect is even more insidious when one considers the internalized effect for racialized physicians who themselves receive the same education and training, absorb both the explicit and silent curricula, whilst formulating their physician identity. They may not know to question why they have offered or withheld certain treatments or referrals and may be shocked to see themselves as contributory oppressors because *they so diligently absorbed their education*.

Amutah et al. (2021) and Deyrup and Graves (2022) propose the following approaches to reducing racialization and improving the use of race in medicine:

- Standardized and granular use of ethnoracial descriptors
- Contextualization of ethnoracial differences in disease as structural and social determinants play a paramount role in observed disease frequencies
- Reformulation of examination questions to de-adopt race-based guidelines and racial heuristics
- Pre-medical admission course on biologic anthropology focused on biology, race and the discordance between human biologic variation and socially defined race
- Focus on structural determinants of health and health disparities in the standard population health course taken in medical schools
- Clinical training content that deemphasizes "classic" vignettes where socially defined race is explicitly linked to disease

The role of the curriculum cannot be emphasized enough in terms of the critical role in unlearning racialization and learning how to use race, health, disease and biosocial context validly. For physicians and residents, the clinical practice guideline and the medical journal constitute important avenues for continued unlearning of medical racialization and racism. Many medical journals are adopting an antiracist stance, however there is much work to be done as the publication of reports on race, racism and health equity are still relatively small compared to the multitude of reports that link minorities with pathology in general.

Deyrup and Graves (2022) note that linking socially defined race and disease is rarely neutral. The reflexive use of race to describe epidemiologic data is imprecise, in that race is used as a proxy for disease and the take home is that race itself puts patients at risk for disease. When racial terms are used to describe epidemiologic data thereby linking minorities with pathology and effectively pathologizing race, it perpetuates continued race-based diagnostic bias (Amutah et al., 2021). We should be clear about what race is a proxy for when we cite race in data as race has been used as a proxy for genetics, socioeconomic status and behavioural risk factors (Amutah et al., 2021). In the setting of publications, the peer review process should include an examination for this erroneous link, otherwise we continue to perpetuate the myth of race constituting disease.

The responsibility to incorporate racism effects on race and ethnicity adjusted data is one that educators need to adopt reflexively (Amutah et al., 2021; Deyrup and Graves). It would be irresponsible to continue to present race-based data without addressing the role of racism and structural factors on the observed outcomes and trends being taught to medical learners.

Personal Reflection

by Crystal Pinto

During my medical training, like many others around me, I absorbed the idea of medicine as a noble profession. The notion that we are, or at least aim to be, selfless healers persists. This idea has continued to gain strength through the course of the current COVID-19 Pandemic and the resultant burdens it placed on healthcare workers. In light of this, it is hard to look at medicine as an institution with a racist history. However, when we look at this history and the ways in which it continues to play out, medicine's blind spots around issues of race can appear sinister.

The current Pandemic also illuminated the significant racial disparities in access to care and recovery. It has been suggested that race-adjustments on spirometers could play a role in the racial disparities in recovery from COVID-19 (Anderson et al., 2021). The race correction factor assumes a 10-15% smaller lung capacity for Black individuals and 4-6% smaller lung capacity for Asian individuals compared with their White counterparts. We also continue to utilize concepts of race and ethnicity in medical research, despite ambiguity about what those terms signify if they are no longer linked to biological constructs, and the consequences of the choice to do so are not benign.

In a case study of the Dynamed Point of Care tool, Singh and Steeves (2020) provide an example of the ways in which an algorithmic tool can present research that uses ambiguous ideas of race and ethnicity in ways that strengthen older ideas of race as being a biological reality. When I am reminded of this aspect of the history of racism in medicine and truly sit with it, it feels a little like sitting in that classroom. I feel that same sense of incomprehension, because it still feels like something is being missed, unnamed or deliberately obscured.

Similarly, when I reflect on my role as psychiatrist, it often gives me pause because of the prescriptive aspects of psychiatric practice. As a psychiatrist, I frequently find myself questioning the role I play in the carceral system that lies at the root of psychiatry. Knowing that involuntary detentions and restraint use disproportionately affect racialized communities, I frequently question whether I am enacting White supremacy through my work. Given the deep ways in which medicine and White supremacy are intertwined, the answer is probably at least partly yes. We need to create space to ask those questions and arrive at the difficult answers.

Pause and Reflect

- How much of the history of racism in medicine is taught in medical schools?
- What types and sources of knowledge, and whose viewpoints have been prioritized in medical education?
- How do previous racist beliefs in medicine continue to impact practice today?

Patient Impacts

The health of racialized minorities continues to lag behind that of non-racialized groups (Cogburn, 2019; Gee et al., 2011). Rates of maternal mortality amongst non-Hispanic Black women in the United States remain significantly higher than non-Hispanic White women (MacDorman et al., 2021) and racial and ethnic disparities persist in significant maternal morbidity (Leonard et al., 2019). Evidence has shown that even at high incomes, a significant racial gap in maternal and infant mortality remains (Kennedy-Moulton et al., 2022).

Indigenous groups similarly face shocking racism in healthcare settings (Allan and Smylie, 2015). There is a long history of forced sterilizations of Indigenous women in North America, both in the context of specific eugenics boards, and as part of a wider attempt at population control (Pegoraro, 2014), with continued reports of coerced sterilization in the 21st Century, for example in Canada (Collier, 2017). In Canada, there have been multiple well-publicized cases of racism against Indigenous patients leading to their deaths (Allan and Smylie, 2015). The exact cause of these disparities continues to raise questions amidst a vigorous discussion of the workings of post-colonial imperialism. Multiple factors are likely at play including the impact of racism as a series of adverse life events that result in physiological and psychological stressors (Berger and Sarnyai, 2015), systemic racism (Yearby, 2018), and the interpersonal interactions between patients and providers (Johnson et al., 2004).

The challenge of racism in medicine affects healthcare in various ways. There is inadequate medical research about the impacts of racism, and the ways in which this negatively impacts the healthcare of racialized patients. There is also a lack of representation of racialized populations in research studies (Food and Drug Administration, 2020). Medical research also has a troubled history when it comes to racialized populations, from the egregious Tuskegee experiments to the less well-known trials of the oral contraceptive pill in Puerto Rico (Barrett, 2019; Shamoo, 2022). The popular view of medical research is that it is color blind and apolitical because it is rooted in facts and evidence; however, the presence of bias in the data collection that forms the very foundation of research raises questions about the validity of findings in relation to racialized populations.

The spirometer as described earlier presents a case in point of biased source data, which in turn generates biased outcomes all the way from diagnoses and treatment options to compensation and insurance for respiratory health conditions. In fact, prominent companies have relied on the plantation era findings of a racial "pulmonary deficit" and its inherent racial bias to block compensation suits by Black employees with lung damage and mesothelioma arising from occupational asbestos exposure (Ellis, 2023; Teixeira, 1999). For example, in the American lawsuit against Owens Corning (previously Owens-Corning Fiberglass), the company submitted that the diminished lung capacity of Black workers was due to naturally lower lung capacity rather than a result of occupational exposure to asbestos (Ellis, 2023; Teixeira, 1999). Lawsuits eventually forced Owens Corning into bankruptcy and an asbestos trust fund was established (Ellis, 2023).

The knowledge imparted to medical students and their subsequent proficiency as physicians in practice is impacted by these racial biases. For example, it has been observed that (i) skin of color is underrepresented in learning materials, and that (ii) some medical practitioners are unable to accurately diagnose skin conditions ranging from common rashes to more serious conditions like skin cancer in racialized patients, with higher rates of later stage diagnoses in patients with darker skin (Abduelmula et al., 2022; Ebede and Papier, 2006; Fenton et al., 2020; Kamath et al., 2021; Narla et al., 2022). This leads to delays in treatment and results in negative patient outcomes.

While overt racism persists in medicine, there is also significant evidence to suggest that many patients experience more subtle forms of racism in their interpersonal interactions with healthcare providers. Multiple studies have shown disparities in patient-provider communication based on race. Schut (2021) demonstrates how racial disparities, independent of socioeconomic factors, can have an impact on patient-provider communication, adherence to treatment and follow up for incidental findings. Other studies have shown that racialized patients are more likely to be interrupted, more likely to have visits that are significantly shorter or have lower word count than those with White patients, and have decreased trust in their relationships with care providers (Cooper et al., 2003; Eggly et al., 2015; Gordon et al., 2006; Johnson et al., 2004; Shen et al., 2018). Healthcare practitioners are also less likely to provide analgesia to racialized patients, including racialized children (Goyal et al., 2015; Guedj et al., 2021).

The quality of the interaction between provider and patient has real and tangible consequences on patient health. Even if the above-mentioned issues of racial disparities in medical education and research did not exist, patient health would still suffer secondary to the racial disparities in communication. This also does not take into account the significant racial disparities in patients' abilities to access care. Multiple aspects of medicine appear to place racialized patients, especially Black and Indigenous patients at a disadvantage.

Clinical Vignette

by Crystal Pinto

Late in my residency training, I saw an Afro-Caribbean woman as an outpatient. She had worked for some time in a setting in which she was the only racialized person. She was frequently on the receiving end of microinsults, felt excluded from conversations in the workplace, and began to believe that her co-workers were deliberately sabotaging her. The first therapist she saw began to question if she was developing paranoia. She stopped seeing that therapist, but became increasingly anxious and depressed. She took a leave of absence from her work. However, she continued to experience depression, and subsequently was seen in the psychiatric clinic in which I worked. Though I was able to name racism as a real experience, and not paranoia, I once made the mistake of implying that I understood her experience. She told me bluntly, "You don't get it. You might think you get it, but you really don't. At least you're not White, so I can say the word racism and you won't try to tell me it's not real. But, you don't get it. Being Black is entirely different. I am perceived differently. I can't be angry, I can't be emotional, I can't even dress down. If I do, people will automatically make all kinds of assumptions about me. My whole life is full of it. It makes it hard to breathe."

Clinical Vignette Analysis

It is sometimes easier to think of racism as a single monolithic experience. However, we know that the experience of racism is quite different for different people. For many, especially within the healthcare system, experiences of racism are often dismissed or ignored. People with no experience of racism may wonder if patients are "imagining things" or "playing the race card." Though I experience racism in some forms, as part of a "model minority" I do not experience it in the same way as Black and Indigenous people do.

I must also grapple with my role as a settler in Canada, a role through which I benefit from and feel like I continue to enact the dispossession and oppression of Indigenous peoples in Canada. In fact, the pervasiveness of racism is often quite difficult to imagine. It often seems easier to believe that the patient in front of us is exaggerating or being dramatic than to accept the full weight and burden of racism in the world around us, and our own role in it. This encounter and others like it continue to prompt reflection on my own ideas about racism, with the recognition that I must be open to hearing about my patients' experiences in order to better understand what I am being told.

Pause and Reflect

- How often do I think about the ways in which racism may impact my patients?
- What does it mean to create a safe space to talk about racism? What is a safe space and how does it look? How do I convey the safe space to racialized patients, coworkers and learners?
- Where I have no kinship with the experience, how can I see with open eyes, hear with listening ears, and reflect with open mind? How will I know when to shut up, when to speak out and when to affirm?
- How do I cultivate the awareness and humility needed to recognize when I am the oppressor, when my clinical practice disseminates microaggressions and when my clinical practice emulates societal bias?
- Are there concrete things I can do in my practice to make my patients feel like their experience is valid and heard?

The Opportunity to Turn the Tide on Racism

The Role of Educational Institutions in Turning the Tide

As dire as the issues of racism in medicine may appear, current trends give us reason to be hopeful. Over the last several years, medical institutions have begun to explicitly acknowledge their racist histories and activate to redress previous injustices. Medical programs have begun to address the exclusions of particular racial groups from their programs. They have acknowledged the provenance of data and innovations obtained through racial experimentation and non-consent, the most notable being the Johns Hopkins Medicine posthumous acknowledgment of Henrietta Lacks. Lacks was an African-American woman whose cancer cells constitute the source of the immortal HeLa cell line, one of the most important cell lines in medical research. In 2020, Johns Hopkins announced plans to construct a research building in Lacks' honour (Johns Hopkins Medicine, 2023).

The inclusion and increase in the proportion of Black and Indigenous doctors is incredibly valuable. Black infant mortality rates plummet when those infants are cared for by Black physicians (Greenwood et al., 2020). Racialized physicians are more likely to practice in underserved and marginalized areas, thereby improving patients' access to care (Marrast et al., 2014). The interpersonal communication between patient and provider improves with racial concordance (Shen et al., 2018). It appears that medicine is poised to acknowledge the issues of racism inherent in its institutions, and this is an essential first step in developing a truly inclusive culture.

The Role of Medical Journals in Turning the Tide

Most medical journals have published special issues or ad hoc special interest sections to capture seminal current events including racially charged events. Unfortunately, this has not coalesced into standing publications on EDI topics. Yet, journals present the key source of rapid and broad information dissemination in the medical field. Journal articles are read for content on the face of things, however, the metadata surrounding journals and their articles is equally important as it captures who is publishing and who the gatekeepers are that decide who should report (see Chapter 1), who is being studied and how they are reported or described. Thus, even the language of reporting and the association between race and reported findings shapes the way clinicians view racialized patients.

The journal presents a forum through which we can use language to shape the academic and clinical climate through intentional use of microaffirmations - *small acts of language that foster inclusion, offer encouragement and build relationships* (Harrison and Tanner, 2018).

Journals provide a venue for closer scrutiny of reporting language, clarification of why race was studied and what race was a proxy for in the study (i.e., social and structural conditions versus true genetic links). For example, when studies reporting on the causes of treatment non-adherence cite racial background or other minority status, readers take away messages about the chief findings, such as treatment accessibility or side effect, and concurrently absorb a correlation between minority patients and non-adherence or a lack of cooperation (Capers et al., 2017; Williams, 2021).

Studies concluding racially disproportionate risks should be probed for structural factors so that the true nature of the relationship is reported. For example, Lukachko and colleagues (2014) note that structural factors such as employment, education and judicial treatment increase Black persons' risk of myocardial infarction. To evaluate this more superficially (e.g., limit the structural analysis to age, race, education level) or report the findings more superficially (e.g., "Black persons have a higher risk of myocardial infarctions"), would preclude an appreciation of the underlying structural factors that shape the observed association.

Being more intentional in how and why race is captured is of the essence if we are to avoid further conflating race, structural factors, behaviour and morbidity. Where structural factors are the chief factor in morbidity and risk behaviour, this should be clearly stated and the fact of race should be acknowledged for what it is: a source of systemic oppression, which in turn exposes subjects to the structural conditions that result in the observed behaviour or outcome being reported. Naming racism for its role in the observed outcomes is essential in the continued recognition of the role of microaggressions on health.

The opportunity to integrate EDI topics into standing journal issues would provide a starting ground for continued discussion and research on strategies. By including more studies that examine the role of structural factors in perpetuating the racial gap in morbidity and mortality, it becomes more incumbent on the scientific community to explore mitigation factors.

Journals can increase the diversity of thought and the diversity of publications by increasing the diversity of their editorial boards. Similarly, decolonizing medical journals requires closer examination of publication bias in terms of the relative success of manuscripts by authors from under-resourced nations, the relative inclusion of manuscripts about marginalized populations and the publication of successful interventions in targeting racism (Ogedegbe, 2020; Williams, 2021).

Medical journals have a shared responsibility in unlearning racial ideology and contributing to an equity-responsive academic and clinical climate. They provide a wide reaching and rapid response platform for knowledge dissemination and dialogue. As such, journals present an ideal venue for ongoing de-adoption of biased research and at the same time providing a forum for constructive dialogue about EDI issues (Ogedegbe, 2020).

❖

To be a racialized person in Medicine, an institution with a long and enduring history of racism, is a profoundly disconcerting experience because one is simultaneously a victim of racism and an agent of this institution.
—Crystal Pinto, 2023

❖

Inclusion Strategies

The spectrum of values, beliefs and experiences that are thought to be vital to the development of a "well-rounded" medical school applicant frequently exclude applicants from the non-dominant culture. Ideas around professionalism, frequently encode Whiteness as the norm. Applicants with adverse life events, shaped by race or other forms of marginalization, are held to the same standards as non-marginalized applicants. Strategies for inclusion would abandon beliefs about "colour blindness" and view the experiences of racialized minorities as being valuable and essential components of the healthcare system, which are currently in short supply. It would involve changing the current definitions of strengths and weaknesses.

The culture of medical education would also need to change to allow for more critical questions about the ways in which current medical institutions maintain the status quo, which continues to privilege Whiteness. To be a racialized person, within a perceived racist institution is a profoundly disconcerting experience, because one is simultaneously a victim of racism and an agent of a racist institution. The risks of this reality are manifold, from silent acceptance of racism in the curriculum to covered ears or a held tongue on observing racist interactions in the clinical setting. Inevitably, the wages of this dual existence becomes one that includes some degree of internalized racism where racialized learners absorb the dominant societal ideology about their ethnoracial biological and/or cultural inferiority (Williams and Mohammed, 2009). The sequelae of this continued experience of discrimination lies in the danger of career dissatisfaction, career non-progression, disengagement and physician turnover (Brown et al., 2021; Johnson, 2017; Nunez-Smith et al., 2009; Palepu et al., 2000; Rodriguez et al., 2014; Rodriguez et al., 2015; Xierali et al., 2021).

Truly inclusive systems create support systems for the people who experience this cognitive dissonance. These support systems would validate the complex emotions that come from this experience. They would allow these complexities to be named without fear of judgement or repercussions. At the current time, these support systems are in short supply and, where they exist, are frequently informal systems that were created by racialized practitioners as a form of survival. Systems cannot become inclusive unless they are willing to allow themselves to be radically reshaped.

Key Takeaways

- Racism is a system of oppression that ascribes superiority and privilege to a dominant majority.
- Race is a social construction that continues to be conflated with biology.
- The persistent history of racism in medicine continues to inequitably distribute risks, placing racialized and other minoritized patients at risk.

- Medical misinformation is rife, including the preponderance of under-representative learning materials, dissemination of information with racialized connotations, erasure or hypervisibility of minorities in the literature, and race correction.
- Physician diversity can lend richness in the care of patients from diverse backgrounds and marginalized communities; however, medicine must first view the experiences of racialized minorities as being valuable and essential components of the healthcare system.
- As dire as the issues of racism in medicine may appear, current trends give us pause for cautious celebration in regard to:
  o explicit acknowledgement of racist histories
  o activation to redress previous injustices
  o restitution for the exclusion of specific racial minorities from medical schools
  o acknowledgement of the provenance of data and innovations obtained through racial experimentation and non-consent
- Health systems have the opportunity to become inclusive and equitable environments by embracing radical reshaping, from the cultural to the structural level, beginning with valuing their diverse healthcare workforce and patients alike.
- Physicians have the opportunity to be active contributors on the journey, through brave conversations, re-evaluation of the medical culture they enable as well as participation in small to big 'p' problem solving within their institutions.

Conclusion

Medicine has a long history of propagating the notion of biological difference between races, from Galen and Avicenna onwards (Byrd and Clayton, 2001). Race is often discussed as a fundamental determinant of human traits and capacities based on an inaccurate conflation of race and biology. These perspectives continue to inequitably distribute risks, placing racialized and other minoritized patients at risk.

Racialized physicians face parallel risks to racialized patients by way of arrested professional development and psychological distress associated with paradoxically becoming agents of racism because of the racist curriculum they encounter and, in turn, disseminate in the form of clinical care. For racialized medical learners, the dual tension or tug of war of demonstrating academic fitness whilst contending with persisting inaccuracies and stereotypes in the curriculum creates vulnerability. The effects of this adverse psychological space cannot be underscored as the effects come to be embodied in various ways, including internalized racism, increased burnout risk and exits from the profession, particularly from academic medicine (Dyrbye, 2021; Esparza et al.; 2022; Gaston-Hawkins, 2020; Liebschutz et al., 2006; Rodriguez, 2015; Rowe et al., 2022; Shanafelt et al., 2016; West et al., 2016; West et al., 2018; Xierali et al., 2021).

The future of the profession depends on a healthy healthcare workforce. Thus, physicians and institutions must jointly shepherd the profession towards a salubrious space of equity, diversity, inclusion and accountability. To grow is to accept a reshaping, from the cultural to the structural level, beginning with valuing today's diverse Western healthcare workforce and patients alike, if we are to approach a semblance of structural integrity.

On a Parting Note...

I can't breathe

Why can't you?

The air, it's so thin, how can I?

Your oxygen mask is dangling right there above your head, just grasp it!

I can't. I can't reach it. It's too high.......and it keeps getting batted away by hands like yours. Then there is that Gordian knot about my ankle?

Of course you can reach the mask! Here, I'll grab you a footstool.

But what if I fall?

No, you won't. If you fall, I fall, we all fall. We all hold each other's footstools steady, and I see you deftly and capably unloosening that knot in ways from which we should all learn.

As change slowly unfolds, an acknowledgment to all the Black men and racialized persons who live in the experience of a toxically placed boot.

© Mariam Abdurrahman, 2023

References

Abduelmula A., Akuffo-Addo E., Joseph M. (2022). The progression of skin color diversity and representation in dermatology textbooks. *J Cutan Med Surg*, 26(5), pp. 523-525.

Allan, B. and Smylie, J. (2015). First Peoples, Second Class Treatment [online]. Available from: https://www.wellesleyinstitute.com/wp-content/uploads/2015/02/Summary-First-Peoples-Second-Class-Treatment-Final.pdf

Amster E. J. (2022). The past, present and future of race and colonialism in medicine. *Canadian Medical Association Journal*, 194(20), pp. E708–E710. https://doi.org/10.1503/cmaj.212103.

Amutah, C., Greenidge, K., Mante, A., Munyikwa, M., Surya, S.L., Higginbotham, E., Jones, D.S., Lavizzo-Mourey, R., Roberts, D., Tsai, J., Aysola, J. (2021). Misrepresenting race - the role of medical schools in propagating physician bias. *N Engl J Med.*, 384(9), pp.872-878. https://doi: 10.1056/NEJMms2025768. Epub 2021 Jan 6.

Anderson, M.A., Malhotra, A. and Non, A.L. (2021). Could routine race-adjustment of spirometers exacerbate racial disparities in COVID-19 recovery? *The Lancet Respiratory Medicine*, 9(2), pp. 124–125. https://doi.org/10.1016/s2213-2600(20)30571-3.

Bailey, Z.D., Feldman, J.M. and Bassett, M.T. (2020). How Structural Racism Works — Racist Policies as a Root Cause of U.S. Racial Health Inequities. *New England Journal of Medicine*, 384(8), pp.768–773. https://doi.org/10.1056/nejmms2025396.

Barrett, L.A. (2019). Tuskegee Syphilis Study of 1932–1973 and the Rise of Bioethics as Shown Through Government Documents and Actions. *DttP: Documents to the People*, 47(4), pp. 11-16. https://doi.org/10.5860/dttp.v47i4.7213.

Batal, M., Chan, H.M., Fediuk, K., Ing, A., Berti, P.R., Mercille, G., Sadik, T. and Johnson-Down, L. (2021). First Nations households living on-reserve experience food insecurity: prevalence and predictors among ninety-two First Nations communities across Canada. *Canadian Journal of Public Health*, 112(S1), pp. 52–63. https://doi.org/10.17269/s41997-021-00491-x.

Beagan, B.L. (2003). Is this worth getting into a big fuss over? Everyday racism in medical school. *Medical Education*, 37(10), pp. 852–860. https://doi.org/10.1046/j.1365-2923.2003.01622.x.

Berger, M. and Sarnyai, Z. (2014). More than skin deep: stress neurobiology and mental health consequences of racial discrimination. *Stress,* 18(1), pp. 1–10. https://doi.org/10.3109/10253890.2014.989204.

Boynton-Jarrett, R., Raj, A., Inwards-Breland, D. J. (2021). Structural integrity: recognizing, measuring, and addressing systemic racism and its health impacts. *EClinicalMedicine,* 36, 100921. https://doi.org/10.1016/j.eclinm.2021.100921.

Brown, C., Daniel, R., Addo, N., & Knight, S. (2021). The experiences of medical students, residents, fellows, and attendings in the emergency department: implicit bias to microaggressions. *AEM education and training,* 5(Suppl 1), pp. S49–S56. https://doi.org/10.1002/aet2.10670.

Burm, S., Deagle, S., Watling, C.J., Wylie, L. and Alcock, D. (2022). Navigating the burden of proof and responsibility: A narrative inquiry into Indigenous medical learners' experiences. *Medical Education.* https://doi.org/10.1111/medu.15000.

Byrd, W.M. and Clayton, L.A. (2001). Race, medicine, and health care in the United States: a historical survey. *Journal of the National Medical Association,* 93(3 Suppl), p.11S34S.

Capers, Q., 4th, Clinchot, D., McDougle, L., & Greenwald, A. G. (2017). Implicit racial bias in medical school admissions. *Academic medicine: journal of the Association of American Medical Colleges,* 92(3), pp.365–369. https://doi.org/ 10.1097/ACM.0000000000001388

Chadha, N., Kane, M., Lim, B., Rowland, B. (2020). Towards the abolition of biological race in medicine: transforming clinical education, research and practice. Berkeley, CA: Institute for Healing and Justice in Medicine [online]. Available from: https://www.instituteforhealingandjustice.org/executivesummary

Chen, C.L., Gold, G.J., Cannesson, M. and Lucero, J.M. (2021). Calling Out Aversive Racism in Academic Medicine. *New England Journal of Medicine,* 385(27), pp. 2499–2501. https://doi.org/10.1056/nejmp2112913.

Cogburn C. D. (2019). Culture, Race, and Health: Implications for Racial Inequities and Population Health. *The Milbank quarterly,* 97(3), 736–761. https://doi.org/ 10.1111/1468-0009.12411.

Collier, R. (2017). Reports of coerced sterilization of Indigenous women in Canada mirrors shameful past. *Canadian Medical Association Journal,* 189(33), pp.E1080– E1081. https://doi.org/10.1503/cmaj.1095471.

Cooper, L. A., Roter, D. L., Johnson, R. L., Ford, D. E., Steinwachs, D. M., Powe, N. R. (2003). Patient-centered communication, ratings of care, and concordance of patient and physician race. *Annals of internal medicine*, 139(11), pp. 907–915. https://doi.org/10.7326/0003-4819-139-11-200312020-00009.

de Bruijn, E.-J. and Antonides, G. (2021). Poverty and economic decision making: a review of scarcity theory. *Theory and Decision*, 92, pp. 5–37. https://doi.org/10.1007/s11238-021-09802-7.

Deyrup, A., & Graves, J. L., Jr (2022). Racial Biology and Medical Misconceptions. *The New England journal of medicine*, 386(6), pp. 501–503. https://doi.org/10.1056/NEJMp2116224.

DuBois W. E. B. (2003). The health and physique of the Negro American. 1906. *American journal of public health*, 93(2), pp. 272–276. https://doi.org/10.2105/ajph.93.2.272.

Dutheil, F., Aubert, C., Pereira, B., Dambrun, M., Moustafa, F., Mermillod, M., et al. (2019). Suicide among physicians and health-care workers: A systematic review and meta-analysis. *PLOS ONE*, 14(12), p. e0226361. https://doi.org/10.1371/journal.pone.0226361.

Dyrbye, L.N., West, C.P., Satele, D., Boone, S., Tan, L., Sloan, J. and Shanafelt, T.D. (2014). Burnout Among U.S. Medical Students, Residents, and Early Career Physicians Relative to the General U.S. Population. *Academic Medicine*, 89(3), pp. 443–451. https://doi.org/10.1097/acm.0000000000000134.

Dyrbye L.N., Satele D., West C.P. (2021). Association of characteristics of the learning environment and US medical student burnout, empathy, and career regret. *JAMA Netw Open*, 4(8), e2119110. https://doi.4:e2119110.10.1001/jamanetworkopen.2021.19110.

Ebede, T., & Papier, A. (2006). Disparities in dermatology educational resources. *Journal of the American Academy of Dermatology*, 55(4), pp.687–690.

Eggly, S., Barton, E., Winckles, A., Penner, L. A., & Albrecht, T. L. (2015). A disparity of words: racial differences in oncologist-patient communication about clinical trials. *Health expectations : an international journal of public participation in health care and health policy*, 18(5), pp.1316–1326. https://doi.org/10.1111/hex.12108.

Ellis, M.E. (2023). Owens Corning and Asbestos [online]. Available from: https://mesothelioma.net/owens-corning/#source3

Espaillat, A., Panna, D.K., Goede, D.L., Gurka, M.J., Novak, M.A., Zaidi, Z. (2019). An exploratory study on microaggressions in medical school: what are they and why should we care? *Perspect Med Educ*, 8(3), pp. 143-151. https://doi: 10.1007/s40037-019-0516-3.

Esparza, C. J., Simon, M., Bath, E., & Ko, M. (2022). Doing the Work-or Not: The Promise and Limitations of Diversity, Equity, and Inclusion in US Medical Schools and Academic Medical Centers. *Frontiers in public health*, 10, 900283. https://doi.org/10.3389/fpubh.2022.900283.

Fadus, M.C., Valadez, E.A., Bryant, B.E., Garcia, A.M., Neelon, B., Tomko, R.L. and Squeglia, L.M. (2021). Racial Disparities in Elementary School Disciplinary Actions: Findings from the ABCD Study. *Journal of the American Academy of Child & Adolescent Psychiatry*, 60(8), pp. 998–1009. https://doi.org/10.1016/j.jaac.2020.11.017.

Fenton, A., Elliott, E., Shahbandi, A., Ezenwa, E., Morris, C., McLawhorn, J., Jackson, J. G., Allen, P., & Murina, A. (2020). Medical students' ability to diagnose common dermatologic conditions in skin of color. *Journal of the American Academy of Dermatology*, 83(3), pp.957–958. https://doi.org/10.1016/j.jaad.2019.12.078.

Food and Drug Administration. (2020). 2015-2019 Drug Trials Snapshots Summary Report [online]. Available from: https://www.fda.gov/media/143592/download

Freimuth, V. S., Quinn, S. C., Thomas, S. B., Cole, G., Zook, E., & Duncan, T. (2001). African Americans' views on research and the Tuskegee Syphilis Study. *Social science & medicine (1982)*, 52(5), pp.797–808. https://doi.org/10.1016/s0277-9536(00)00178-7.

Gaston-Hawkins, L. A., Solorio, F. A., Chao, G. F., & Green, C. R. (2020). The silent epidemic: causes and consequences of medical learner burnout. *Current psychiatry reports*, 22(12), p.86. https://doi.org/10.1007/s11920-020-01211-x.

Gee, G. C., & Ford, C. L. (2011). Structural racism and health inequities: Old issues, new directions. *Du Bois review: social science research on race*, 8(1), pp. 115–132. https://doi.org/10.1017/S1742058X11000130.

Gordon, H. S., Street, R. L., Jr, Sharf, B. F., Souchek, J. (2006). Racial differences in doctors' information-giving and patients' participation. *Cancer*, 107(6), pp.1313–1320. https://doi.org/10.1002/cncr.22122.

Goyal, M.K., Kuppermann, N., Cleary, S.D., Teach, S.J. and Chamberlain, J.M. (2015). Racial Disparities in Pain Management of Children with Appendicitis in Emergency Departments. JAMA Pediatrics, 169(11), p.996. https://doi.org/10.1001/jamapediatrics.2015.1915.

Greenwood, B.N., Hardeman, R.R., Huang, L. and Sojourner, A. (2020). Physician–patient racial concordance and disparities in birthing mortality for newborns. *Proceedings of the National Academy of Sciences*, 117(35), pp. 21194-21200. https://doi.org/10.1073/pnas.1913405117.

Grubbs V. (2020). Precision in GFR reporting: let's stop playing the race card. *Clin J Am Soc Nephrol,* 15(8), pp.1201-1202. https://doi: 10.2215/CJN.00690120.

Guedj, R., Marini, M., Kossowsky, J., Berde, C.B., Kimia, A.A. and Fleegler, E.W. (2021). Racial and ethnic disparities in pain management of children with limb fractures or suspected appendicitis: A retrospective cross-sectional study. *Frontiers in Pediatrics,* 9. https://doi.org/10.3389/fped.2021.652854.

Guillory, J.D. (1968). The Pro-Slavery Arguments of Dr. Samuel A. Cartwright. *Louisiana History: The Journal of the Louisiana Historical Association* [online], 9(3), pp. 209–227. Available from: http://www.jstor.org/stable/4231017

Hall, J. M., Fields, B. (2015). "It's Killing Us!" Narratives of Black adults about microaggression experiences and related health stress. *Global qualitative nursing research,* 2, 2333393615591569. https://doi.org/10.1177/2333393615591569.

Hankinson, J.L., Odencrantz, J.R., Fedan, K.B. Spirometric reference values from a sample of the general U.S. population. (1999). *Am J Respir Crit Care Med,* 159, pp.179–187. https://doi:10.1164/ajrccm.159.1.9712108.

Hariharan, B., Quarshie, L.S., Amdahl, C., Winterburn, S. and Offiah, G. (2021). Experiencing racism within medical school curriculum: 2020 ICCH student symposium. *Patient Education and Counseling,* 105 (7), pp. 2599-2602. https://doi.org/10.1016/j.pec.2021.12.018.

Harrison, C., and Tanner, K. D. (2018). Language Matters: Considering Microaggressions in Science. *CBE life sciences education,* 17(1), fe4. https://doi.org/10.1187/cbe.18-01-0011.

Hassouneh, D., Lutz, K.F., Beckett, A.K., Junkins, E.P. and Horton, L.L. (2014). The experiences of underrepresented minority faculty in schools of medicine. *Medical Education Online,* 19(1), p .24768. https://doi.org/10.3402/meo.v19.24768.

Henry, N. (2021). Racial Segregation of Black Students in Canadian Schools. *The Canadian Encyclopedia* [online]. Available from: https://www.thecanadian encyclopedia.ca/en/article/racial-segregation-of-black-students-in-canadian-schools

Johns Hopkins Medicine. (2023). The Legacy of Henrietta Lacks [online]. Available from: https://www.hopkinsmedicine.org/henriettalacks/

Johnson, R. L., Roter, D., Powe, N. R., Cooper, L. A. (2004). Patient race/ethnicity and quality of patient-physician communication during medical visits. *American journal of public health,* 94(12), pp. 2084–2090. https://doi.org/ 10.2105/ajph.94.12.2084.

Johnson, T. (2017). The minority tax: an unseen plight of diversity in medical education. *IM Diversity* [online]. Available from: https://imdiversity.com/ diversity-news/the-minority-tax-an-unseen-plight-of-diversity-in-medical-education/

Jones, C.P. (2002). Confronting institutionalized racism. *Phylon*, 50 (1), pp. 7-22. https://doi:10.2307/4149999.

Kaiser, J. (2021). NIH director apologizes for 'structural racism,' pledges actions. https://doi: 10.1126/science.abh3223.

Kalifa, A., Okuori, A., Kamdem, O., Abatan, D., Yahya, S. and Brown, A. (2022). 'This shouldn't be our job to help you do this': exploring the responses of medical schools across Canada to address anti-Black racism in 2020. *CMAJ*, 194(41), pp.E1395–E1403. https://doi.org/10.1503/cmaj.211746.

Kamath, P., Sundaram, N., Morillo-Hernandez, C., Barry, F., & James, A. J. (2021). Visual racism in internet searches and dermatology textbooks. *Journal of the American Academy of Dermatology*, 85(5), 1348–1349.

Kennedy-Moulton, K., Miller, S., Persson, P., Rossin-Slater, M., Wherry, L. and Aldana, G. (2022). Maternal and infant health inequality: New evidence from linked administrative data. *NBER Working Paper Series*. https://doi.org/ 10.3386/w30693.

Khan, R., Apramian, T., Kang, J.H., Gustafson, J. and Sibbald, S. (2020). Demographic and socioeconomic characteristics of Canadian medical students: a cross-sectional study. *BMC Medical Education*, 20(1), p. 151. https://doi.org/ 10.1186/s12909-020-02056-x.

Leonard, S.A., Main, E.K., Scott, K.A., Profit, J. and Carmichael, S.L. (2019). Racial and ethnic disparities in severe maternal morbidity prevalence and trends. *Annals of Epidemiology*, 33, pp. 30–36. https://doi.org/10.1016/j.annepidem .2019.02.007.

Levey AS, Titan SM, Powe NR, Coresh J, Inker LA. (2020). Kidney disease, race, and GFR estimation. *Clin J Am Soc Nephrol*, 15(8), pp. 1203-1212. doi: 10.2215/CJN.12791019. Epub 2020 May 11.

Liebschutz, J.M., Darko, G.O., Finley, E.P., Cawse, J.M., Bharel, M. and Orlander, J.D. (2006). In the minority: black physicians in residency and their experiences. *Journal of the National Medical Association*, 98(9), pp. 1441–8.

Lucey, C.R. and Saguil, A. (2020). The Consequences of Structural Racism on MCAT Scores and Medical School Admissions. *Academic Medicine*, 95(3), pp.351–356. https://doi.org/10.1097/acm.0000000000002939.

Lujan, H.L. and DiCarlo, S.E. (2018). Science reflects history as society influences science: brief history of 'race,' 'race correction,' and the spirometer. *Advances in Physiology Education*, 42(2), pp. 163–165. https://doi.org/10.1152/advan. 00196.2017.

Lukachko, A., Hatzenbuehler, M. L., & Keyes, K. M. (2014). Structural racism and myocardial infarction in the United States. *Social science & medicine (1982)*, 103, pp. 42–50. https://doi.org/10.1016/j.socscimed.2013.07.021.

MacDorman, M.F., Thoma, M., Declcerq, E. and Howell, E.A. (2021). Racial and Ethnic Disparities in Maternal Mortality in the United States Using Enhanced Vital Records, 2016–2017. *American Journal of Public Health*, 111(9), pp. e1–e9. https://doi.org/10.2105/ajph.2021.306375.

Marrast, L. M., Zallman, L., Woolhandler, S., Bor, D. H., & McCormick, D. (2014). Minority physicians' role in the care of underserved patients: diversifying the physician workforce may be key in addressing health disparities. *JAMA internal medicine*, 174(2), 289–291. https://doi.org/10.1001/jamainternmed.2013.12756.

Mateo, C.M. and Williams, D.R. (2021). Racism: a fundamental driver of racial disparities in health-care quality. *Nature Reviews Disease Primers*, 7(1), p.2 0. https://doi.org/10.1038/s41572-021-00258-1.

McCord, C., Freeman, H.P. (1990). Excess mortality in Harlem. *N Engl J Med*, 322(3), pp. 173-177.

Merriam Webster (2022). Definition of racism [online] *Merriam-webster.com*. Available from: https://www.merriam-webster.com/dictionary/racism

Narla, S., Heath, C. R., Alexis, A., Silverberg, J. I. (2022). Racial disparities in dermatology. *Archives of dermatological research*, 1–9. https://doi.org/10.1007/ s00403-022-02507-z.

National Institute of Health (NIH). (2021). Ending structural racism [online]. Available from: https://www.nih.gov/ending-structural-racism

Nieblas-Bedolla, E., Christophers, B., Nkinsi, N. T., Schumann, P. D., Stein, E. (2020). Changing How Race Is Portrayed in Medical Education: Recommendations from Medical Students. *Academic medicine : journal of the Association of American Medical Colleges*, 95(12), 1802–1806. https://doi.org/10.1097/ACM.000000 0000003496.

Nunez-Smith, M., Pilgrim, N., Wynia, M., Desai, M. M., Bright, C., Krumholz, H. M., & Bradley, E. H. (2009). Health care workplace discrimination and physician turnover. *Journal of the National Medical Association*, 101(12), 1274–1282. https://doi.org/10.1016/s0027-9684(15)31139-1.

Odoms-Young, A. and Bruce, M.A. (2018). Examining the Impact of Structural Racism on Food Insecurity. *Family & Community Health*, 41(2), pp. S3–S6. https://doi.org/10.1097/fch.0000000000000183.

Ogedegbe, G. (2020). Responsibility of medical journals in addressing racism in health care. *JAMA Netw Open*, 3(8), e2016531. doi: 10.1001/jamanetwork open.2020.16531.

OHCHR. (2022). Indigenous peoples face growing challenges to access safe water [online]. Available from: https://www.ohchr.org/en/stories/2022/10/indigenous-peoples-face-growing-challenges-access-safe-water

Osseo-Asare A., Balasuriya L., Huot S.J., et al. (2018). Minority resident physicians' views on the role of race/ethnicity in their training experiences in the workplace. *Jama Netw Open*, 1:e182723. https://doi: 10.1001/jamanetworkopen.2018.2723.

Paine, L., de la Rocha, P., Eyssallenne, A. P., Andrews, C. A., Loo, L., Jones, C. P., Collins, A. M., Morse, M. (2021). Declaring racism a public health crisis in the United States: cure, poison, or both? *Frontiers in public health*, 9, 676784. https://doi.org/10.3389/fpubh.2021.676784

Palepu, A., Carr, P. L., Friedman, R. H., Ash, A. S., & Moskowitz, M. A. (2000). Specialty choices, compensation, and career satisfaction of underrepresented minority faculty in academic medicine. *Academic medicine: journal of the Association of American Medical Colleges*, 75(2), 157–160. https://doi.org/10.1097/00001888-200002000-00014

Parekh, R.S., Perl, J., Auguste, B., Sood, M.M. (2022). Elimination of race in estimates of kidney function to provide unbiased clinical management in Canada. *Canadian medical association journal*, 94(11), pp.E421-E423. https://doi: 10.1503/cmaj.210838.

Pegoraro, L. (2014). Second-rate victims: the forced sterilization of Indigenous peoples in the USA and Canada. *Settler Colonial Studies*, 5(2), pp. 161–173. https://doi.org/10.1080/2201473x.2014.955947.

Pierce, C. (1970). Offensive mechanisms. In: Barbour, F.B. eds. *The Black Seventies*. Boston, MA: Porter Sargent, pp. 265-82.

Pierce, C. (1995). Stress analogs of racism and sexism: Terrorism, torture, and disaster. In C. Willie, P. Rieker, B. Kramer, & B. Brown (Eds.), *Mental health, racism, and sexism* (pp. 277–293). Pittsburgh, PA: University of Pittsburgh Press.

Ripp, K., Braun, L. (2017). Race/ethnicity in medical education: an analysis of a question bank for Step 1 of the United States Medical Licensing Examination. *Teach Learn Med.*, 29(2), pp.115-122. doi: 10.1080/10401334.2016.1268056. Epub 2017 Jan 4.

Roach, P., Ruzycki, S.M., Hernandez, S., Carbert, A., Holroyd-Leduc, J., Ahmed, S. and Barnabe, C. (2023). Prevalence and characteristics of anti-Indigenous bias among Albertan physicians: a cross-sectional survey and framework analysis. *BMJ Open*, 13(2), p. e063178. https://doi.org/10.1136/bmjopen-2022-063178.

Roberts, J.H., Sanders, T. and Wass, V. (2008). Students' perceptions of race, ethnicity and culture at two UK medical schools: a qualitative study. *Medical Education*, 42(1), pp. 45-52.   https://doi.org/10.1111/j.1365-2923.2007.02902.x.

Rodriguez, J. E., Campbell, K. M., Fogarty, J. P., & Williams, R. L. (2014). Underrepresented minority faculty in academic medicine: a systematic review of URM faculty development. *Family medicine*, 46(2), pp.100–104.

Rodríguez, J.E., Campbell, K.M. & Pololi, L.H. (2015). Addressing disparities in academic medicine: what of the minority tax?. *BMC Med Educ*, 15(6). https://doi.org/10.1186/s12909-015-0290-9.

Rowe, S.G., Stewart, M.T., Van Horne, S., Pierre, C., Wang, H., Manukyan, M., Bair-Merritt, M., Lee-Parritz, A, Rowe, M.P., Shanafelt, T, Trockel, M. (2022). Mistreatment experiences, protective workplace systems, and occupational distress in physicians. *JAMA Netw Open*, 5(5):e2210768. https://doi: 10.1001/jamanetworkopen.2022.10768.

Schernhammer, E.S. and Colditz, G.A. (2004). Suicide rates among physicians: A quantitative and gender assessment (meta-analysis). *American Journal of Psychiatry*, 161(12), pp. 2295–2302. https://doi.org/10.1176/appi.ajp.161.12.2295.

Schut, R.A. (2021). Racial disparities in provider-patient communication of incidental medical findings. *Social Science & Medicine*, 277, p. 113901. https://doi.org/10.1016/j.socscimed.2021.113901.

Shamoo, A.E. (2022). Unethical medical treatment and research in U.S. Territories. *Accountability in Research*, 24 Jan 2022, pp. 1-14. https://doi.org/ 10.1080/08989621.2022.2030720.

Shanafelt, T. D., Mungo, M., Schmitgen, J., Storz, K. A., Reeves, D., Hayes, et al. (2016). Longitudinal study evaluating the association between physician burnout and changes in professional work effort. *Mayo Clinic proceedings*, 91(4), pp.422–431. https://doi.org/10.1016/j.mayocp.2016.02.001.

Shen, M.J., Peterson, E.B., Costas-Muñiz, R., Hernandez, M.H., Jewell, S.T., Matsoukas, K. and Bylund, C.L. (2018). The effects of race and racial concordance on patient-physician communication: A systematic review of the literature. *Journal of racial and ethnic health disparities*, 5(1), pp.117–140. https://doi.org/10.1007/s40615-017-0350-4.

Singer, M. (1994). AIDS and the health crisis of the U.S. urban poor: the perspective of critical medical anthropology. *Soc Sci Med,* 39, pp. 931-48.

Singh, S. and Steeves, V. (2020). The contested meanings of race and ethnicity in medical research: A case study of the DynaMed Point of Care tool. *Social Science & Medicine*, 265, p. 113112. https://doi.org/10.1016/j.socscimed.2020.113112.

Sue, D. W. (2005). Racism and the conspiracy of silence. *Counseling Psychologist,* 33, *pp.* 100–114.

Sue, D.W., Capodilupo, C., Torino, G., Bucceri, J., Holder, A.B., Nadal, K.L., et al. (2007). Racial microaggressions in everyday life: implications for clinical practice. *American psychologist,* 62, pp.271–286.

Texeira, E. (1999). Racial basis for asbestos lawsuits?; Owens Corning seeks more stringent standards for blacks. *The Baltimore Sun* [online] 25 March 1999. Available from: https://www.baltimoresun.com/news/bs-xpm-1999-03-25-9903250041-story.html

Thomas J.M. (2020). *Diversity Regimes: Why Talk Is Not Enough to Fix Racial Inequality at Universities.* New Brunswick, NJ: Rutgers University Press. https://doi: 10.36019/9781978800458.

Tsai, J., Ucik, L., Baldwin, N., Hasslinger, C., George, P. (2016). Race matters? Examining and rethinking race portrayal in preclinical medical education. *Acad Med,* 91, pp.916-920.

United States Department of Energy (USDE). (2019). Human Genome Project Information [online]. https://web.ornl.gov/sci/techresources/Human_Genome/index.shtml

Vyas, D.A., Eisenstein, L.G., Jones D.S. (2020). Hidden in plain sight - reconsidering the use of race correction in clinical algorithms. *N Engl J Med.,* 383(9), pp.874-882. https://doi: 10.1056/NEJMms2004740.

Wheeler, M., de Bourmont, S., Paul-Emile, K., Pfeffinger, A., McMullen, A., Critchfield, J. M., & Fernandez, A. (2019). Physician and trainee experiences with patient bias. *JAMA internal medicine*, 179(12), pp.1678–1685. https://doi.org/10.1001/jamainternmed.2019.4122.

West, C. P., Dyrbye, L. N., Erwin, P. J., & Shanafelt, T. D. (2016). Interventions to prevent and reduce physician burnout: a systematic review and meta-analysis. *Lancet (London, England)*, 388(10057), pp.2272–2281. https://doi.org/10.1016/S0140-6736(16)31279-X.

West, C. P., Dyrbye, L. N., & Shanafelt, T. D. (2018). Physician burnout: contributors, consequences and solutions. *Journal of internal medicine*, 283(6), pp.516–529. https://doi.org/10.1111/joim.12752.

Wikipedia. (2023a). *List of unarmed African Americans killed by law enforcement officers in the United States* [online]. Available from: https://en.wikipedia.org/wiki/List_of_unarmed_African_Americans_killed_by_law_enforcement_officers_in_the_United_States

Wikipedia. (2023b). *Death of Joyce Echaquan* [online]. Available from: https://en.wikipedia.org/wiki/Death_of_Joyce_Echaquan

Williams, D. R., & Mohammed, S. A. (2009). Discrimination and racial disparities in health: evidence and needed research. *Journal of behavioral medicine*, 32(1), 20–47. https://doi.org/10.1007/s10865-008-9185-0.

Williams, M. (2021). Racial microaggressions: critical questions, state of the science, and new directions. *Perspectives on psychological science,* 16(5), pp.880-885.

Willoughby, C.D.E. (2018). Running Away from Drapetomania: Samuel A. Cartwright, Medicine, and Race in the Antebellum South. *Journal of Southern History,* 84(3), pp. 579–614. https://doi.org/10.1353/soh.2018.0164.

Wong G., Derthick A.O., David E.J., Saw A., Okazaki S. (2014). The *what*, the *why*, and the *how*: a review of racial microaggressions research in psychology. *Race Soc Probl.,* 6(2), pp.181-200. doi: 10.1007/s12552-013-9107-9. Epub 2013 Oct 24.

Wright, R.J. (2011). Epidemiology of stress and asthma: from constricting communities and fragile families to epigenetics. *Immunology and Allergy Clinics of North America,* 31, pp.19-39.

Xierali, I. M., Nivet, M. A., Syed, Z. A., Shakil, A., & Schneider, F. D. (2021). Recent trends in faculty promotion in U.S. medical schools: implications for recruitment, retention, and diversity and inclusion. *Academic medicine : journal of the Association of American Medical Colleges,* 96(10), pp.1441–1448. https://doi.org/10.1097/ACM.0000000000004188.

Yearby, R. (2018). Racial Disparities in Health Status and Access to Healthcare: The Continuation of Inequality in the United States Due to Structural Racism. *American Journal of Economics and Sociology,* 77(3-4), pp. 1113–1152. https://doi.org/10.1111/ajes.12230.

Yudell, M., Roberts, D., DeSalle, R. and Tishkoff, S. (2016). Taking race out of human genetics. *Science,* 351(6273), pp. 564–565. https://doi.org/10.1126/science.aac4951.

Young, S. L., Bethancourt, H. J., Frongillo, E. A., Viviani, S., & Cafiero, C. (2023). Concurrence of water and food insecurities, 25 low- and middle-income countries. *Bulletin of the World Health Organization,* 101(2), pp.90–101. https://doi.org/10.2471/BLT.22.288771.

Chapter 11
Smokescreens: Sanitized Racism through Race Correction, Tolerance and Privilege

Mariam Abdurrahman, MD, Sabrina Agnihotri, MD, PhD, Crystal Pinto, MD, Chase McMurren, MD, Marissa Joseph, MD

❖

"Tolerance and apathy are the last virtues of a dying society"
—Aristotle, nd

❖

Abstract: This chapter examines insidious brands of racism, including tolerance and race correction. Race correction is explored as a clinically sanitized form of racism with strong historical origins in colonialism. Tolerance is examined for its intricate role in constructing and amplifying "otherness" such that it propagates a socially sanitized form of discrimination and various configurations of racism despite its initial evolution as an antidote to intolerance. Furthermore, the impact of this dynamic is examined, with a focus on the burnout link, minority taxation and the tolerance-privilege interaction. Privilege is examined in so far as it perpetuates the status quo. Tolerance is posited as a philosophically flawed virtue, existing only when difference or diversity is present such that a dominant majority engages in the toleration of minority groups through a mixed mechanism of devaluation and non-interference. Through reflective exercises, the merit-privilege link is examined.

Keywords: *devaluation, diversity, minority tax, non-interference, otherness, power imbalance, privilege, racism, tolerance, toleration*

Introduction

In multicultural and diverse societies, intolerance – a lack of respect for practices or beliefs other than one's own – has been recognized as one of the most common forms of human rights violations and abuse (Council of Europe, 2023). Intolerance breeds discrimination because individual and group differences are perceived as less favourable when compared to those holding a majority position. Although intolerance and discrimination can arise from perceived dissimilarities across any number of attributes, such as age, gender, religion, and disability, the focus of this section will be on the differences associated with belonging to a racialized minority group when compared to the dominant majority.

If left unopposed, racial intolerance can deprive one of the freedom of expression needed to reach their full potential, on a personal level and as a contributing member of society. By reason then, would not the practice of tolerance, as an equally opposing force against intolerance, prove to be a worthy solution to such indignity? Indeed, in an effort to reduce intergroup conflict within ethno-racially and otherwise diverse societies, the concept of tolerance, or act of toleration, has been publicly decreed by international organizations, such as the United Nations Culture of Peace Declarations (UNESCO, 1995; Witenberg, 2000).

These proclamations by the United Nations and like bodies encapsulate tolerance as an active attitude and responsibility of the individual to accept that human beings are "naturally diverse in their appearance, situations, speech, behaviour and values [and] have the right to live in peace and to be as they are," without the imposition of others' views (UNESCO, 1995, p 9). From this perspective, the positive attributes of practiced tolerance as a barrier to discrimination are clear, including protection from violence, provisions for the freedom to express one's cultural identity and, as a baseline, ensure that diverse groups can collaborate in the face of irreconcilable differences (Vogt, 1997; Verkuyten et al., 2019).

There is growing recognition regarding the intricate role tolerance plays in constructing and amplifying "otherness" that allows many insidious forms of racism to propagate. In medicine, the "otherness" may be incorporated in insidious forms such as race correction where perceived differences receive a race adjustment factor in spite of the recognition that race and biology are distinct entities, as discussed extensively in Chapter 10. In effect, medicine is still operating behind various smokescreens (see Figure 11.1), which allow the sanitization of racism, whether through race correction (also known as race norming), tolerance or inability to recognize the privilege-tolerance dynamic, which are further discussed in this chapter. Figure 11.1 illustrates the complex interaction of the constitutive elements of clinically sanitized racism, which exist on a background of broader structural and systemic discrimination. Eradicating one element from Figure 11.1 is not adequate or effective as the other constituent elements continue to interact and fill the void. This speaks to the need for concerted action at all levels, lest the persistence of structural elements that facilitate racism, described by some as *racism without the racists* (Cordeiro-Rodrigues and Ewuoso, 2022; Gee and Ford, 2011; Feagin and Bennefield, 2014). An idealized system of social structures may not have consciously racist people operating or overseeing the infrastructure, but it can still produce racially disparate outcomes because structural elements have already been arranged in a way that systematically favours some groups over others.

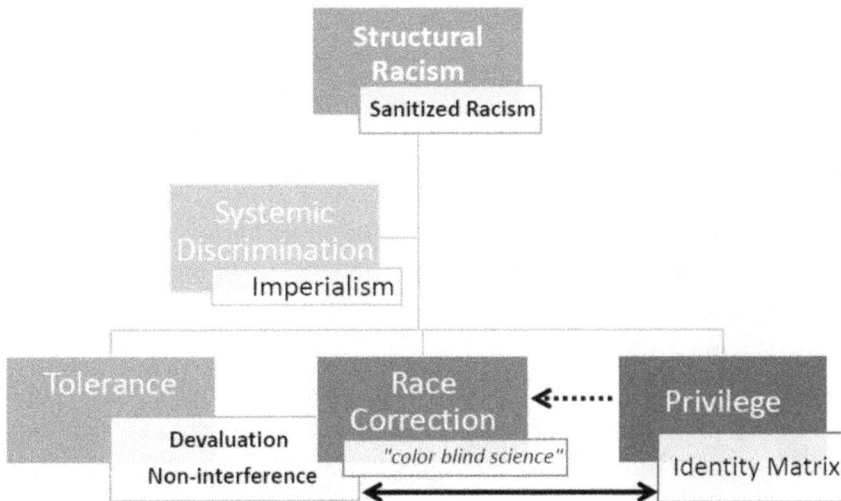

Figure 11.1. *Complex interaction of the constituent elements of clinically sanitized racism, which exist on a background of broader systemic discrimination. As evident in the diagram, eradicating any single element is not adequate or effective as the other constituent elements continue to interact and fill the void.*

The Issues

Sanitized Racism in the Form of Race Correction

❖

"the Creator's will in regards to the negro [declares] him to be a submissive knee-bender"
—Cartwright, 1854

❖

Algorithms and correction factors are key tools in the fabric of clinical practice and may in fact inform almost all aspects of diagnosis, evaluation and treatment depending on the medical subspecialty. Prior to the recent discourse on race adjustments, corrective factors were regarded as "standard" aspects of clinical care and are deeply embedded within clinical practice guidelines. Despite the recognition that race and biology are not synonymous, the origins of many race correction factors appear to stem from social constructions of racial difference, thus the authors contend that race correction embodies a clinically sanitized brand of racism. Nephrology and respirology present the two most recent areas of ongoing dialogue on the origin and impact of race correction, as further elaborated below. Consider estimates of lung function and the spirometer- how widely known is it that its origins date back to plantation era slavery? How many respirologists are aware of the sinister origins of the spirometer?

Samuel Cartwright, an American physician in the antebellum South, reviewed U.S. President Thomas Jefferson's writings on the respiratory function of slaves, including a reported "deficit" in vital capacity and Jefferson's conclusion that forced labor was a way to "vitalize the blood" of deficient Black slaves (Lujan and DiCarlo, 2018). Cartwright carried out his own study and also observed a 20% difference in spirometry results between Whites and enslaved Blacks. He concluded that this was a racial deficit of Blacks, which gave credence to Jefferson's idea that forced labor improved the pulmonary function of slaves (Cartwright, 1851). He went so far as to justify slavery based on the biological differences between races including differences in pain sensation and lung capacity (Guillory J, 1968, pp 209-227). In fact, by Jefferson and Cartwright's logic, slavery was what kept Black individuals alive. This slavery era work, which was entirely without scientific rigour, spawned the widespread practice of race-correction in pulmonary function tests (Braun, 2014; Braun, Wolfgang and Dickersin, 2013; Lujan and DiCarlo, 2018). This work continues to influence the practice of pulmonary medicine in the form of race-adjustments on most modern spirometers (Lujan and DiCarlo, 2018).

The index studies on which today's spirometers are built do not appear to recognize context, in that there is no acknowledgment that social factors such as poverty and environmental exposures likely play a greater role in pulmonary capacity despite clear evidence that the social determinants of health and context exert a far greater influence on health status than do race, culture, and ethnicity (Lujan and DiCarlo, 2018). As early as 1906, W.E.B. Du Bois had concluded that race was not a scientific category and that differences in health outcomes between races were a consequence of social inequality, yet medicine in the early 21st century continues to use the idea of race and racial differences both in research and in clinical practice (Yudell et al., 2016, pp 564-564; Vyas et al., 2020, p 874). The impact of race correction in lung function can be quite extensive in reach. The racial correction has been used to deny worker's compensation and settlement claims for occupational respiratory exposures, as exemplified by the Owens Corning lawsuits described in Chapter 10.

Like estimates of pulmonary function, renal function estimates are also afflicted by racial undertones. Lab requisitions for estimated glomerular filtration rate (eGFR) require an indication as to whether the patient is Black as the eGFR includes an upward race correction factor for Black persons (Parekh et al., 2022). The origin of the correction is based on observations that at a given GFR, relative to Whites, Blacks had slightly higher levels of creatinine, a muscle protein metabolite. The increased creatinine was attributed to controversial reports of Black persons having higher muscle mass than White persons (Grubbs, 2020; Parekh et al., 2022). To date, no studies have provided any conclusive evidence that Blacks indeed have higher muscle mass than Whites (Grubbs, 2020). Despite the lack of evidence, race and biology were once again conflated and adopted into standard clinical practice. The net effect of the upward race correction factor is an overestimation of renal function by up to 10%, which has real implications including delayed diagnosis of chronic kidney disease, late referral for renal transplantation and overall poorer outcomes for Black patients (Parekh et al., 2022). The estimated glomerular filtration rate (eGFR) remains the subject of vigorous debate and the UK National Institute for Health and Care Excellence as well as the US National Kidney Task Force have recommended the removal of race from eGFR estimates. Local uptake has been variable but encouraging for the de-adoption of eugenic influences in clinical practice.

Presumed differences in pulmonary and renal function have resulted in the severity of disease being underestimated in Black patients (Delgado et al., 2021; Grubbs, 2020). This issue is not confined to respirology and nephrology, and is evident in cardiology, cardiac surgery, obstetrics, transplantation and general internal medicine as demonstrated by Vyas and colleagues (2020). In these specialties, the most common method of race adjustments take the form of discounted or upward corrected scores for therapeutics, surgical procedures and disease severity risk scoring. Vyas and colleagues (2020) note that "many of these race-adjusted algorithms guide decisions in ways that may direct more attention or resources to White patients than to members of racial and ethnic minorities". The scoring almost invariably shows a trend that favours White patients over patients of other ethnoracial groups in terms of eligibility for procedures and therapeutics. This deeply embedded method of differentially assigning privilege and, therefore, assigning harm occurs despite the average physician's belief that they do no harm and serve patients equitably.

The practice of race correction is long-standing and so deeply buried as to be undetectable and reflexive, a problem that will likely continue as long as we laud science as being color blind, apolitical, noble and rational. While today's medical trainees and practicing physicians may agree that racial bias has no place in healthcare, they may not know the relevant historical precepts and the etiology of clinical practices that shape both the art and science of medicine today. Appreciation of these issues is necessary to better understand the fraught space occupied by racialized colleagues and the forces that introduce and maintain racial ideology in clinical practice. Furthermore, for racialized learners and practicing physicians, the dual process of pursuing medicine concurrent with absorbing the racial messaging in the training and clinical practice environment creates a cognitive dissonance that may prove to be too noxious. The contribution of racism to burnout has been discussed and is again reiterated here given the high rates of burnout in medicine. The need to build an equity-responsive climate in medicine is a priority for patients and providers alike.

Professional Vignette

by Mariam Abdurrahman

As I drove to work one quiet misty morning in 2021, I was only half-listening to the news on the radio. I noted in passing a phrase I was not familiar with: race norming. Wondering what it might be, I made a mental note to look it up and carried on with my commute unaware of the connotations of the term. The news loop replayed again later and this time I listened raptly to the coverage of the National Football League (NFL) race norming scandal. The scandal pertained to settlement claims for cognitively impaired American football players who had sustained chronic traumatic encephalopathy (CTE) in the course of their sports career. I had never heard of "race norming". I had completed neuropsychiatry and geriatrics rotations during residency training, yet there was never a mention of racial score adjustment tools when I attended memory clinics.

Professional Vignette Analysis

On exploring race norming further, I learned that in this case, it was based on a race corrected neuropsychological assessment (Belson, 2020/2021/2021; Possin et al., 2021). Coverage of the NFL race norming matter identified that the Heaton Norms were adapted into the manual utilized for assessing Black players submitting compensation claims for cognitive impairment (Belson, 2020). The Heaton Norms adjust neurocognitive scores for racial and ethnic differences, amongst other demographic variables; the Norms were developed to reduce the risk of false positives and the harms that can arise from this (Norman et al., 2011).

The race norming process rests on an assumption of lower premorbid cognition in Black players despite the fact that biologically-based racial differences in intelligence have long been debunked (Possin et al., 2021). The Human Genome Project identified a 0.1% difference in humans at the DNA level but these differences do not align with socially constructed race categories (USDE, 2019). The race norming process is in fact a crude proxy for lifelong social experiences (Possin et al., 2021). Race norming obscures what is actually being measured, which is the social determinants of cognitive health, including the impact of marginalization on cognition.

I found the basis of race norming to be distressing and repugnant as the association between repetitive concussive trauma, sub-clinical concussive trauma and early dementia has been recognized for near a century now, and in fact the key risk groups are those engaging routinely in contact sports and physical combat. Furthermore, the pathophysiology does not differ between races; the inflammatory cascade and resultant cerebral deposition of proteins, neurofibrillary tangles, and cerebral atrophy are pathognomonic of chronic traumatic encephalopathy (Mez et al., 2017). Aside from the obvious assumptions made about the cognitive capacity of Black players, what other assumptions were made in adapting race norming into occupational settlements? This was an ostensibly level playing field in which the inciting injuries were repeatedly unfolding.

A hit to the head is a hit to the head, right? Not according to the NFL's race correction methodology which was predicated on the fact that sports players have variable intellectual potential based on demographic variables. It seems strange that an instrument can become racially animated, using faulty assumptions to generate settlement rather than accounting for the actual occupational injury and the impact on the life currently being lived, the future years of functional ability lost, and the potential years of life lost. The physicians and neuropsychologists conducting the evaluations could have elected to exclude the race adjustment factor. However, while it was not mandatory for physicians to consider a player's race when evaluating a claim, the League often appealed evaluations that did not use race-based benchmarks (Belson, 2021).

As I ruminated about contemporary variations of medical racism, I wondered where else versions of race norming might be playing out clinically and whether any consideration is given to the implicit biases inherent in the process. I considered the medical profession again and our prima facie creed to do no harm. Surely, this instrument is the antithesis of that principle. In this case, racial primacy operates through a clinical tool that has only served to further propagate assumptions about the value of life in the other lane relative to the dominant in-group. The resultant harm to racialized persons is manifold in that it ensures a premature finish line compounded by having started well behind in the racially demarcated lines of privilege.

Race norming is a palpable factor in the health outcomes of people of color as it shapes access to healthcare resources, diagnosis and treatment. Although the lawsuit against the NFL brought the issue of cognitive race norming to light, race norms are entrenched in other areas of medicine, including heart failure risk scoring, as well as renal function adjustments, and spirometry cut-offs, amongst many other clinical areas (Vyas et al., 2020), as previously discussed. On June 2, 2021, the National Football League (NFL) announced it would discontinue the use of race norming (Canada and Carter, 2021).

Race norms are ostensibly devised to account for innate differences, however the results of the Genome Project refute the utility of race correction, as the 0.1% DNA difference within the human species does not map to socio-politically defined race categories (USDE, 2019; Venter et al., 2001). Who examines the examiner? When such a tool is being devised or adjusted from a general tool, does the adjuster (examiner) reflect on their implicit biases and which ones may be at play in devising or adjusting the instrument? What are the assumptions made and how are they evaluated for bias? At the individual level, as a physician I wonder about the race corrected instruments and practices I may perpetuate and I wonder why I did not learn about the origins during my medical education. Why did I not think to ask? Is it sufficient to blame my education? As a hospital-based physician, how many race-adjusted tests am I blindly using?

❖

To tolerate someone else is an act of power; to be tolerated is an acceptance of
weakness
—Walzer, 1997

❖

Sanitized Racism in the Form of Tolerance

Tolerance can be viewed as a philosophically flawed virtue, existing only when difference or diversity is present. For it is only when we are presented with diversity that our range of acceptance is truly tested (Witenberg, 2000; Witenberg, 2001; Van Doorn, 2014); thus, the act of tolerance implies that an individual may have characteristics that are disliked or involve negative feelings; and simultaneously that any differences must be rendered palatable (Vogt, 1997; Walzer, 1997).

In practice, tolerance can represent a patronizing acceptance of others that does not give way for developing respect or appreciation of differences. Within a society, the perceived majority tends to hold an imbalance of power, with the inherent ability to determine whether a racialized minority will be tolerated, and which rules or norms the minority group need to satisfy in order to be tolerated and allowed to participate.

Devaluation and Non-interference as Mechanisms of Tolerance-Based Racism

Brown (2006) described two key mechanisms underlying the association between tolerance and racism: devaluation and non-interference. Through devaluation, the practices or beliefs embodied by a racialized minority may be seen as distasteful, deviant or undesirable by the dominant majority. To be seen as tolerated by the majority group, often White or Westernized in culture, implicitly affirms an objection to the beliefs and practices of the minority group and imputes a sense of superiority to the majority. As such, being tolerated can be framed as a benevolent act that may leave the racialized minority feeling indebted to the majority and unable to express their identity freely (Major et al., 2013; Meyer, 2003; Verkuyten et al., 2019).

Non-interference (i.e., passively endured tolerance) can also serve as a medium through which toleration can bolster racism. It can be utilized to support inequality by reinforcing the dominance of those exerting tolerance, suggesting to the minority that safety only exists when their culture is largely kept within their private spheres, thus, only accepting majority-driven practices as permissible in public. Such acts reinforce social alienation experienced by racialized minorities, providing limited opportunity to establish a sense of belonging as one's true self. Therefore, through continued non-interference, toleration can serve as a pathway for racialized minorities to ignore conflict with the majority and experience being tolerated as an act of generosity when permitted to express any aspect of their identity (Insel, 2019). Tolerance in effect is a power imbalance between a magnanimous majority in-group and the endured minority.

Through tolerance, both devaluation and non-interference can be utilized as forms of psychological oppression. Like racial microaggressions, racially based toleration often presents in an ambiguous form. In turn, this uncertainty can leave those in the minority to monitor their daily interactions with hypervigilance, negatively impacting physical and psychological health (Honohan, 2013; Lovett, 2010; Major et al., 2013; Meyer, 2003). For example, Derks and Scheepers (2018) demonstrated maladaptive cardiovascular effects experienced by those subjected to such subtle discriminations, as well as an impaired self-regulation of healthy behaviours resulting from covert stigmatization. In addition, several studies have illustrated similar cognitive ramifications, such as decreased task motivation and undermining one's self-confidence (Mendoza-Denton et al., 2010; Sechrist et al., 2004). The chapter discussing model minorities (Chapter 8) provides further discussion.

Clinical Vignette

Anisha is a second-year internal medicine resident currently completing a clinical rotation in outpatient cardiology at a busy Canadian hospital. She is Canadian, though self-identifies as being of Southeast Asian descent and practices Hinduism. She arrives to work one morning excited to share with her staff supervisor and resident colleagues, most of whom are White, news of the upcoming major religious holiday of Diwali, or the Festival of Lights. As a practicing Hindu, she has never before asked to have the day off to celebrate Diwali. She ponders why this may be, while considering the similarities between Diwali and the holiday of Christmas, a protected day of celebration by the majority of individuals at her workplace. Anisha quickly pushes the thought away, reminding herself to feel grateful to be able to celebrate the holiday in any form as a Canadian citizen.

In recent years, Anisha has connected more with her faith, but she often hides any visual signs of this from her supervisor and colleagues at work. After much reflection, Anisha cannot find the exact words to describe why she feels this way. She cannot identity any specific instances of being made to feel overtly uncomfortable or prohibited to engage in her religious practices. However, she recalls several interactions with resident colleagues and staff supervisors who appeared to joke about the "number of gods" and "funny songs" they attributed with the practice of Hinduism. During these times, she recalls laughing along with her colleagues, despite ignoring a physical feeling of discomfort. These repeated interactions left her with a sense of being ostracized, not being accepted by her White colleagues unless parts of her identity are concealed. Eventually, she began comparing what visits to her temple were like in comparison with going to church, services she had seen numerous times on TV since childhood. She questioned why the services at the temple she visited could not simply be done in English, why they sat on the floor instead of in pews, and why she needed to remove her shoes.

Regardless, on this day, Anisha approaches the staff clinic supervisor to request the day of Diwali off this year to celebrate. Her supervisor, Dr. Doe, initially informs her that the day off would not be an option given how busy the service is and that "nothing is as big as Christmas!" Anisha attempts to describe the meaning and importance of the holiday to her supervisor, who asks no questions and does not demonstrate any signs of interest. Dr. Doe eventually interrupts Anisha, stating that he must attend a meeting, and declines the request for time off. Anisha finds herself thinking "that's okay, he was nice enough to hear about the silly day, I should just be thankful my family and I can practice Diwali in Canada at all!"

Clinical Vignette Analysis

The above vignette illustrates the subtle ways in which the practice of tolerance can lead to further marginalization of racialized minorities. The stem begins by highlighting the hesitancy Anisha feels with acknowledging the importance of a religious celebration. This is contrasted with the natural acceptance of traditions belonging to the racialized majority and expressed gratitude for living in a country that has tolerated her family to a degree of allowing them to celebrate the day. Here, we see a pathway through which the toleration/tolerated dynamic evolves, which prevents Anisha from expressing herself freely and emphasizes her sense of otherness.

Anisha also struggles with her feelings of discomfort that arose from the devaluation by her colleagues directed towards the perceived differences in her religious practices. She appears to accept these behaviours as humorous, while also acknowledging a feeling of uncertainty in relation to whether they are truly of a racist nature. Anisha questions her own identity, which, as described earlier in this chapter, can lead to numerous deleterious physical and mental health outcomes over time. Anisha then attempts to engage with her supervisor, who demonstrates no curiosity regarding Diwali and appears uninterested in learning more about her religion. In this scenario, Dr. Doe's inaction can be seen as an act of oppression that places Anisha in the role of "lesser than" and "othered". Anisha conforms to the silent rules of non-interference by excusing Dr. Doe's behaviour and instead chastises herself for wanting more. Once again, she conforms by suppressing her otherness in the public sphere, and instead, expresses extreme gratitude for being tolerated.

Pause and Reflect

Self-Reflection: Asking Questions in Racially Diverse Settings

Curiosity and inquiry represent ways in which we can further our understanding of the diversities that exist in our society when done in a thoughtful, reflective and sensitive way. When asking others such questions, it may be beneficial to consider:

- Including words such as "typically," "usually," when asking about other cultures to take pressure off the individual to answer in absolutes.
- Asking open-ended questions that open up discussion and encourage problem-solving.
- Being open, sincere and genuinely interested in what the other person is saying.
- Explaining why you are interested and using a neutral tone of inquiry.
- Thinking about the underlying assumptions you may be making in generating your question and why you are asking it.

The Impact of Tolerance in Medicine

The impact of tolerance in medicine is wide ranging and exerts a toll on minoritized physicians. We begin by examining how tolerance is experienced by racialized physicians, then examine the physician burnout link, the concept of the minority tax and the sequelae of minority taxation.

In cosmopolitan Western settings, the presence of minorities in healthcare settings has been growing, but remains relatively low with poorer career progression when compared to their non-minority counterparts. In the United Kingdom, approximately 42% of National Health Service (NHS) physicians identified as Black or belonging to an ethnic minority group, but represented less than 14% of all senior managerial positions (NHS Workforce Race Equality Standard, 2022). Similarly in the US, only 28% of practicing physicians identified as Black or belonging to an ethnic minority group, and less than half of this figure was associated with medical leadership positions in both academic and hospital settings (Association of American Medical Colleges, 2019; Crews and Wesson, 2018). In Canada, it has been estimated that approximately one-third of physicians are from racialized minority groups (Khan et al., 2020).

Beginning as early as medical school, mounting evidence suggests that subtle and recurring forms of racism, such as tolerance, serve as an obstacle to the success of physicians from minority backgrounds. Kristoffersson et al. (2021) investigated the clinical experiences of Swedish medical students who self-identified as minorities and found that they reported regularly encountering subtle adverse treatment with ambiguous racist undertones. These incidents included aspects of devaluation and non-interference inflicted by supervisors, peers, various healthcare staff, and patients. However, they seldom thought of these events as representing intentional racism, and as such, hesitated to refer to themselves as having been victims of such discrimination. Additionally, despite feeling isolated and without support, the students simultaneously expressed gratitude "…for how well they have been received in medical education, thereby confirming the White majority who so tolerantly welcomed them – to an education they have the same right to as everyone else" (p. 6). These experiences of isolation, oppression and discrimination are concerning for the evolution of cynicism, disengagement and burnout, a prevalent problem in medicine today (Dyrbye, 2021; Esparza et al.; 2022; Gaston-Hawkins, 2020; Rodriguez, 2015; Rowe et al., 2022; Shanafelt et al., 2016; West et al., 2018; West et al., 2018; Xierali et al., 2021).

❖

"I sit on a man's back choking him and making him carry me, and yet assure myself and others that I am sorry for him and wish to lighten his load by all means possible… except by getting off his back."
— Leo Tolstoy, 1886

❖

The Burnout Link

Issues of exclusion related to race do not end with medical education and training. Racialized physicians continue to struggle with discrimination as they enter practice. Evidence suggests that racialized medical students face discrimination in the process of matching to a residency program, and then again in the residency programs themselves. These can be experienced in various ways, but certainly contribute to self-doubt and for some, a desire to leave medicine (Liebschutz et al., 2006; Esparza et al.; 2022; Rodriguez, 2015; Xierali et al., 2021). Residency is a formative period for professional identity, and the constant struggles with discrimination and self-doubt have a significant impact on the development of this identity.

In their narrative inquiry into the experience of Indigenous medical learners, Burm et al. (2022) describe the "tug-of-war" between identities as medical trainees and as Indigenous persons, and the ways in which this impacts individuals' sense of belonging. In their narrative inquiry, participants described struggling with experiences of racism where they felt pressured to respond to questions about their academic fitness for medical school as well as persisting inaccuracies and stereotypes in the curriculum. Within the Canadian context, it has been shown that there is significant anti-Indigenous bias among physicians, and the ways in which concerns about "reverse racism" and difficulties talking about racism impact the ability to address these biases (Roach et al., 2023). As such, the burden of correcting erroneous assumptions is even greater, as it can pose additional challenges to forming collegial relationships with peers and superiors.

Racialized minority faculty can also face choices around engagement versus disengagement, as they learn the rules of the system of which they are a part (Hassouneh et al., 2014.) They are keenly aware of their own role in making the system navigable for students and residents who look up to them; while this can be a source of pride and meaning, it can also contribute an additional burden. Furthermore, there is often an expectation that they would naturally contribute to diversity initiatives by the institution, which has been described as a contemporary head tax or "minority tax" (Johnson, 2017). Hassouneh and colleagues (2014) speak of the process of surviving and thriving, which reflects an interplay between the extent of the exclusion and the process of living one's values.

For racialized minorities, the process of medical education can feel like a gauntlet to be survived. The more one learns of the system, the more one becomes aware that the system was designed to exclude racialized people. Surviving this system often involves turning a blind eye to this and finding ways to fit into the dominant culture. Doing so often means ignoring the values of justice that may have driven one to medicine in the first place.

Finding a balance between being included in the dominant group and remaining true to one's own values is vital to thriving in this environment. That balance must the navigated individually by racialized physicians who continue to experience harm by institutions that were built, and are maintained, with the tools of White supremacy, settler colonialism, capitalism, and patriarchy (Esparza et al., 2022).

Medical training and the practice of medicine are psychologically hazardous professions, with the most lethal risk evident in the increased rates of suicide in the profession relative to the general population (Dutheil et al. 2019; Schernhammer and Colditz, 2004). The elevated rates of stress, anxiety and psychological distress amongst medical learners, trainees and physicians in practice are well documented (Dyrbye et al., 2014). For racialized minority students, the burden may be even greater when the effects of racial microaggression are taken into account.

The sequelae of microaggressions are noteworthy given the epidemic levels of burnout in medicine. The adverse effects of microaggressions have been reported to include anger, depression, skepticism and disengagement, fatigue and hopelessness (Espaillat et al., 2019; Hall and Fields, 2015; Osseo-Assare, 2018; Wong et al., 2014). Interestingly, these sequelae comprise of the three factors that broadly make up burnout as illustrated in Figure 11.2a: depletion or exhaustion, negativity or cynicism, and loss of professional efficacy. These adverse effects of microaggression are postulated to contribute to the leaky pipeline of minority exits from academia and medical leadership (Figure 11.2b).

Burnout

Microaggressions

- ☐ Exhaustion

- ☐ Cognitive load of invalidation: displacement of generative cognitive space by microaggression-related fatigue and negative affect states

- ☐ Depersonalization: cynicism, detachment

- ☐ Disconnection: scepticism, cynicism, hopelessness, hypervigilance protection

- ☐ Reduced professional accomplishment

- ☐ Reduced professional effectiveness: erosion of confidence, professional doubt and withdrawal, paradoxical stereotype threat

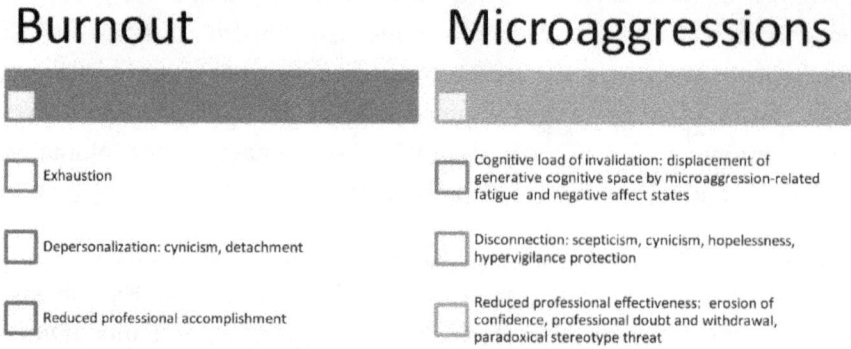

Figure 11.2a *Conceptual overlap between burnout and the sequelae of microaggressions*

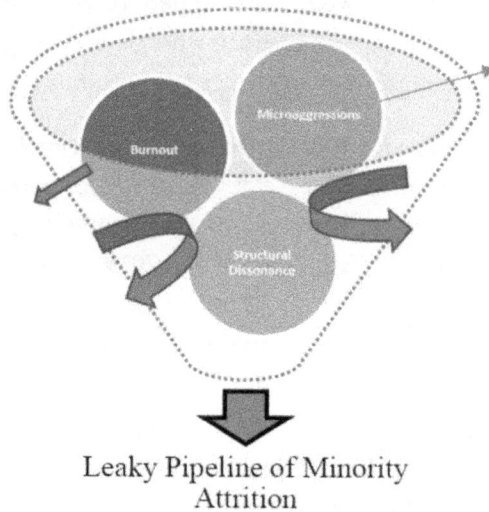

Leaky Pipeline of Minority
Attrition

Figure 11.2b. *Interaction between burnout, microaggressive climates and the leaky pipeline*

The effect of each physician withdrawal and risk of more to come is concerning for the health impacts on the exiting physician and the health system sequelae. In addition, each exit imparts a notable effect on further EDI advancement in medicine as each minority exit constitutes a failed opportunity at building an equity-responsive environment. It bodes poorly for the diversity required to offer care to an increasingly diverse patient population, particularly when minoritized physicians must in turn pay a minority tax of sorts for their very presence in the profession.

The Minority Tax

The currency of tolerance and apparent inclusion presents a heavy burden, payable by a minority tax as there is an unspoken, and at times delegated expectation of minorities to serve as diversity champions or "the face of the brand", mentors for minority trainees and contributors to institutional diversity initiatives (Esparza et al., 2022; Johnson, 2017). The minority tax comprises of an array of additional duties, expectations and challenges that accompany being an exception within a cisgender White male-dominated institutional environment; the minority tax is complex and constitutes a key source of inequity in the profession (Esparza et al., 2022; Johnson, 2017).

The additional duties levied in the minority tax are often not compensated but consume much time and may interfere with the "higher yield" or traditionally recognized work that typically sets physicians on the pathway for promotion; the inverse relation with promotion is much discussed on the academic medicine front (Esparza et al., 2022; Rodriguez, 2015; Xierali et al., 2021). In combination with the minority tax, the daily experiences of racial oppression and discrimination lead to a dangerous sequelae of disengagement, burnout and exit of minoritized physicians (Drybye, 2021; Esparza et al.; 2022; Rodriguez, 2015; Xierali et al., 2021); these sequelae are even more concerning in the context of the COVID19 Pandemic impacts on the physician and healthcare workforce. The weight of minority taxation bears heavy on the profession. Burnout stemming from minority taxation and concurrent experiences of discrimination constitute a key loss to the physician's personal and professional community.

In the bid to demonstrate moving beyond tolerance to true inclusivity, institutions may miss the mark and in their zeal, establish diversity initiatives that become more performative than tangible. When diversity devolves to institutional re-branding, rather than a core value or set of practices, the burden becomes manifold for minority learners and physicians who then contend with a combination of overt racism, implicit biases, and minority taxation (Esparza et al., 2022). Their professional experiences may come to be marked by the psychic tensions of being complicit in the dynamic and acting as institutional agents of racism, yet having limited agency over the system as a whole.

In keeping with the evident flaw to "diversity regimes" (Thomas, 2020), Esparza and colleagues (2022) note that "the placement of responsibility on a select few—rather than the entirety of institutional, departmental, and programmatic leadership—is neither sustainable nor equitable". Nor does this recognize the responsibility and accountability due of each member of the institution. As such, the minority tax can be dangerously transactional in *tolerant* settings, a quid pro quo that levies minority physician entry and presence in exchange for institutional efforts to demonstrate diversity.

Ripple Effects of Toleration

Invalidation of one's experience of being a victim of racist or discriminatory practices has been found to lead to further marginalization of practicing physicians from minority backgrounds (Beagan, 2003; Dickins et al., 2013; Odom et al., 2007; Sandoval et al., 2020). Repeated practices conveying hidden racist, hostile or derogatory insults based on tolerated differences in cultural/ethnic backgrounds have also been found to negatively impact racialized minority medical and nursing students' mental and physical health (Ackerman-Barger et al., 2020). These findings highlight critical training gaps that could assist physicians with identifying covert racism, such as acts of toleration, skills to manage such discrimination and awareness of supports to access.

Finally, little attention has been given to understanding the role of tolerance in patient-physician interactions and how it may impact patient care. Demographic studies have repeatedly found that physicians who are part of racialized minorities tend to treat traditionally underserved patients and serve in areas of physician shortage (Beagan, 2003; Essed, 1991; Kristoffersson et al., 2021; Leyerzapf and Abma, 2017). Thus, physicians who are most likely to have experienced the damaging effects of tolerance and sanitized racism go on to treat patients who have likely faced similar discrimination. Although minoritized physicians and patients may share experiences of discrimination and oppression, physicians generally inhabit a relatively greater space of privilege. This potential commonality can be harnessed to support the patient-physician alliance and trust-building within marginalized patient populations, with subsequent improved patient treatment adherence and outcomes (Shen et al., 2018), particularly where the physician's privilege is used to promote an equity-responsive environment. This is the central thrust of an ally's work: action to end the form of oppression that gives them privilege (Bishop, 1994, pg. 3).

Physicians occupy a space of privilege in Western medicine, no matter their social background. The relative privilege of the physician's status can be used to bridge the equity gap in any number of ways from within the exam room to the interprofessional workspace and for those involved with medical education, the classroom and bedside. Privilege and tolerance travel together, as the power imbalance in the toleration dynamic comes from a dominant majority being in the space of privilege that "allows" co-existence through non-interference; ideally this state of affairs evolves to a space of mutual respect and authentic inclusivity, rather than one of fear. The role of privilege is further explored in the subsequent section on *A Head Start*.

Personal Reflection: On Privilege, Passing and Hearing Fear

by Chase McMurren

My name is Chase. I live and work in Tkarón:to | GichiKiiwenging, though come from Lethbridge, which is on traditional Siksikaitsitapi | Blackfoot Confederacy Territory and is covered by Treaty 7. My clan is the Turtle and my spirit name is Water Song Medicine Keeper. My ancestors are Métis, Celtic, French and Ukrainian. I am privileged to practice (colonial [bio])medicine & provide integrative acupuncture-assisted medical psychotherapy, primarily for physicians and artists struggling with grief and overwhelm. I also have a home-visiting practice for long-living people with advanced illness who wish to die at home. I am honoured to serve as the Indigenous Health Theme Lead in the MD Program and the Indigenous Practitioner Liaison within the Office of Indigenous Health in the Temerty Faculty of Medicine at the University of Toronto.

As a cis-gendered, English-speaking, "white-passing" man, I have been given all sorts of unearned privilege. When people see me, they have no reason to suspect that I am Indigenous.

One dubious privilege of being white-coded is access to certain candid conversations. As I do not appear stereotypically Indigenous, I've been caught in or found myself within earshot of conversations on wards & in classrooms about the perceived unfairness of Indigenous-focused MD admission pathways & whether Indigenous learners fairly earn their spots in medical school. As a medical student, I often felt sheepish about disclosing my Indigenous identity because of the unkind, demeaning ways I'd heard people opine. Whether people knew the details of Indigenous application streams or not, I often got hints that people felt it was unfair & that spots were being taken away from "more deserving candidates." I don't think this has changed very much. It is rare for me to speak with an Indigenous physician colleague or medical student who hasn't experienced some sort of unabashed questioning of whether "people like us" deserve to be where we are.

While the people with these opinions may begrudgingly tolerate efforts to train Indigenous physicians, I wonder about the impact of unexamined emotions like fear, resentment, guilt & shame. (Of note, less than 1% of physicians in Canada identify as Indigenous. Until 1961, an Indigenous person needed to give up their Indigenous identity & rights in order to become a physician in Canada.)

How can we each create the conditions for turning toward the discomfort of getting to know the parts of ourselves that are scared & feel threatened?

❖

privileges are a type of power that can be harnessed to address the structural inequities encountered in day-to-day experiences
—Shim & Vinson, 2021 p.9

❖

A Head Start: Privilege, Trajectories and Finish Lines

Social ills like racism have an enduring and insidious effect on health and self-actualization. The self-actualization of racialized groups is complex in that a selection of disadvantageous choices and limitations can only produce an incomplete trajectory of innate potential. When one considers both the start and finish line of actualization for minority groups, the concept of a *double lag* is quickly apparent, with the starting line being well behind and the finish line also being foreshortened relative to dominant groups in society.

The self-actualization race itself is one fraught with obstacles for those belonging to the most marginalized groups due to the well systematized checkpoints that arrest progress. In contrast, the most privileged may be surprised to learn that what they view to be merit may in fact be an extension of privilege. Privilege matters, not solely because of the inherent power it confers but because that power can be instrumental to change.

Maslow's hierarchy of human needs (i.e., physiologic, safety, love/belonging, esteem, and self-actualization) is well known and has been proposed as a potential framework for the pursuit of wellness in medicine (Hale et al., 2019). However, even a brief reflection on this hierarchy reveals that these needs are not met equally for all, and that marginalized communities face much greater challenges meeting their most basic needs. Inequities in food and water security are well documented in Indigenous communities, low-income settings and racialized communities (Batal et al., 2021; OCHCHR, 2022; Odoms-Young and Bruce, 2018; Young et al., 2022). With inequities in such fundamental needs like food and water, it is evident that individuals born in such settings have some obstacles to surmount before they even get to the starting line that would place them in line for opportunities to advance themselves to their full potential.

Although we have already discussed the challenges that members of racialized minorities experience with achieving a sense of belonging in medical institutions, it is important to note that the feeling of "not-belonging" begins much earlier for racialized minorities. As Berger and Sarnyai (2014) demonstrate, the experience of racism has a profound effect on the neurobiology of those targeted by it and significantly impacts self-esteem. Thus, the concept of the late starting line (i.e., access to basic needs) and premature finish line (i.e., interrupted or arrested trajectory to self-actualization) is evident on considering these notable differences encountered by racialized persons and marginalized communities.

Individuals who drew their first and subsequent breaths in spaces where their physiologic needs were consistently met are likely to experience a briefer journey to self-actualization. Although this does not guarantee self-actualization, it does mean that energy is not depleted on securing basic needs. In the subsequent trajectory to self-actualization, challenges are negotiated with a combination of social capital, problem-solving skills and personal strengths, and it is common to believe at the end that successes are based on these merits without a distinction of the background privilege. It is common to be proud of good decisions that have been made, the ways in which complex problems have been navigated, and the resultant achievement of positions of power and influence. Often this pride is not accompanied by recognition of the fact that the cognitive and emotional capacities required to navigate the process are strongly influenced by the resources conferred by the circumstances of birth and the privilege of being able to skip over a number of steps in the hierarchy of needs, thus some have an advanced starting line and a shorter race, so to speak.

The recognition that what was perceived as merit may have in fact been a consequence of privilege may be psychologically daunting. In fact, it may threaten self-esteem and induce feelings of guilt, shame and paradoxical anger that present as defensiveness. However, recognition that privilege comes with power can be powerful in itself as it provides an opportunity to deconstruct and relinquish some privilege in order to bridge the equity gap. In so doing, those dwelling in the peripheries of the identity matrix

(Figure 15.1) have equitable access to opportunities enjoyed in the center and those existing in the center space of the matrix are responsible for participating in the solution. The moral imperative for change is shared by all.

Pause and Reflect: the privilege versus merit exercise
What is my greatest source of privilege at present? What advantages does it give me? In what ways have I engaged in the dynamic of toleration along my trajectory to present privilege states? What privileges and merits brought me to this career juncture? What were my options at the time I chose this career direction? Were there any social or societal constraints? At what points in my career journey did my privilege exceed that of peers with similar merits?

Once you complete the questions in the reflective exercise, move onto the second part of the exercise which is captured in Figure 11.3.

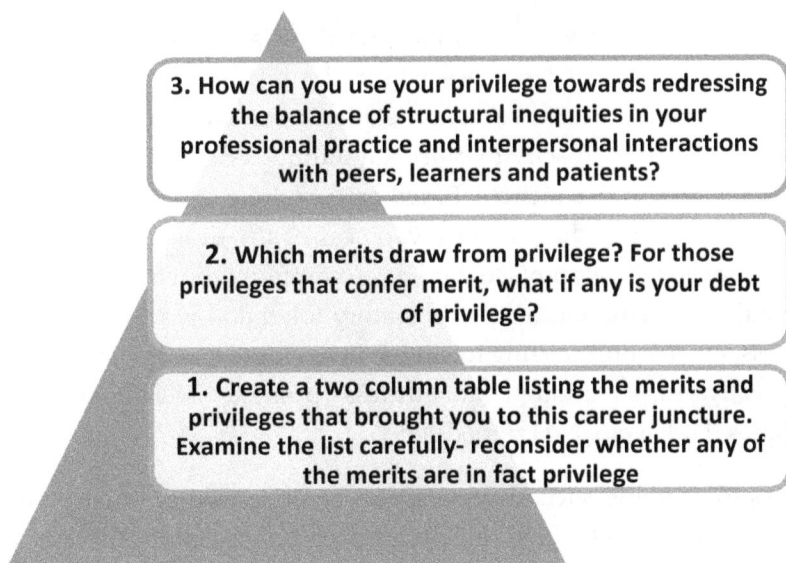

3. How can you use your privilege towards redressing the balance of structural inequities in your professional practice and interpersonal interactions with peers, learners and patients?

2. Which merits draw from privilege? For those privileges that confer merit, what if any is your debt of privilege?

1. Create a two column table listing the merits and privileges that brought you to this career juncture. Examine the list carefully- reconsider whether any of the merits are in fact privilege

Figure 11.3. *The privilege-merit pyramid is designed to facilitate disentangling privilege from merit. Begin at the base of the pyramid and progress sequentially from Steps 1 to 3. Once complete, your pyramid will likely include a relatively small base of exclusive merits, upon which sit a broad layer of privileged merits (i.e., interdependence) and finally at the pinnacle, a sense of transferable privileges, which may range from the interpersonal to the local systemic and possibly broader level, depending on the extent of influence and power you hold.*

The idea behind this exercise is to understand that merit and privilege bleed into each other; that what we instinctively view as merit is often conflated with privilege. By definition, this constitutes a source of power that we can consciously draw on as we attempt to cast a fresh eye on our professional climate in order to better recognize microaggressions, question structural inequities and attempt to reduce our contribution to systematized discrimination. The pyramid in Figure 11.3 concurrently reflects a hierarchy of responsibilities for recognition and distributive justice in regards to power relations. The pinnacle addresses an inflection point for the transfer of privilege.

The Opportunity

Awareness and Response to Tolerance-Based Racism

The difficulty in addressing tolerance-based racism encountered within medicine and society at large lies within the insidious and ambiguous nature of such incidents. However, as detailed in this chapter, toleration for the tolerated has the capacity to cause a multitude of deleterious physical and psychological consequences. Based on this alone, it is imperative that we develop strategies that confer awareness of the discourses that exist across educational, workplace and/or community environments that continue the perpetuation of discriminatory toleration practices. Without awareness, we risk normalizing toleration behaviours that do not appear to be explicitly racist, though nonetheless promote racially-motivated inequalities (DiAngelo, 2011; Essed, 1991).

Strategies to promote such awareness can be organized at micro-, meso- and macroscopic levels. First, at a microscopic level, self-reflection and developing a critical eye towards one's own implicit biases and the roles we may play to enact toleration can serve as a powerful vantage point. As discussed by Beagan (2003), by learning to challenge each other to uphold and maintain curiosity regarding our diversities and acknowledging our own power and privilege can help bridge issues of racism and cultural differences. When combined with other institutional and organizational efforts, implicit bias training at the individual level can also impact meaningful change (Kang and Kaplan, 2019).

Second, at a mesoscopic level, several suggested strategies within medical education and clinical training settings have been proposed, including:

i.   involving medical educators to develop and implement curricula about cultural hierarchies and everyday racism;
ii.   bystander training for students and faculty to help with recognition of subtle forms of racism and exclusion;
iii. training on how to support victims; instilling policies geared towards marking toleration as unacceptable behaviour;
iv.   supporting diversity and allyship initiatives; and,
v.   creating safe spaces for those of racialized minority backgrounds to congregate and reflect on their experiences together (Ackerman-Barger et al., 2020; Beagan, 2003).

To this end, Sandoval et al. (2020) developed a two-hour workshop for preclinical medical and dental students to help with their preparation of responding to microaggressions and covert racism in the workplace. Their results demonstrated significant improvement in learners' self-reported perceived difficulty with identifying and responding to racial intolerance and awareness of institutional support systems from pre- to post-workshop participation.

Lastly, enacting change at macroscopic levels, through hospital and government policy makers, healthcare networks and community organizations can reduce the structural inequities that promote the devaluation and non-interference that underlie toleration. As highlighted by Verkuyten et al. (2020), establishing social justice requires political and government spheres to systematically investigate their own complexities and paradoxes that contribute to toleration and evoke intolerance. Involving diverse perspectives at this level through inclusive hiring practices also provides an opportunity to engage racialized groups with lived experiences of toleration who may otherwise remain unseen and unheard.

Inclusion Strategies

Parting the Smokescreen of Toleration: Awareness, Recognition and Action

As outlined previously, effective inclusion strategies should be systemic, spanning across the efforts of the individual, educators, policy makers and government, amongst other organizational structures whose influence can topple the structural inequities that perpetuate racial discrimination. Given that the recognition of tolerance as a form of sanitized racism has only recently entered the discourse, it follows that current emphasis may best be placed on developing resources and supports targeting education and awareness strategies.

Inclusion of the traditionally oppressed voices of racialized minorities would serve as a key strategy for understanding tolerance and discrimination in action. Seeking the perspectives of such groups, from patients, medical learners, practicing physicians, and organizational leadership, would reflect a diversity of viewpoints and broaden our understanding of the experiences of the tolerated. Concurrently, learning what the experience of toleration looks like can facilitate the *tolerater's* ability to recognize the ways in which they contribute to the dynamic. In addition, building a stronger foundational understanding of how tolerance impacts physicians and patients alike can lead to creating stronger physician-patient alliance and improved patient outcomes.

Pause and Reflect

This exercise outlines sample questions aimed to promote self-reflection, awareness and skill development relating to tolerance-based racism encountered by medical professionals.

Sample Questions for Individual Medical Learner Self-Reflection on Tolerance

- In what ways might my day-to-day social interactions perpetuate "otherness"?
- Has belonging to certain social groups ever effected my sense of belonging in medical school or as physician?
- Do I look like who I imagine a patient would assume is their physician? Why or why not?

Sample Medical Education Level Reflective Questions

- What cultural hierarchies do you believe exist within our medical system?
- What action can I take as a learner encountering tolerance-based racism in clinical settings?
- What resources exist within the medical education setting to report, discuss or educate myself regarding tolerance-based racism?

Sample Clinical Leadership Level Reflective Questions

- What is this institution's history and does it support any hierarchies based on social identity?
- Does the institution have any policies that espouse or perpetuate magnanimity towards any minority groups?
- How are the policies on social "coexistence" framed? Does the language inadvertently perpetuate "otherness" of any groups?

Key Takeaways

- The medicine of race correction can perpetuate oppression and be dangerously inaccurate.
- Racialized physicians experience concurrent burdens of racism and a superimposed minority tax.
- Positive attributes of tolerance as a barrier to discrimination include protection from violence, provisions for the freedom of identity expression and collaboration in the face of irreconcilable differences.
- Negative attributes of tolerance stem from the construction and amplification of "otherness" which facilitates the propagation of racism.

- Privilege hides behind the smokescreen of tolerance as the key dynamic of tolerance is a power imbalance between a magnanimous majority in-group and the endured minority.
- Addressing toleration first begins by closely examining the ways in which we engage in toleration whether at the bedside, at the podium or elsewhere in the medical ecosystem.
- Learning what the experience of toleration looks like can facilitate the tolerater's ability to recognize the ways in which they contribute to the dynamic.
- Physician burnout is at epidemic levels. For minoritized physicians, added danger arises from a continued dynamic of toleration, minority taxation and concurrent racial oppression.
- Effective inclusion strategies require multilevel action to collectively shift the dynamic, ease the burden of the minority tax and shift away from zealous but performative diversity regimes to authentic engagement and action on inclusivity.

Conclusion

Tolerance is a complex concept that evolved as an antidote to intolerant attitudes and actions in the face of rising diversity. There is growing recognition regarding the intricate role that tolerance plays in constructing and amplifying "otherness" that allows many insidious forms of racism to propagate. The smokescreen of tolerance can deter the recognition of racism for what it is. It is so effective as to confer on racialized minorities the dubious and intolerable privilege of being tolerated.

Dispelling toleration requires the recognition that privilege itself can act as a blinder to oppression, with many daily rote actions replaying the dynamic of devaluation through non-interference. These interactions between power, privilege, tolerance and racism play a profound role in the self-actualization of minorities, particularly as it can be difficult to name toleration. Given that the recognition of tolerance as a form of sanitized racism has only recently been identified, current emphasis may best be placed on developing resources and supports targeting education and recognition of the very dynamic and its insidious subtext.

Inclusion of traditionally silent and silenced voices is essential to understanding tolerance and discrimination in action. Seeking the perspectives of such groups, from patients, medical learners, practicing physicians, and organizational leadership, would reflect a diversity of viewpoints and broaden our understanding of the experiences of the tolerated. In addition, addressing tolerance-based racism first begins by closely examining the ways in which we engage in toleration whether at the bedside, at the podium or elsewhere in the power structures of the medical ecosystem.

On a Parting Note...

Here

I am here.

Do you see me?
Do you hear me?
Do you know me?

I am them.
Do you see them?
Do you hear them?
Do you know them?

They are.
We are.

Listen.
Learn.
Know.

Be humble.
Be open.

Be here.

© Marissa Joseph, 2023

References

Ackerman-Barger, K., Boatright D., Gonzalez-Colaso R., Orozco R., and Latimore, D. (2020). Seeking inclusion excellence: Understanding racial microaggressions as experienced by underrepresented medical and nursing students. *Academic Medicine: Journal of the Association of American Medical Colleges*, 95(5), pp. 758–763. https://doi.10.1097/ACM.0000000000003077.

Association of American Medical Colleges. (2019). Diversity in Medicine: Facts and Figures 2019 [online].

Batal, M., Chan, H.M., Fediuk, K., Ing, A., Berti, P.R., Mercille, G., et al. (2021). First Nations households living on-reserve experience food insecurity: prevalence and predictors among ninety-two First Nations communities across Canada. *Canadian Journal of Public Health*, 112(S1), pp.52–63. https://doi.org/10.17269/s41997-021-00491-x.

Beagan, B. (2003). "Is this worth getting into a big fuss over?" - Everyday racism in medical school'. *Medical Education*, 37, pp. 852–60. https://doi.10.1046/j.1365-2923.2003.01622.x.

Belson, K. (2020). Black Former N.F.L. Players Say Racial Bias Skews Concussion Payouts August 25, 2020 [online]. Available from: https://www.nytimes.com/2020/08/25/sports/football/nfl-concussion-racial-bias.html

Belson, K. (2021). N.F.L. Asked to Address Race-Based Evaluations in Concussion Settlement March 9, 2021 [online]. Available from: https://www.nytimes.com/2021/03/09/sports/football/nfl-concussions-settlement-race.html

Belson, K. (2021). N.F.L. Plan Filed to Scrap Race as Factor in N.F.L. Concussion Settlement October 20, 2021 [online]. Available from: https://www.nytimes.com/2021/10/20/sports/football/nfl-concussion-settlement-race.html.

Bishop, A. (1994). Becoming an ally: Breaking the cycle of oppression. Halifax: Fernwood Publishing.

Berger, M. and Sarnyai, Z. (2014). 'More than skin deep': stress neurobiology and mental health consequences of racial discrimination. *Stress*, 18(1), pp.1–10. https://doi.org/10.3109/10253890.2014.989204.

Braun L, Wolfgang M, Dickersin K. (2013). Defining race/ethnicity and explaining difference in research studies on lung function. *Eur Respir J*, 41(6), pp. 1362-70. https://doi:10.1183/09031936.00091612. Epub 2012 Aug 9.

Braun L. Breathing race into the machine: the surprising career of the spirometer from plantation to genetics. (2014). Minneapolis, MN: University of Minnesota Press. https://doi:10.5749/minnesota/9780816683574.001.0001.

Brown, W. (2006). *Regulating Aversion: Tolerance in the Age of Identity and Empire.* Princeton NJ: Princeton University Press Available at: https://press. princeton.edu/books/paperback/9780691136219/regulating-aversion

Burm, S., Deagle, S., Watling, C.J., Wylie, L. and Alcock, D. (2022). Navigating the burden of proof and responsibility: A narrative inquiry into Indigenous medical learners' experiences. *Medical Education.* https://doi.org/10.1111/medu.15000.

Canada, T. and Carter, C. (2021). The NFL's racist 'race norming' is an afterlife of slavery [online] July 8, 2021. Available from: https://www.scientific american.com/article/the-nfls-racist-race-norming-is-an-afterlife-of-slavery/

Cartwright S. (1851). Report on the diseases and physical peculiarities of the Negro race. *N Orleans Med Surgical J,* (7), pp. 691-715.

Cartwright, S. A. (1851). "Diseases and peculiarities of the negro race" [online]. DeBow's Review. XI. Available https://www.pbs.org/wgbh/aia/part4/ 4h3106t.html

Cordeiro-Rodrigues, L., & Ewuoso, C. (2022). Racism without racists and consequentialist life-maximizing approaches to triaging. Bioethics, 36(3), pp. 243–251. https://doi.org/10.1111/bioe.13009.

Council of Europe. (2023). Discrimination and tolerance [online]. Available from: https://www.coe.int/en/web/compass/discrimination-and-intolerance

Crews, D. and Wesson, D. E. (2018). Persistent bias: A threat to diversity among health care leaders. *Clinical Journal of American Society of Nephrology,* 13(11), pp. 1757-1759. https://doi.10.2215/CJN.07290618.

Delgado, C., Baweja, M., Crews, D.C., Eneanya, N.D., Gadegbeku, C.A., Inker, et al. (2021). 'A unifying approach for GFR estimation: recommendations of the NKF-ASN task force on reassessing the inclusion of race in diagnosing kidney disease', *Journal of the American Society of Nephrology,* 32, pp. 2994–3015.

Derks, B. and Scheepers, D. (2018). Neural and cardiovascular pathways from stigma to health. In B. *Major, J. F. Dovidio, & B. G. Link (Eds.), The Handbook of Stigma, Discrimination and Health.* England: Oxford, pp. 241–264.

DiAngelo, R. (2011). White Fragility. *International Journal of Critical Pedagogy,* 3(3), pp. 54–70.

Dickins, K., Levinson, D., Smith, S.G., Humphrey, H.J. (2013). The minority student voice at one medical school: Lessons for all? *Academic Medicine: Journal of the Association of American Medical Colleges*, 88(1), pp. 73–79. https://doi.10.1097/ACM.0b013e3182769513.

Du Bois, WEB. (1903). *The Souls of Black Folk: Essays and Sketches.* Chicago: A.G. McClurg & Co.

Du Bois, W. E. B. (2003). The health and physique of the Negro American. 1906. *American journal of public health*, 93(2), 272–276. https://doi.org/10.2105/ajph.93.2.272.

Dutheil, F., Aubert, C., Pereira, B., Dambrun, M., Moustafa, F., Mermillod, M., et al. (2019). Suicide among physicians and health-care workers: A systematic review and meta-analysis. *PLOS ONE*, 14(12), p.e0226361. https://doi.org/10.1371/journal.pone.0226361.

Dyrbye, L.N., West, C.P., Satele, D., Boone, S., Tan, L., Sloan, J. and Shanafelt, T.D. (2014). Burnout among U.S. medical students, residents, and early career physicians relative to the General U.S. Population. *Academic Medicine*, 89(3), pp.443–451. https://doi.org/10.1097/acm.0000000000000134.

Dyrbye L.N., Satele D., West C.P. (2021). Association of characteristics of the learning environment and US medical student burnout, empathy, and career regret. *JAMA Netw Open*. https://doi.4:e2119110. 10.1001/jamanetwork open.2021.19110.

Espaillat A, Panna DK, Goede DL, Gurka MJ, Novak MA, Zaidi Z. (2019). An exploratory study on microaggressions in medical school: what are they and why should we care? *Perspect med educ*, (3), pp. 143-151. https://doi:10.1007/s40037-019-0516-3.

Esparza, C. J., Simon, M., Bath, E., & Ko, M. (2022). Doing the work-or not: the promise and limitations of diversity, equity, and inclusion in US medical schools and academic medical centers. *Frontiers in public health*, 10, 900283. https://doi.org/10.3389/fpubh.2022.900283.

Essed, P. (1991). *Understanding Everyday Racism: An Interdisciplinary Theory.* Thousand Oaks, CA, US: Sage Publications, Inc.

Faber, S. C., Khanna Roy, A., Michaels, T. I., & Williams, M. T. (2023). The weaponization of medicine: Early psychosis in the Black community and the need for racially informed mental healthcare. *Frontiers in psychiatry*, 14, 1098292. https://doi.org/10.3389/fpsyt.2023.1098292.

Feagin, J., & Bennefield, Z. (2014). Systemic racism and U.S. health care. Social science & medicine (1982), 103, pp. 7–14. https://doi.org/10.1016/j.socscimed.2013.09.006.

Gaston-Hawkins, L. A., Solorio, F. A., Chao, G. F., & Green, C. R. (2020). The silent epidemic: causes and consequences of medical learner burnout. *Current psychiatry reports*, 22(12), p. 86. https://doi.org/10.1007/s11920-020-01211-x.

Gee, G. C., & Ford, C. L. (2011). Structural racism and inequities: Old issues, new directions. Du Bois review: social science research on race, 8(1), pp. 115–132. https://doi.org/10.1017/S1742058X11000130.

Grubbs V. (2020). Precision in GFR reporting: let's stop playing the race card. *Clin J Am Soc Nephrol*, 15(8), pp. 1201-1202. https://doi: 10.2215/CJN.00690120.

Guillory, J.D. (1968). The pro-slavery arguments of Dr. Samuel A. Cartwright. *Louisiana History: The Journal of the Louisiana Historical Association* [online], 9(3), pp.209–227. Available from: http://www.jstor.org/stable/4231017

Hale, A. J., Ricotta, D. N., Freed, J., Smith, C. C., & Huang, G. C. (2019). Adapting Maslow's hierarchy of needs as a framework for resident wellness. *Teaching and learning in medicine*, 31(1), 109–118. https://doi.org/10.1080/10401334.2018.1456928.

Hall, J. M., & Fields, B. (2015). "It's killing us!" Narratives of Black adults about microaggression experiences and related health stress. *Global qualitative nursing research*, 2, 2333393615591569. https://doi.org/10.1177/2333393615591569.

Hassouneh, D., Lutz, K.F., Beckett, A.K., Junkins, E.P. and Horton, L.L. (2014). The experiences of underrepresented minority faculty in schools of medicine. *Medical Education Online*, 19(1), p.24768. https://doi.org/10.3402/meo.v19.24768.

Honohan, I. (2013). Toleration and non-domination. In: Dobbernack, J. and Modood, T., eds. *Hard to Accept: New Perspectives on Tolerance, Intolerance and Respect*. London: Palgrave Macmillan, pp. 77–100. https://doi.10.1057/9780230390898_4.

Insel, A. (2019). Tolerated but not equal. *Philosophy and Social Criticism*, 45(4), pp. 511–515. https://doi.10.1177/0191453719831332.

Johnson, T. (2017). The minority tax: An unseen plight of diversity in medical education. *IM Diversity* [online]. Available from: https://imdiversity.com/diversity-news/the-minority-tax-an-unseen-plight-of-diversity-in-medical-education/

Kang, S.K. and Kaplan, S. (2019). Working toward gender diversity and inclusion in medicine: myths and solutions. *The Lancet*, 393(10171), pp. 579–586. DOI: 10.1016/S0140-6736(18)33138-6.

Khan, R., Apramian T., Kang, J.H., Gustafson, J., and Sibbald, S. (2020). Demographic and Socioeconomic Characteristics of Canadian Medical Students: A Cross-Sectional Study. *BMC Medical Education*, 20(1), pp. 151. https://doi.10.1186/s12909-020-02056-x.

Kristoffersson, E., Rönnqvist, H., Andersson, J., Bengs, C., and Hamberg, K. (2021) "It was as if I wasn't there" – Experiences of everyday racism in a Swedish medical school. *Social Science & Medicine*, 270, pp. 113678. https://doi.10.1016/j.socscimed.2021.113678.

Leyerzapf, H. and Abma, T. (2017) Cultural minority students experiences with intercultural competency in medical education. *Medical Education*, 51(5), pp. 521–530. https://doi.10.1111/medu.13302.

Liebschutz, J.M., Darko, G.O., Finley, E.P., Cawse, J.M., Bharel, M. and Orlander, J.D. (2006). In the minority: black physicians in residency and their experiences. *Journal of the National Medical Association*, 98(9), pp.1441–8.

Lovett, F. (2010). Cultural accommodation and domination. *Political Theory*, 38(2), pp. 243–267. https://doi.10.1177/0090591709354870.

Lujan, H.L. and DiCarlo, S.E. (2018). Science reflects history as society influences science: brief history of 'race,' 'race correction,' and the spirometer. *Advances in Physiology Education*, 42(2), pp.163–165. https://doi.org/10.1152/advan.00196.2017.

Major, B., Mendes, W. and Dovidio, J. (2013). Intergroup relations and health disparities: A social psychological perspective. *Health Psychology : Official Journal of the Division of Health Psychology, American Psychological Association*, 32, pp. 514–24. https://doi.10.1037/a0030358.

Mendoza-Denton, R., Downey, G., Purdie, V.J., Davis, A., and Pietrzak, J. (2010). Group-value ambiguity: Understanding the effects of academic feedback on minority students' self-esteem. *Social Psychological and Personality Science*, 1, pp. 127–135.

Meyer, I.H. (2003). Prejudice, social stress, and mental health in lesbian, gay, and bisexual populations: Conceptual issues and research evidence. *Psychological Bulletin*, 129(5), pp. 674–697. https://doi.10.1037/0033-2909.129.5.674.

Mez, J., Daneshvar, D. H., Kiernan, P. T., Abdolmohammadi, B., Alvarez, V. E., Huber, B. R., et al. (2017). Clinicopathological evaluation of chronic traumatic encephalopathy in players of American football. *JAMA, 318*(4), 360–370. https://doi.org/10.1001/jama.2017.8334.

NHS Workforce Race Equality Standard. (2022). *2022 data analysis report for NHS trusts* [online]. Available from: https://www.england.nhs.uk/publication/nhs-workforce-race-equality-standard-2022/

Norman, M. A., Moore, D. J., Taylor, M., Franklin, D., Jr, Cysique, L., Ake, C., Lazarretto, D., et al. (2011). Demographically corrected norms for African Americans and Caucasians on the Hopkins Verbal Learning Test-Revised, Brief Visuospatial Memory Test-Revised, Stroop Color and Word Test, and Wisconsin Card Sorting Test 64-Card Version. *Journal of clinical and experimental neuropsychology, 33*(7), pp. 793–804. https://doi.org/10.1080/13803395.2011 .559157.

Odom, K.L. Roberts, L.M., Johnson, R.L., and Cooper, L.A. (2007). Exploring obstacles to and opportunities for professional success among ethnic minority medical students. *Academic Medicine, 82*(2), pp. 146–153. https://doi.10.1097/ ACM.0b013e31802d8f2c.

Odoms-Young, A. and Bruce, M.A. (2018). Examining the impact of structural racism on food insecurity. *Family & Community Health, 41*(2), pp.S3–S6. https://doi.org/10.1097/fch.0000000000000183.

OHCHR. (2022). Indigenous peoples face growing challenges to access safe water. [online] Available from: https://www.ohchr.org/en/stories/2022/10/indigenous-peoples-face-growing-challenges-access-safe-water

Osseo-Asare, A., Balasuriya, L., Huot, S. J., Keene, D., Berg, D., Nunez-Smith, M., Genao, I., Latimore, D., & Boatright, D. (2018). Minority resident physicians' views on the role of race/ethnicity in their training experiences in the workplace. *Jama Netw Open*, 1, e182723. https://doi: 10.1001/jamanetworkopen.2018.2723

Parekh RS, Perl J, Auguste B, Sood MM. (2022). Elimination of race in estimates of kidney function to provide unbiased clinical management in Canada. CMAJ, 194(11), pp. E421-E423. https://doi: 10.1503/cmaj.210838.

Possin, K. L., Tsoy, E., & Windon, C. C. (2021). Perils of race-based norms in cognitive Testing: The case of former NFL players. *JAMA neurology, 78*(4), 377–378. https://doi.org/10.1001/jamaneurol.2020.4763.

Roach, P., Ruzycki, S.M., Hernandez, S., Carbert, A., Holroyd-Leduc, J., Ahmed, S. and Barnabe, C. (2023). Prevalence and characteristics of anti-Indigenous bias among Albertan physicians: a cross-sectional survey and framework analysis. *BMJ Open*, 13(2), p.e063178. https://doi.org/10.1136/bmjopen-2022-063178.

Rodriguez, J. E., Campbell, K. M., Fogarty, J. P., & Williams, R. L. (2014). Underrepresented minority faculty in academic medicine: a systematic review of URM faculty development. *Family medicine, 46*(2), pp. 100–104.

Rodriguez, J.E., Campbell, K.M. & Pololi, L.H. (2015). Addressing disparities in academic medicine: what of the minority tax?. *BMC Med Educ,* 15(6). https://doi.org/10.1186/s12909-015-0290-9.

Rowe, S. G., Stewart, M. T., Van Horne, S., Pierre, C., Wang, H., Manukyan, M., Bair-Merritt, M., Lee-Parritz, A., Rowe, M. P., Shanafelt, T., & Trockel, M. (2022). Mistreatment experiences, protective workplace systems, and occupational distress in physicians. *JAMA network open,* 5(5), e2210768. https://doi.org/10.1001/jamanetworkopen.2022.10768

Sandoval, R.S., Sandoval, R.S., Afolabi, T., Said, J., Dunleavy, S., Chatterjee, A., and Ölveczky D. (2020). Building a tool kit for medical and dental students: Addressing microaggressions and discrimination on the wards. *MedEdPORTAL : The Journal of Teaching and Learning Resources,* 16, pp. 10893. DOI: 10.15766/mep_2374-8265.10893.

Schernhammer, E.S. and Colditz, G.A. (2004). Suicide rates among physicians: A quantitative and gender assessment (meta-analysis). *American Journal of Psychiatry,* 161(12), pp.2295–2302. https://doi.org/10.1176/appi.ajp.161.12.2295.

Sechrist, G.B., Swim, J.K. and Stangor, C. (2004). When do the stigmatized make attributions to discrimination occurring to the self and others? The roles of self-presentation and need for control. *Journal of Personality and Social Psychology,* 87, pp. 111–122. https://doi.10.1037/0022-3514.87.1.111.

Shanafelt, T. D., Mungo, M., Schmitgen, J., Storz, K. A., Reeves, D., Hayes, S. N., Sloan, J. A., Swensen, S. J., & Buskirk, S. J. (2016). Longitudinal study evaluating the association between physician burnout and changes in professional work effort. *Mayo Clinic proceedings, 91*(4), pp.422–431. https://doi.org/10.1016/j.mayocp.2016.02.001.

Shen, M.J., Peterson, E.B., Costas-Muñiz, R., Hernandez, M.H., Jewell, S.T., Matsoukas, K. and Bylund, C.L. (2018). The effects of race and racial concordance on patient-physician communication: A systematic review of the literature. *Journal of racial and ethnic health disparities,* 5(1), pp.117–140. https://doi.org/10.1007/s40615-017-0350-4.

Shim, R. S., Vinson, S. Y. eds. (2021). Social injustice and mental health. In *Social injustice and mental health.* Washington, DC: APA Publishing.

Thomas J.M. (2020). *Diversity Regimes: Why Talk Is Not Enough to Fix Racial Inequality at Universities*. New Brunswick, NJ: Rutgers University Press. https://doi: 10.36019/9781978800458.

Tolstoy, L. (1886). Writings on Civil Disobedience and Nonviolence. New York, NY: Bergman Publishers, 1967.

United Nations Educational, Scientific and Cultural Organization (UNESCO). (1995). *Declaration of Principles on Tolerance [online]*. Available at: https://unesdoc.unesco.org/ark:/48223/pf0000151830

United States Department of Energy (USDE). (2019). Human Genome Project Information [online]. https://web.ornl.gov/sci/techresources/Human_Genome/index.shtml

Van Doorn, M. (2014). The nature of tolerance and the social circumstances in which it emerges. *Current Sociology*, 62, pp. 905–927. https://doi.10.1177/0011392 114537281.

Venter, J. C., Adams, M. D., Myers, E. W., Li, P. W., Mural, R. J., Sutton, G. G., Smith, H. O., et al. (2001). The sequence of the human genome. *Science (New York, N.Y.)*, 291(5507), 1304–1351. https://doi.org/10.1126/science.1058040.

Verkuyten, M., Yogeeswaran, K. Adelman, L. (2019). Intergroup toleration and its implications for culturally diverse societies. *Social Issues and Policy Review*, 13, pp. 5–35. https://doi.10.1111/sipr.12051.

Verkuyten, M., Yogeeswaran, K. Adelman, L. (2020). The negative implications of being tolerated: tolerance from the target's perspective. *Perspectives on Psychological Science*, 15, pp. 544–561. https://doi.10.1177/1745691619897974.

Vogt, W.P. (1997). *Tolerance & Education. Learning To Live with Diversity and Difference*. New York: SAGE Publications.

Vyas, D. A., Eisenstein, L. G., Jones, D. S. (2020). Hidden in plain sight - reconsidering the use of race correction in clinical algorithms. *The New England journal of medicine*, 383(9), pp. 874–882. https://doi.org/10.1056/NEJMms2004740.

Walzer, M. (1997). *On Toleration*. New Haven: Yale University Press.

West, C. P., Dyrbye, L. N., Erwin, P. J., Shanafelt, T. D. (2016). Interventions to prevent and reduce physician burnout: a systematic review and meta-analysis. *Lancet (London, England)*, 388(10057), pp. 2272–2281. https://doi.org/10.1016/S0140-6736(16)31279-X.

West, C. P., Dyrbye, L. N., Shanafelt, T. D. (2018). Physician burnout: contributors, consequences and solutions. *Journal of internal medicine, 283*(6), pp. 516–529. https://doi.org/10.1111/joim.12752.

Williams E. A. (2008). Gags, funnels and tubes: forced feeding of the insane and of suffragettes. *Endeavour, 32*(4), 134–140. https://doi.org/10.1016/j.endeavour.2008.09.001.

Witenberg, R. (2000). Do unto others: Toward understanding racial tolerance and acceptance. *Journal of College and Character,* 1(5), pp. 2. DOI: 10.2202/1940-1639.1283.

Witenberg, R. (2001). The Development of Tolerance. In: Augoustinos, M. and Reynolds, K., eds. *The Psychology of Prejudice and Racism.* Thousand Oaks, CA: Sage Publishing.

Wong G., Derthick, A.O., David, E.J., Saw, A., Okazaki, S. (2014). The *what,* the *why,* and the *how*: a review of racial microaggressions research in psychology. *Race Soc Probl,* 6(2), pp. 181-200. https://doi: 10.1007/s12552-013-9107-9. Epub 2013 Oct 24.

Wright, R.J. Epidemiology of stress and asthma: from constricting communities and fragile families to epigenetics. *Immunology and Allergy Clinics of North America,* 31, pp. 19-39.

Xierali, I. M., Nivet, M. A., Syed, Z. A., Shakil, A., Schneider, F. D. (2021). Recent trends in faculty promotion in U.S. medical schools: implications for recruitment, retention, and diversity and inclusion. *Academic medicine: journal of the Association of American Medical Colleges, 96*(10), pp. 1441–1448. https://doi.org/10.1097/ACM.0000000000004188.

Young, S. L., Bethancourt, H. J., Frongillo, E. A., Viviani, S., & Cafiero, C. (2023). Concurrence of water and food insecurities, 25 low- and middle-income countries. *Bulletin of the World Health Organization, 101*(2), pp.90–101. https://doi.org/10.2471/BLT.22.288771.

Yudell, M., Roberts, D., DeSalle, R. Tishkoff, S. (2016). Taking race out of human genetics. *Science,* 351(6273), pp. 564–565. https://doi.org/10.1126/science.aac4951.

Chapter 12
Disability, Diversity and Inclusion in Medicine

Meera Joseph, MD, Richard Hae, MD

❖

"If we are to achieve a richer culture, rich in contrasting values, we must recognize the whole gamut of human potentialities, and so weave a less arbitrary social fabric, one in which each diverse human gift will find a fitting place."
—Margaret Meade

❖

Abstract: Despite ongoing work to promote diversity within the healthcare workforce, there continues to be underrepresentation of physicians and other healthcare workers who have visible and invisible disabilities. Bias towards persons with disabilities continues to prevail, leading to inequalities in healthcare delivery to persons with disabilities compared to those without. This chapter explores ableism in medicine, the value of diversity in the healthcare profession and strategies to promote inclusivity of persons with disabilities in the medical profession.

Keywords: ableism, barriers, disability, medical model, social model, temporarily able bodied.

Introduction

The term *disability* is broad and can include physical, sensory, learning, psychological, and chronic health conditions (Gault et al., 2020). A disability may affect or limit a person's movements, their senses, the way in which they communicate, or the way in which they learn (Wolbring and Lillywhite, 2001). It may or may not be visible, and it may be a permanent condition, or one that is temporary. A person may be born with a disability, or acquire it later in life. It is also not uncommon to have more than one disability. In a survey of medical students (Miller et al., 2009), five categories of disabilities were reported: (1) specific learning difficulties; (2) mental health challenges; (3) sensory impairment; (4) chronic illness; and (5) mobility problems.

A 2012 Canadian Survey on Disability (Statistics Canada, 2017) estimated that 13.7% of Canada's population, age 15 and older, reported having a disability; however, only 11.2% of practicing physicians report having a disability (Moulton, 2017). In the United States, approximately 20% of the population reported having a disability, with only 2% of physicians reporting one (DeLisa and Thomas, 2005). A similar gap exists when looking at reporting of disability amongst medical students, with only 3% of U.S. medical students reporting a disability in 2016 (Meeks and Herzer, 2016). Therefore, it is important to ask why the prevalence of disability in the medical profession is lower than what is seen in the general population.

Does medicine have a recruitment or selection bias against persons with disability? If the population rates of disability are also present in the profession, it raises further questions about the source of the gap in prevalence rates. Is the reporting of disability discouraged in medicine? Is there a lack of awareness amongst the general population that a disability does not preclude one from studying medicine? Are medical learners and physicians in practice underreporting disabilities out of shame, fear of implications and/or lack of recognition amongst other reasons? Are disabilities not accommodated well enough in the medical system to promote equitable representation? What is the impact of the lack of representation of physicians with disabilities on the healthcare system? What are the barriers faced by persons with disabilities within the medical system? The chapter will explore these inquiries in due course.

Hesitancy amongst medical students and physicians in disclosing a disability has been previously reported, with rates of disclosure by staff and students amongst the lowest for medicine and dentistry compared with other STEM (sciences, technology, engineering, and mathematics) disciplines, such as the biological sciences (Kuper et al., 2021; Joice and Tetlow, 2021). Several reasons for underreporting have been identified, including: implicit bias towards disability in the medical system; fear of disclosure in the high-stakes culture of medicine; conflict of interest in the process of requesting accommodations; and lack of trust in disability resource providers (Meeks et al., 2018). Those who do identify as having a disability face many challenges in the medical education system such as: difficulties with work, assessment, and attendance; finding support for clinical placements; bullying, negative attitudes and discrimination; and a fear that having a disability would preclude them from practicing medicine (Miller et al., 2009).

What is concerning is that not only is there a gap in the prevalence of disabilities in the medical profession compared to the general population, there is also a gap in the quality of care provided to those with disabilities compared to those without (Joseph et al., 2018). Despite attempts to promote fairness and inclusivity within medicine, beliefs that those with disabilities need to be "fixed" (Hogan, 2019) continue to persist in the medical culture which leads to false assumptions about patients with disabilities, which ultimately result in negative care experiences and adverse health outcomes (Bunbury, 2019).

It is also important to recognize that ability is a temporal and relative quality but the 'normative' stance in medicine has hindered a shift towards a more inclusive field for providers, pupils and patients alike. Although many may live without disability for the majority of their lives, as life events and the effects of aging accrue, disability is bestowed in varying degrees. As such, we really lead lives of temporary able-bodiedness (Janz, 2021). The greatest shift in inclusion might be gained with an intentional shift to an outlook of temporarily able bodied in the education and training of physicians and other healthcare providers. Shifting the medical culture and broader societal view towards this stance may set us in the right direction towards greater inclusivity.

Recently there has been a welcome shift to creating a workforce that is more inclusive of physicians with disabilities, along with a worldwide call for systems change. This includes removing systemic barriers to trainees with disabilities, providing education on disability in medical school, addressing ableist views and strengthening inclusive practices (Singh and Meeks, 2023). The Accessible Canada Act (ACA) was also passed in 2019 with the intention to create a barrier-free Canada by 2040 (Accessible Canada Act, 2019). Despite these widespread calls for action, there is still a long way to go in generating awareness of the barriers to disability inclusion in medicine, and creating change in this space. This chapter explores ableism in medicine, the value of disability in healthcare, barriers and stereotypes faced by patients with disabilities, and strategies to be more inclusive and welcoming of people with disabilities.

❖

"Abled does not mean enabled. Disabled does not mean less abled."
—Khang Kijarro Nguyen, n.d.

❖

The Issues

Ableism in Medicine

Disability scholar Fiona Kumari Campbell defines ableism as "a network of beliefs, processes and practices that produces a particular kind of self and body (the corporeal standard) that is projected as the perfect, species-typical and therefore essential and fully human" (Campbell, 2001). Disability then, is cast as a "diminished state of being human" (Campbell, 2001; Janz, 2019). In other words, ableism is the discrimination against people with disabilities based on a belief that those who are "able bodied" are superior and those who have disabilities require "fixing".

The historic "medical model" of disability was rooted in ableist thinking, viewing disability as a pathology or impairment that required treatment or a "fix" (Hogan, 2019). The "medical model" is often experienced as "the tragedy model of disability" by persons with disabilities who encounter pity, patronization and the experience of being overlooked during medical encounters as healthcare providers often converse at them or with the able-bodied person present if they are accompanied to appointments (Foxman, 2021).

In the past, the medical model of disability was believed by many physicians and, unfortunately, led to mistreatment of people with disabilities, including involuntary institutionalization and forced medical procedures. Institutionalization and forced procedures may no longer be prevalent, however, incorrect assumptions and attitudes in medicine about the lives, experiences, values, preferences and expectations of people with disabilities continue to prevail (Marzolf et al., 2022). In one study, 82% of physicians believed the quality of life of people with disabilities is either "a little worse" or "a lot worse" than those without (Iezonni et al., 2021). The many consequences of such attitudes will be explored later in this chapter, but it is difficult to imagine how a physician who holds such beliefs can make recommendations in the best interest of the patient. For example, would a physician who believes that people with disabilities have a poor quality of life be more likely to recommend a conservative approach to management?

In contrast to the "medical model", the "social model" of disability views disability as a problem resulting from the interaction of social and environmental conditions with a person's impairment (Hogan, 2019). In other words, people are disabled not because of a condition that requires fixing, but by systemic barriers in society. To contrast the two models, if a patient has difficulty getting up on an examination table due to a mobility limitation, the medical model of disability would try to fix the person's mobility so that they are able to get up on the examination table, whereas the social model of disability would suggest that the examination table should be adjustable to accommodate for the mobility limitation. While the social model has many merits and emphasizes the importance of recognizing and removing barriers, reality falls between the two models. There are some disabilities, such as chronic health conditions, which do require treatment. In addition, the person's environment should be able to accommodate for any differences in ability that result from the condition.

> **Pause and Reflect**
>
> Think back to an encounter with a patient who had a disability. Was your focus on treating the disability or finding ways to remove barriers which made the disability more pronounced? What are some changes in the environment which could have made it easier for them to utilize the environment more optimally?

The Opportunity

The Value of Disability in Healthcare

Diversity among physicians is essential to address attitudinal barriers, combat bias, and build empathy within the medical system (Marzolf et al., 2022). When people with disabilities are viewed as subjects to be studied and treated, negative attitudes and false stereotypes will continue. When people with disabilities are colleagues, it helps one to realize the implicit bias that exists toward ableism, both towards colleagues and patients, thereby improving the delivery of healthcare. When medicine mirrors the population it serves and physicians with disabilities are seen, medical culture is more likely to be responsive and inclusive of persons with disabilities.

An Australian survey of the general community was administered by Morgensen and Hu (2019) to understand perspectives on medical students and practitioners with disability. Most respondents believed that a person with a disability or chronic illness should be encouraged to pursue a career in medicine, and that being inclusive of persons with disabilities in the healthcare workforce would be advantageous for many reasons.

First, the lived experience of healthcare professionals with a disability brings empathy to the profession in a way that cannot be brought by those without the experience of living with a disability. For example, care providers with a disability understand what it is like to navigate the complexities of the healthcare system and may face many of the barriers and difficulties in access encountered by patients with disabilities (Morgensen and Hu, 2019). Clinicians and researchers with disabilities remind us that we should not be making assumptions based on functionality and stereotype (Meeks et al., 2020). Similarly, the increased rapport and informed care that is provided may also result in patients being more likely to adhere to recommendations from their providers (Meeks et al., 2020).

Secondly, increasing the numbers of physicians with disabilities will also help clarify that impairment does not equate with incapacity. Having colleagues with disabilities will help reduce the sense of "them" (the patients with a disability) and "us" (the able-bodied doctors on whom they rely for their good health) and will challenge the unconscious bias that goes along with that divide (Fitzmaurice et al., 2021).

Third, having peers with disabilities will help prepare medical students to treat patients with disabilities. In a survey of U.S. medical students, 81% of students reported inadequate competence to treat patients with disabilities. The authors posit that competence would be improved by interaction with peers and colleagues with disabilities (Fitzmaurice et al., 2021).

Finally, the health professions need to represent the population they serve (Meeks et al., 2020). Lack of diversity in medical education programs comes at a high cost to patient outcomes and loss of potential medical innovations. "The philosophy of disability inclusion must be adjusted from one where disabled trainees are viewed as problematic and having to 'overcome' disability to one where institutions anticipate and welcome disabled trainees as a normative part of a diverse community" (Singh and Meeks, 2023). Too often, conversations about the "*accommodation* of learners with disabilities" is framed in the context of the system bending to give the affected learners the *opportunity* to participate rather than the more inclusive goal of meeting the rights of each diverse member of the learning community. Accommodation need not be a dirty word when it is appropriately discharged as a duty and a right, rather than an act of magnanimity and tolerance.

❖

"Just because a man lacks the use of his eyes doesn't mean he lacks vision"
—Stevie Wonder, n.d.

❖

Clinical Vignette

Cathy Turnbull is a 25-year-old female who is being seen by Dr. Kim in his family practice. Layla is a medical student who is working with Dr. Kim that day. Cathy has been a patient of Dr. Kim's since birth, and he has had the privilege of getting to know her quite well over the years. Cathy has Trisomy 21 syndrome and hypertension, and this appointment was made by her mother for a routine check-up. After doing a blood pressure check, and reassuring Cathy and her mother that things are under control, Dr. Kim quickly reviews her vaccination status and realizes that she is due for her tetanus booster. After administering the vaccine, he tells Cathy and her mother that he will arrange for follow-up in approximately one year.

After Cathy and her mother leave, Layla reflects on her experience with another 25-year-old female she saw with Dr. Kim that week, and asks why that other patient was asked about sexual history, Papanicolaou testing, and vaccination for HPV, but Cathy was not. Dr. Kim realizes in that moment, that he assumed based on Cathy's disability that she would not be sexually active, and therefore failed to provide her with the same standard of care as his other young, female patients.

Clinical Vignette Analysis

Patients with disabilities face many barriers to receiving healthcare, including equitable access to reproductive care (Joseph et al., 2018). Attitudinal barriers exist amongst physicians, including beliefs that disabled women are asexual and that disabled women who are single are celibate. There is also a presumption that women with disabilities cannot be mothers, even if the disability has no impact on a women's reproductive system. These perceptions lead to an absence or hesitancy amongst physicians in providing a woman with a disability about information regarding contraception, sexually transmitted diseases and routine screening such as for cervical cancer. Physicians also perceive that disabled women are heterosexual.

The vignette emphasizes the importance of improving disability education and awareness in medical training. Without it, many inequities in the delivery of healthcare to persons with disabilities will go unnoticed, as in the case of Cathy and Dr. Kim. Having increased representation of medical students and physicians with disabilities will bring awareness to some of these issues, and ultimately improve patient care.

Did You Know?
There are many healthcare disparities faced by people with disabilities (Joseph et al., 2018): • Patients with disabilities face many structural barriers in healthcare settings such as, exam tables that do not adjust, doors that are not automatic • Women with major mobility limitations face lower rates of Papanicolaou testing compared to other women • Women with disabilities experience lower rates of screening for breast cancer with mammography • Women with learning disabilities and mobility limitations are less likely to receive information about sexual health

Pause and Reflect on Your Clinical Experiences
• Think about a clinical encounter you had where you treated a patient with a disability. This encounter can involve any physical, sensory, intellectual, or psychiatric disability. What was the main reason for the clinical encounter? Reflect on your clinical history taking and think about what types of questions you asked. • Now think about another clinical encounter that you may have experienced with a similar chief complaint. Were the questions you asked similar in the two scenarios? Did you omit any questions about the patient's history of the presenting illness, medical history, or social history in either case? Reflect on whether you made any assumptions about the patient with the disability that led you to omit any questions that you asked the patient without the disability. Was there a possibility that you could have missed any important diagnoses based on your history taking?

Pause and Reflect on Your Clinical Experiences

- Similarly, think about how you performed the physical exam on the patient with the disability. Did you perform all aspects of the physical exam that you performed on the patient without the disability? If not, what were some of the reasons that you decided to omit these aspects of the physical exam? Was it physically challenging to fully examine the patient with the disability? What aspects of the clinical encounter made it difficult to perform a complete physical exam (e.g., physical environment, ability to follow instructions, time limitations)? Reflect on whether you feel anything could have been missed based on the differences in how the physical examination was performed.

- Looking at the above examples, do you feel that any important diagnoses could have been missed based on the history taking or physical examination findings that may have been omitted?

The purpose of this exercise is to challenge the assumptions you may have made in the history taking and to get you to think about whether the same standard of care is being provided to patients with and without disabilities. Sometimes a question that you feel may have an obvious answer may surprise you when asked. There may also be times where it can be difficult to examine a patient because of a physical or sensory disability, but it is important that these patients receive the same standard of care when specific tests or maneuvers are indicated. For example, there may be challenges in performing a full neurologic exam in someone who has a hearing impairment as we often provide verbal cues to give patients instructions to follow during the examination. Providing them with written instructions may be more challenging and time consuming, but we have a legal obligation to ensure that we are not omitting things or providing a different standard of care when important information is required by examination.

Inclusion Strategies

❖

"I can't change the direction of the wind, but I can adjust my sails to always reach my destination."
—Jimmy Dean

❖

Strategies to Promote Disability Inclusion in Medicine

Disability inclusion in medicine must start with ensuring the inclusion of medical students with disabilities. There was a call by Meeks et al. (2018) to: (1) address access and admissions for individuals with disabilities to individual medical schools and ensure standardization across all programs; (2) engage disability experts and individuals with disabilities in advisory committees; and (3) integrate disability into equity, diversity and inclusion (EDI) initiatives, language and policies. The following are some strategies to promote inclusion of medical students with disabilities.

Change how we think of "qualified": To promote disability inclusion, we must first ask ourselves what it means to be "qualified" (Meeks et al., 2018). With the emergence of competency-based medical education, there has been a shift towards an outcomes-based approach to training, where learners must demonstrate achievement of certain patient-centered outcomes to qualify for completion of training or progression to the next stage. However, medical students, resident physicians, and practicing physicians include individuals who may have impaired vision, mobility limitations, attention-deficit disorders, who are hearing-impaired, who require the use of wheelchairs etc. Therefore, an individual's ability to meet all requirements of a training program will be multi-factorial (Meeks et al., 2018).

As an example, a nephrology training program may list the insertion of temporary dialysis lines as a competency in nephrology training. However, for a resident physician who is blind, achieving this competency would be challenging. Not all nephrologists practice in centers where they are expected to insert temporary dialysis lines, and assistance for dialysis line insertions can be provided by other services, such as interventional radiology, internal medicine or critical care. Therefore, program directors and education leaders must closely review and determine which technical standards are flexible or adaptable and which are immutable with respect to the competencies such that students with disabilities are able to meet the requirements of the program. This can be done on a case-by-case basis with the assistance of individuals who have expertise in disabilities (Meeks et al., 2018).

Eliminate outsourcing of the disability resource role: Within a university system, disability resources are often outsourced to the main undergraduate campus, instead of being housed within the medical school. These offices are often physically distant from the medical school campus, have limited hours, employ personnel with limited knowledge of the medical curriculum, and take an unreasonable amount of time to respond with a decision regarding accommodation (Meeks et al., 2018). This can make the process of requesting for accommodations or other resources challenging for medical learners with disabilities.

To remove these barriers and complexities, medical schools should consider having disability resource personnel with dedicated training on the medical curriculum, housed within the medical school building (Meeks et al., 2018). Ideally, this would be a person who is an expert in disability, but at the very least, disability experts should be consulted in creating policies and resources for accommodation and adjudication. Investing resources into this area would emphasize to prospective students with disabilities that the school is truly invested in their success.

Become familiar with technology that can help meet technical requirements: Amplified and visual stethoscopes, standing wheelchairs, dictation and magnification software, and automated cardiopulmonary resuscitation (CPR) devices are a few of the technologies that can allow learners and physicians who are deaf, have spinal cord injuries, or have visual disabilities to pursue medical education and practice in a clinical setting (Meeks et al., 2018). Often, educators are unaware of the resources available, making them uncertain of what can be achieved and how.

Deans and program directors should be aware of the technologies available, and have the resources and ability to access them for learners in need. It may be instructive for all deans and medical program directors to take accessibility and ableism training with refreshers being a core component of their tenures.

Remove any conflicts of interest: A major structural barrier to student disability disclosure occurs when there is a conflict of interest in the process of requesting accommodations. An example of how a conflict of interest can be created is when a person who reviews the student's request for accommodations also sits on a committee to evaluate the student's promotion or evaluation. If the student perceives a conflict of interest, they may be more hesitant to request accommodations out of fear that it will have an impact on their academic performance and career. Those who participate on committees that adjudicate disability determination also may not have a full knowledge of best practices or relevant laws related to the provision of appropriate accommodations for students with disabilities. In these scenarios, students may hesitate to disclose a disability, fearing potential bias or discrimination in the evaluative process. Taken together, students may be disincentivized from disclosing their disability or seeking accommodations when they perceive a conflict of interest in the disclosure process (Meeks et al., 2021).

Establish trust: Trust between students, trainees and their medical school is critical. When disability resource providers are unfamiliar with the medical curriculum and accommodations that may be required in a clinical setting, a learner's trust in the school to meet their disability-related needs can be undermined. This lack of expertise sends the message that accommodating disability-related barriers and commitments to disability inclusion are not a high priority for the medical school. A lack of personnel to support these needs may communicate that medical students cannot be disabled and do not require accommodations, perpetuating long-standing ableist views. This informs the climate around disability disclosure and stigma, and run counter to the stated commitments to diversity, equity and inclusion by medical education programs (Meeks et al., 2021).

Professional Vignette

By Meera Joseph

I was the senior fellow physician on a busy internal medicine service, with over 30 patients admitted under one attending physician. Three times a week, we would meet with the attending physician for team rounds, where we would go around and see each patient under our care, as a team. I came into work on a Monday morning, exhausted after a weekend of call, dreading team rounds that day. The attending physician, Dr. Smith, was known for his athleticism and his commitment to promoting healthy habits – I knew from others that this translated to making his team take the stairs instead of the hospital elevators. With patients distributed across seven floors, Dr. Smith made it clear to us that morning that he would not allow his team to be "lazy" and that we would be taking the stairs during team rounds. There would be no excuse to take the elevator while we were with him.

As we were making our way up seven flights of stairs, I stopped to catch my breath for a second and noticed that Jim, one the medical students on the team, was lagging behind the rest of us who were struggling to keep up with Dr. Smith. None of us commented on Jim's slow pace, but we also did not try to wait for him as he made his way up the stairs. Rounds were started without him, and he caught up to us when possible.

Later that day, I made an offhanded comment to Jim about how I would not need to work out when I got home after climbing stairs all morning. Jim seemed to hesitate for a moment, but then disclosed to me that he had a diagnosis of ankylosing spondylitis which decreased the range of motion in his hips and knees. This was not noticeable in his gait, but due to pain and decreased mobility, it had an impact on how quickly and easily he was able to climb stairs. He shared with me that he was hoping for a reference letter from Dr. Smith, but did not speak up out of fear that Dr. Smith may think less of Jim's abilities to practice medicine if the disability was disclosed.

I was caught off guard as Jim shared his story with me. Looking at Jim, I could never have guessed that he had a mobility limitation. Because his disability was not visible, both Dr. Smith and I had made the false assumption that Jim would be able to climb stairs. I stopped for a moment to think about all the other conditions, which may not be visible, but could make the task of climbing seven flights of stairs difficult for a person. Did we have a team member with asthma? Was there anyone with vascular disease who was put in pain from climbing stairs? I realized in that moment that I never stopped to consider disabilities that may not be visible. I had also assumed that as healthcare providers, we were all equally able, and that it was only the patients who had challenges and functional limitations. I immediately felt guilty about these assumptions that were clearly rooted in ableism. I apologized to Jim and shared with him that I would tell Dr. Smith tomorrow that we had to take the elevator.

It bothered me to think that Jim did not feel safe enough to disclose his disability without thinking that he may be jeopardizing his career or chance at a residency spot. Jim was extremely bright and clearly excelling in medical school. A mobility limitation would not be something that would hold him back in a career in medicine. But when I stopped to think, I realized that I could not think of one attending physician with a disability that I knew of. I could see how that lack of representation would make Jim feel unsure of how his disability would be perceived by the medical community.

The following day, I told Dr. Smith that I would be taking the elevator to conserve energy during rounds, and asked if any other team members wanted to join me. I was joined by Jim and two other junior residents. I encouraged Jim to be more open about his experiences so that we could all learn from him and his experiences. When we saw a patient with osteomyelitis of the spine, Jim opened up to the team about his diagnosis and provided suggestions on how we could make the physical examination more comfortable for that patient with back pain. Like me, Dr. Smith was taken aback when Jim shared his story. For the remainder of the week, although nothing was said, Dr. Smith joined us on the elevator.

The following year, I ran into Jim while on service for cardiology. Jim had matched to residency in internal medicine, and was on his first rotation on the clinical teaching unit. I congratulated him on his match, and wondered if he had received a letter of recommendation from Dr. Smith.

Professional Vignette Analysis

Jim changed the way I think of disability and made me reflect on the assumptions I make about others. He also showed me the value of being a person with a disability in healthcare and the wonderful perspective it brings to the care we provide for others. Because of Jim, I stop and think about the barriers I may be creating for others, and try my best to create a work-environment that is inclusive of everyone.

Pause and Reflect

What do I Bring to this Issue? An Exercise in Self-Reflection
- Have you ever felt uncomfortable asking about a peer or colleagues' disability? What was it that made you feel uncomfortable?
- What barriers have you created for learners or colleagues with disabilities?
- How can you create a more inclusive work-environment for medical trainees and healthcare workers of all abilities?

Key Takeaways: Physicians as Change Makers

- Physicians must embrace the opportunity to be change makers and leaders in disability inclusion.
- It is critical to eliminate the stereotype of the tragedy model that views people with disabilities as requiring "fixing" or as being incapable.
- Colleagues with disabilities add value to medical education and healthcare. They can provide valuable input that improves patient care experiences and outcomes. Looking like the population we serve is powerful in terms of the patient care experience and outcomes.
- As change makers, physicians can influence the medical admissions system, encouraging routine review of admission standards for disability inclusion.
- Students with disabilities should be provided with clear and accessible information about accommodations, and it should be done in a way that is free of any conflicts of interest.
- Disability resource professionals should be hired or consulted as disability inclusion processes and resources are created.

- Keeping abreast of innovations in accessibility and intentionally including disability resource professionals at the front and centre of temporal, spatial and clinical practice design is essential to promoting inclusivity.
- Normalizing help-seeking behaviors amongst physicians and learners is critical to eliminating stigma within the profession about disability.
- Advocacy for the incorporation of a disability curriculum in medical education is essential to improving the capacity to care for those with disabilities and to bring awareness to the health inequities experienced by persons with disability.
- In keeping with a shift in the medical curriculum, reframing attitudes and intentionally building capacity for an inclusive environment begins with both the formal and silent curriculum in medicine. An intentional adoption of a temporarily able-bodied outlook is important if we are to build the capacity to expect and respect variation in the human condition, seek and welcome innovations that promote inclusivity, and thus, learn and work within an inclusive healthcare workforce.

Conclusion

There are many opportunities for the inclusion of persons with disabilities in medicine, both as providers and patients. We need to start thinking of disability within a positive construct rather than a construct of deficit historically seen with the lens of "the tragedy model of disability". As illustrated in the quality of life surveys conducted amongst physicians, disability is still largely seen as a state of being less than whole, which has impacts on disclosure by learners and physicians, concurrent with adverse impacts on the care experiences and outcomes for patients with disabilities.

Shifting our outlook to one of temporary able bodiedness and incorporating the spectrum of disabilities is necessary and just. Being "able bodied" by *normative* standards is a dynamic state that is subject to life events and ageing. It behooves us to shift our outlook on the inherent range of human abilities if we are to transform medicine and healthcare to inclusive environments that respect and equitably adapt for the spectrum of disabilities in learners, colleagues and patients with whom we work.

On a Parting Note...

The doctor will see you now...

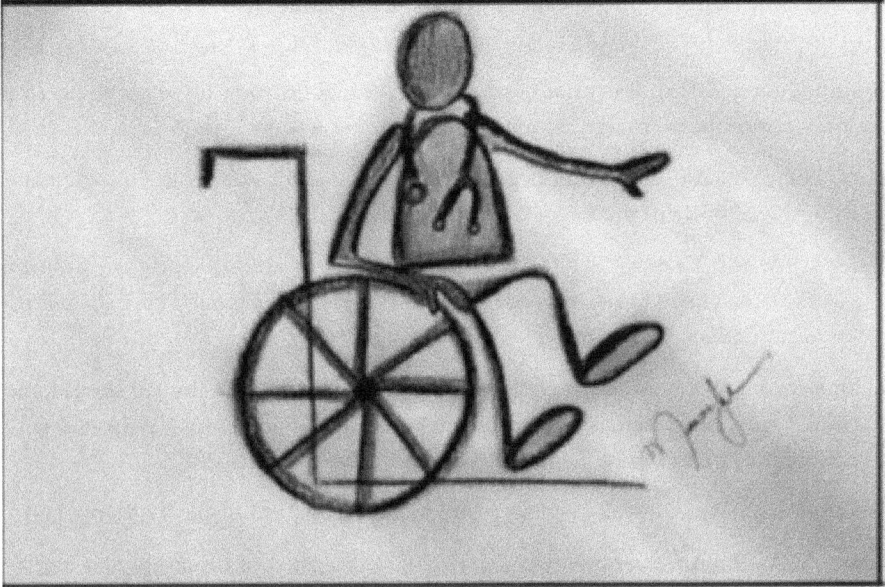

Original artwork by first author, Meera Joseph

References

Bunbury, S. (2019). 'Unconscious bias and the medical model: How the social model may hold the key to transformative thinking about disability discrimination'. *International Journal of Discrimination and the Law*, 19(1), pp. 26-47.

Brainy Quote. (2023). Potentialities [online]. Available from: https://www.brainy quote.com/quotes/margaret_mead_132704

Campbell, F.A. (2001). 'Inciting Legal Fictions-Disability's Date with Ontology and the Abieist Body of the Law'. *Griffith Law Review*, 10(1), pp. 42.

DeLisa, J.A. and Thomas, P. (2005). 'Physicians with disabilities and the physician workforce: a need to reassess our policies'. *American Journal of Physical Medicine & Rehabilitation*, 84(1), pp. 5-11.

Fitzmaurice, L., Donald, K., Wet, C. and Palipana, D. (2021). 'Why we should and how we can increase medical school admissions for persons with disabilities'. *The Medical Journal of Australia*, 215(6), pp. 249-251.

Foxman, S. (2021). 'Does ableism seep into medical care?'. *Dialogue*, 17(4), pp. 11-13.

Gault, M.A., Raha, S.S. and Newell, C. (2020). 'Perception of disability as a barrier for Canadian medical students'. *Canadian Family Physician*, 66(3), pp. 169-171.

Government of Canada. (2019). *Consolidated Federal Laws of Canada, Accessible Canada Act* [online]. Available from: https://laws-lois.justice.gc.ca/eng/acts/a-0.6/

Hogan, A.J., (2019). 'Social and medical models of disability and mental health: evolution and renewal'. *Canadian Medical Association Journal*, 191(1), pp. E16-E18.

Iezzoni, L.I., Rao, S.R., Ressalam, J., Bolcic-Jankovic, D., Agaronnik, N.D., Donelan, K., Lagu, T. and Campbell, E.G. (2021). 'Physicians' perceptions of people with disability and their Health care: Study reports the results of a survey of physicians' perceptions of people with disability'. *Health Affairs*, 40(2), pp. 297-306.

Janz, H.L. (2019). Ableism: the undiagnosed malady afflicting medicine. *Canadian Medical Association Journal*, 191(17), pp. E478-E479.

Janz, H.L. (2021). 'You may be TAB'. *CPSO Dialogue*, 17(4), p. 14.

Joice W., and Tetlow, A. (2021). Disability STEM data for students and academic staff in higher education 2007-08 to 2018-19 Royal Society [online]. Available from: https://royalsociety.org/-/media/policy/topics/diversity-in-science/210118 -disability-STEM-data-for-students-and-staff-in-higher-education.pdf

Joseph, M., Saravanabavan, S. and Nisker, J. (2018). 'Physicians' perceptions of barriers to equal access to reproductive health promotion for women with mobility impairment'. *Canadian Journal of Disability Studies*, 7(1), pp. 62-100.

Kuper, H., Shakespeare, T., Soto, C. and Booth, S. (2021). 'Low numbers of disabled doctors mean potential loss of insightful care for everyone'. *British Medical Journal*, p.1

Marzolf, B.A., McKee, M.M., Okanlami, O.O. and Zazove, P. (2022). 'Call to action: Eliminate barriers faced by medical students with disabilities'. *The Annals of Family Medicine*, 20(4), pp. 376-378.

Meeks, L.M. and Herzer, K.R. (2016). 'Prevalence of self-disclosed disability among medical students in US allopathic medical schools'. *Journal of the American Medical Association*, 316(21), pp. 2271-2272.

Meeks, L.M., Herzer, K. and Jain, N.R. (2018). 'Removing barriers and facilitating access: increasing the number of physicians with disabilities'. *Academic Medicine*, 93(4), pp. 540-543.

Meeks, L.M., Maraki, I., Singh, S. and Curry, R.H. (2020). 'Global commitments to disability inclusion in health professions'. *Lancet (London, England)*, 395(10227), pp. 852-853.

Meeks, L.M., Poullos, P. and Swenor, B.K. (2020). 'Creative approaches to the inclusion of medical students with disabilities'. *AEM Education and Training*, 4(3), p. 292.

Meeks, L.M., Case, B., Stergiopoulos, E., Evans, B.K. and Petersen, K.H. (2021). 'Structural barriers to student disability disclosure in US-allopathic medical schools'. *Journal of Medical Education and Curricular Development*, 8, 23821205211018696.

Miller, S., Ross, S. and Cleland, J. (2009). 'Medical students' attitudes towards disability and support for disability in medicine'. *Medical Teacher*, 31(6), pp. e272-e277.

Mogensen, L. and Hu, W. (2019). '"A doctor who really knows...": a survey of community perspectives on medical students and practitioners with disability'. *BMC Medical Education*, 19(1), pp. 1-10.

Moulton D. (2017). 'Physicians with disabilities often undervalued'. *Canadian Medical Association Journal*, 189(18), pp. E678–E679.

Singh, S. and Meeks, L.M. (2023). 'Disability inclusion in medical education: towards a quality improvement approach'. *Medical Education*, 57(1), pp. 102-107.

Statistics Canada. (2017). *Canadian Survey on Disability, 2012.* Available from: https://www150.statcan.gc.ca/n1/daily-quotidien/ 150313/dq150313b-eng.htm

Wolbring, G. and Lillywhite, A. (2021). 'Equity/Equality, Diversity, and Inclusion (EDI) in Universities: The Case of Disabled People'. *Societies*, 11(2), p. 49.

Part 3.
Opening Eyes and Opening Minds: Leading with Equity,
Diversity and Inclusion

Chapter 13
Critical Allyship

Tara La Rose, PhD, Albina Veltman, MD

❖

"Being an ally is just the first step, the simplest one, it is the space wherein the privileged began to accept the flawed dynamics that make for inequality. Being a good ally is not easy, it's not something you can jump into…"
— Mikki Kendall, 2020

❖

Abstract: This chapter considers allyship as a way of engaging in social change making with equity-deserving groups in the context of healthcare and medical practice. Perspectives of critical allyship as a way of working collaboratively with marginalized and oppressed people is discussed. Critical reflexivity is framed as part of the process of becoming and ally and is explored as a key element in change making. The importance of praxis, the use of reflection in action and reflection on action as a means of honing the application of theory in practice, is considered as a process supporting allies' self-education. Finally, healthcare advocacy is presented as part of the holistic function of allyship in change making. Questions and reflective activities are included to support healthcare professionals' preparedness for beginning the allyship journey and for maintaining engagement in allyship practice.

Keywords: *ally, allyship, critical allyship, critical reflexivity, lived/living experience, post- structuralism, showing up, social justice*

Introduction

Allyship is a way of engaging in social change making and advocacy practice in collaboration with equity-deserving groups and with individuals experiencing marginalization and oppression. This discussion of allyship focuses on medical contexts where healthcare professionals seek to engage actively with groups and individuals to create change within health systems and within the broader social and economic contexts supporting these care contexts.

Perspectives of allyship and critical allyship as collaboration are discussed in detail throughout the chapter. Case vignettes are used to support reflection and engagement with complexities of healthcare settings as ways of considering the many competing demands that allies face in practice. Furthermore, this chapter explores critical reflexivity as a key element in change making and the importance of praxis as a process for supporting allies' self-education and healthcare advocacy. Questions and reflective activities are included to support healthcare professionals preparing for engagement in the practice of critical allyship. Allyship may be practiced across contexts with patients, with peers, with learners and within the community both in and outside of the professional healthcare role. In this framing of allyship, what is most important is the understanding that allyship requires action, the integration of critical self-reflection and reflexivity in practice as well as ongoing commitment.

In the Canadian context, scholar Ann Bishop (1994) was one of the first authors to write about the concept of allyship as a means of responding to social justice issues and oppression to create systemic change. Since this time, many more authors have written and continue to write about the concept of allyship today (Arif et al., 2022; Baines, 2022; Nixon, 2019; Sumerau et al., 2021). Nonetheless, the book *Becoming an Ally* (1994) remains a seminal text, addressing the complexity of working across difference, and understanding allyship as a form of anti-oppressive practice. Bishop (2015) defines an "ally" as:

...a member of an oppressor group who takes action to end the form of oppression that gives them privilege... (pg. 3).

This definition highlights the ally's willingness to give up some access to privilege to promote change in systems and processes in order to enhance access to resources for those they seek to support (ibid, pg. 5). While this core concept remains an important part of allyship, understandings of allyship have evolved and are now more complex. In particular, there is now heightened recognition of the centrality of identity and increasing challenges to the idea of a singular understanding of identity. In addition, perspectives have shifted from framings of privilege and power relations as a kind of *zero-sum game* in scholarship from the 1990s to a greater focus on framing identities as multiple, intersecting, and overlapping as well as interlocking and complex in contemporary contexts. Power relations are understood as dynamic and ever-present and as operating on multiple levels simultaneously; these perspectives are consistent with contemporary post-structural perspectives (Baines, 2017; Bishop, 2020; Nixon, 2019).

The Issues

Exploring the issues through vignettes...

Professional Vignette

Dr. Francine Grant is a trans-identified psychiatrist who works in a large urban healthcare system. Francine transitioned after entering into professional practice and worked hard to educate her colleagues and hospital administration about how best to understand her transition, her trans identity and how to work with patients *like* her. Francine is an ambitious woman who has worked hard to achieve her goals at work, as well as seeking out medical leadership opportunities at the local, national and international level. With an increased awareness of equity, diversity and inclusion (EDI) principles and concern for effective care and treatment for trans-identified patients within the field of medicine, she has become an important professional advocate and a popular invited speaker in the medical community, and the community at large. As a result, Francine receives more than 100 requests per year to speak at local, national, and international events, some focused specifically on medicine and healthcare, while others are focused more generally on human rights and empowerment for the trans community.

Francine believes that attending these sessions is important, but it is impossible for her to accept all the requests. When Francine says "no" to her local colleagues, she is sometimes criticized for seeing herself as "too important" for her local community where she "got her start". In other cases, people critique her for always being the one to speak on the issues suggesting that other people be invited to speak -- but usually these detractors have no suggestions about whom else to invite. When Francine politely declines speaking requests outside of the local area, she is sometimes offered higher speaking fees or other "perks" to try to entice her to attend. This makes Francine feel disrespected and like her life experience is a commodity.

Francine sometimes complains to her friends that she feels overwhelmed, emotionally exhausted and resentful that her identity as a trans woman seems to "trump" all her other accomplishments. While she thinks it is great that people are concerned about trans issues, she sometimes feels like systems administrators and medical leaders think that simply asking Francine to speak is enough – that her presence for a couple of hours somehow makes healthcare safe for trans people -- and therefore, that the other healthcare professionals do not have to take on the work of trans allyship and systemic change. She feels like she is being asked to do the work for an entire health system.

Clinical Vignette

Dr. Vida has a long history of working in family medicine in rural and remote communities. Dr. Vida chose these opportunities in part because she came from a low-income immigrant family, and she was concerned about being able to pay off several hundred thousand dollars in student loans when she finished her medical education in addition to supporting her family. To increase her income in the early years of her practice, Dr. Vida took a special contract that paid her supplemental income while studying, in return for her commitment to complete a minimum number of years of service in rural and remote health districts - a requirement she has now far exceeded.

When Dr. Vida started her practice, she discovered that she loved working in her assigned community. In particular, Dr. Vida really liked the fact that she felt her own experiences of accessing healthcare as a racialized person helped inform her practice in rural and remote communities. She remembered some of the negative judgement her family received when her mother, as new comer, had supplemented mainstream healthcare with traditional/cultural remedies. This made her cautious about how she approached patients who had their own traditional ways of supporting good health and who had lacked access to mainstream medicine for extended periods of time before her arrival in the community. Dr. Vida was also somewhat angry about the lack of local resources and the fact that many of the resources that were made available through the health system were out of date and/or insufficient – commonly referred to by patients as "big city leftovers".

Another challenge that Dr. Vida experienced was patients' resistance to referrals to other healthcare professionals. Patients often became upset and angry when referrals were made because referrals almost always required patients to leave the community. While Dr. Vida realized that the cost and energy of travelling over 300 miles to see a specialist and get certain types of diagnostic tests completed was expensive for patients, she felt that consultations with other healthcare professionals were necessary and important – and her ethical duty. However, Dr. Vida also noticed that some patients did not follow through on the referrals she made. Others waited until they were in a real crisis before coming to see her and then coming only on the insistence of their families…some with great hesitancy, anger and/or mistrust. When Dr. Vida questioned patients about this, she was told that they "didn't want to get sent down south…" or that "people don't come back" when they leave the community to get healthcare in a larger center. Dr. Vida was frustrated by these responses and believed they were mostly untrue…. She felt that in some way she was being blamed for the limited resources available in the community and the need to make outside referrals…but what choice did she have?

Vignette Analysis

These two vignettes invite us into a conversation about the concept of allyship or alliance within the health and social care/social welfare sectors. While the term ally may generally be associated with military protection by nation states that share and engage in bilateral agreements (Cambridge Dictionary, 2023); the meaning shifts significantly when considering this within the context of healthcare practices. The ideal of allyship or the concept of "becoming an ally" to patients focuses on purposeful collaboration among those providing and accessing healthcare services, working together towards institutional and systemic change (Bishop, 2020). Allyship describes engagement and support to marginalized individuals and groups where the individual providing the support does not share an identity (or aspects of identity) with those who are engaged in a struggle over rights, freedoms, and access to resources (Baines, 2022; Bishop, 2020; Nixon, 2019).

Dr. Francine Grant understands the experience of trans identified people because she is a trans woman – but her social standing as a doctor means that even in her experience of marginalization there is privilege because Francine has the knowledge and financial resources to effectively negotiate the healthcare system in a way that someone who is not a doctor may not. Francine also understands the challenges of system changes in the psychiatric community, in the medical community, more generally, and in the context of the healthcare system, more broadly.

Her multiple identities work together to allow her to bridge the divide between the trans community and medicine/healthcare in particular ways. While Francine honours her capacity to build bridges, she also understands the importance of challenging the complacency that exists within the healthcare community and hopes to do more to create change and get other people involved in the process. Francine's capacity for critical reflection also points to her own need for self-care and to ensure that there she takes care of her needs rather than allow her role as an ally and bridge builder to result in exhaustion, potentially leading to burnout, which will mean Francine is no longer able to do the work she loves and to potentially create a better healthcare environment for trans people.

Similarly, Dr. Vida's own life experiences, through critical reflection and critical reflexivity provided her with insights into the challenges faced by rural and remotes communities. Her capacity to draw on her own experiences is likely a part of what made the challenge of working in this setting appealing to her. However, Dr. Vida also used critical reflexivity and praxis to go beyond her own experiences and to consider how responses to her treatment and care recommendations (for example referrals) were received and interpreted by patients. These responses were understood by Dr. Vida as telling her something about how patients interpreted her advice and also suggested that she needs to know more about the underlying systemic issues. Understanding the hidden meanings of her actions and the interpretations of these actions based on patient experiences provided Dr. Vida with a broader scope for change making.

Understanding Allyship

As mentioned previously, Ann Bishop was one of the first authors to write about the concept of allyship in her seminal work, *Becoming an Ally* (1994). Bishop (1994) defines allyship as a means of responding to social justice issues and oppression with a focus on systemic change making. The scholarship on allyship has grown and expanded since Bishop's initial publication, with many more authors writing about allyship in a contemporary context (Arif et al., 2022; Baines, 2022; Nixon, 2019; Sumerau et al., 2021). While the scholarship continues to evolve, the concept of allyship still emphasizes the close relationship between oppression and privilege (Bishop, 1994).

Contemporary perspectives of allyship draw on critical theories from traditions such as the Chicago School and radical/structural/Black feminism thought. The perspectives lean as heavily on the work of pioneering adult educators like Paulo Freire (2020) and Miles Horton (1990), who boldly suggested that people who experience marginalization and oppression understand deeply and intimately how systems work, and how these systems work against some people. Post-structural understandings of power are also important to reframing power and resistance as complicated processes present in most interactions between and among people (Baines, 2017; Nixon, 2019). Allyship also understands competition and individualism as contributing to oppression. Therefore, it is safe to suggest that in order to help eliminate oppression, a move away from individualism and a return to collectivism and collaboration is necessary (Baines, 2017; Bishop, 2020).

One of the consistent understandings present in allyship scholarship is the rejection of "experts" and "expertise" (Baines et al., 2022; Bishop, 2020). Instead, allyship requires a focus on relationships through which power sharing occurs, knowledge is constructed, and where diversity results in a wide range of epistemological orientations such as the idea of lived/living experience and the importance of these personal experiences (Arif et al., 2022; Sumerau et al., 2021; Wong and Vinsky, 2021).

Medical practitioners have particular expertise about specific subjects (e.g., diagnosis, biology, pharmacology); similarly, patients have experience living with particular health and wellness issues and navigating healthcare systems. Thus, when service providers and service recipients work together as allies, they are engaging in relationship building for the purpose of building shared understanding leading to shared action (Arif et al., 2022; Baines, 2022; Bishop, 2020; Nixon, 2019; Vinsky and Prevatt-Hyles, 2021).

Allyship is concerned with responding to the issues and concerns that present in the moment, as well as challenging the sources of these problems and engagement in prevention -- in some ways this is what healthcare is all about (Baines et al., 2022).

As an ally, service providers emphasize the capacity and capabilities of service users and support the empowerment of allies. Baines et al. (2022) suggests that "service users' lived experiences offer important insights and energy for them to challenge oppression against themselves by catalyzing and facilitating these processes..." (p. 10).

To make the most of these capacities, allies have a role to play in creating the spaces, places and time to support marginalized and oppressed people to create their own knowledge and understanding (Arif et al., 2022; Baines et al., 2022; Nixon, 2019). In a healthcare context, this might look like supporting a community groups' request to hold regular meetings in a healthcare space, or advocating for hiring a peer support staff member who can help patients navigate the system.

Allies have a role in creating change in the systems in which they operate or work; these are places where marginalized and oppressed people may not have the same level of access. To do this, allies require the capacity to engage in critical reflexive analysis in order to support these goals (Wong and Vinsky, 2021).

The Opportunity

What are the opportunities for creating change with critical allyship?

Critical Allyship

Contemporary critical understandings of allyship draw heavily on critical perspectives. As a result, critical allyship integrates lived experiences while also reflecting on the significance of structural factors as requiring the energy and response of allies. Baines et al. (2022) suggest that relationship, collaboration, and consistency are important aspects of successful allyship. Critical allyship emphasizes the action aspect of allyship, rather than simply seeing allyship as an identity based solely on awareness of issues and an openness to listening (Nixon, 2019; Sumerau et al., 2021).

Practical Activities for Becoming an Ally

Much of the critical allyship literature focuses on allyship as an ongoing, active, and participatory process (Arif et al., 2021; Baines, 2022; Nixon, 2019; Sumerau et al., 2021). Bishop (2015) frames allyship as a process of "becoming", always partial and incomplete, something that requires individuals to strive to achieve repeatedly, because of the changing nature and complexity of context and because of the multiple, over-lapping and intersecting realities of marginalization and oppression.

Allyship is also described as a form of "praxis" requiring those striving to achieve alliance to engage in a process of reflection in action and on action simultaneously (Baines et al., 2022; Bishop, 2020; Wong and Vinsky, 2021; Vinsky and Prevatt-Hyles, 2021). Committing and protecting time and resources dedicated to promoting and supporting these relationships are also important elements in making allyship a reality.

Critical reflexivity is fundamental to the process of praxis, and therefore, is a core element in the work of allyship. Critical reflection or knowledge of self is the first step in this process, but it is not enough to support critical allyship. Knowing who you are informs critical reflexivity, which is further concerned with the notion of context as a highly complex and multi-modal process. Context is imbued with the process of convergence which creates new layers of context as processes, places, people, histories, values, and beliefs come together in our daily interactions. Individuals who want to become critical allies must understand themselves, the context that they bring to their allyship, and how these work together to produce dynamic outcomes when they interact with other people who also bring themselves and their values, histories, beliefs, and understandings to the interaction.

When critical allies enter into these processes, their reflection moves from an individual process to one that is about connectedness and relationship. Through connection with others and discussion of the meaning of context, the norms, goals, objectives (and their sources) become implicated in how and whether the individual is able, prepared, willing and/or wanted as an ally. Some authors complicate the idea of critical reflection suggesting that it is a process that must link us back to social, professional, and contextual benchmarks (Baines, 2017; La Rose, 2017; Vinsky and Prevatt-Hyles, 2021; Taylor and White, 2001; Wong and Vinsky, 2021). These authors suggest that it is only through group processes that the answers to these rhetorical questions may be realized, in that the group is able to reflect on and consider whether actions and engagement meet the norms and expectations embedded in the group itself and in the broader social context.

Pause and Reflect

While this all sounds very complicated, beginning with your own experiences is perhaps the best place to start. Many authors have suggested that self-questioning is an important place to begin in the process of allyship (Vinsky and Prevatt-Hyles, 2021; Taylor and White, 2001; Wong and Vinsky, 2021). Drawing on this long history of questioning, considering how you have come to be in this process of becoming a critical ally is one way to begin to understand the conscious and subconscious contexts that come with you into these interactions. Drawing on questions developed by Bishop (1994/2020), we have devised a reflective exercise consisting of questions for allies working in the healthcare sector to consider and reflect upon.

- What are your own experiences of allyship and collaboration in your role as a healthcare provider? Who has supported you in a time of need? How has this support presented itself? Who have you chosen to support? How have you demonstrated support? Take a moment to reflect and consider these questions:
  - What strengths and challenges do you bring to the process of allyship? What additional knowledge or resources do you need to succeed in supporting patients in your role as a healthcare professional?
  - What do you know about the health and social care system(s) you work in? What spaces and places for allyship have you identified within these systems? What spaces remain unknown or inaccessible and why?

Once you have an overview of allyship in your healthcare role generally, deeper reflection about you in your role and the context of your role in individual interventions becomes important. These understandings help critical allies to deeply consider the way in which their identity, role, and their interaction with patients can be spaces for creating deeper relationships and understandings that enhance allyship or potentially foreclose these opportunities. Eric Shragge (2007), a longstanding community organizer in Quebec, Canada, suggests that this deeper concept of critical reflexivity begins with 3 important questions which we have adapted to the healthcare context:

1) Who am I?
2) Who am I as a [medical/healthcare professional]?
3) Who am I in this interaction/intervention?

The first question requires sharing or making conscious something about ourselves and how we see ourselves. The second question asks practitioners to think about ourselves in the professional role that we have taken on: what kind of healthcare professional are you, and within that category, what kind of professional are you? For example, if you are a psychiatrist, are you following the teachings of Sigmund Freud, or are you more aligned with Carl Jung? What training schemas do you bring to practice from the school where you received your education? What theories have you little exposure/experience with? What theories do you embrace and what theories do you reject? And to each of these questions you may also want to ask *why*?

When considering the question: *Who am I in this interaction/intervention?*, reflecting on the framework that you enter into through the context of your role is important. Working in an emergent context, like emergency department service is different from working in a clinic that provides ongoing/long-term voluntary service for example as a primary healthcare provider; understanding the difference in these roles is part of engaging appropriately with patients. Similarly, completing a mandatory visit for an insurance investigation is different than providing services to a person who comes seeking support for what they perceive to be a new and evolving problem. Understanding the purposes and goals of the intervention tells you something about your role and should therefore inform the way in which you interact with the patient and the manner in which allyship may develop in/from these interactions. Understanding your role allows you to demystify the techniques and practices you use as you work with patients.

In addition to Shragge's three questions, there are a few critical questions for further consideration that may help you to think more deeply about your healthcare professional education and the educational scheme that you bring to practice. These two additional questions shed some light on what is commonly understood as the silent or hidden curriculum in medicine (Pourbairamian et al., 2022) and the presence of situated knowledge that creates an intertextuality that flows from the formal curriculum into healthcare professionals' daily practice (Sakamoto and Pinter, 2005) (see Chapters 2-4).

These questions are:

- Who am I as an alumnus of X Medical School/Post-Secondary Program?
- Can I trust my education?

These questions invite those seeking to become allies to reflect on the origins of the knowledge and beliefs embodied as part of formal education as well as reminding us that learning is temporal in nature. What we learn as correct and desirable in time and place, is just that, bound in time and place while knowledge is something that changes, is built upon and may be challenged by new and emerging perspectives.

The temporal nature of professional education has the potential to shape how we understand some of the marginalized and oppressed groups with whom healthcare professional are seeking alliance. The temporal and proximal realities of where we get our education are significantly influenced by the sociopolitical context of the institution in which we received our medical education and training and when we received our education (see Chapters 1-4). Professional schools shape their curriculum around a set of values and beliefs articulated in the school's mission and mandate. Schools respond to community values, needs and wants, and to the needs, wants and values of governors, government, alumnae and funding bodies. These change from time to time and from place to place.

There are many examples of significant changes in the practice of medicine and the understandings of truths, facts and knowledge within healthcare curriculum. Changes in what we understand as the truths, facts and knowledges within education change what we believe and the way we practice – but it requires exposure to this "new" material in order to make these changes possible. This often means that healthcare professionals need to unlearn and relearn as they undertake ongoing professional development activities. Some examples of these types of changes include the promotion of eugenics and the forced sterilization of developmentally disabled, Indigenous and Black people – which is now understood as based on faulty science and as criminal in nature (Dyck, 2013); the framing of LGBTQ+ identities as mental illness and the resulting incarceration, forced hospitalization and treatment of LGBTQ peoples – which is now understood as unethical and harmful (Rose, 2016); the presumption of predispositions to certain stigmatized mental health issues among racialized individuals and the over diagnosis of psychotic disorders in these populations – which continues to be a challenge in practice in spite of statistical, experiential and scientific evidence to the contrary (Schwartz and Blankenship 2014).

For many decades science has maintained that its virtue comes from its unique and ubiquitous capacity to eliminate bias and to create objective facts and knowledge. Increasingly, in a post-structural world we are embracing the idea that science simply introduces new forms of bias and that all knowledge has situated meaning bound by context and interpretation (May, 2021). Allies think about context and the poly-contextual nature of our understanding as they travel both in terms of locality and temporality, and seek out additional professional development in order to maintain good professional currency. Be willing to sometimes let go of what you thought you knew.

Building on these ideas of the poly-contextual nature of what we know and how we know it, the issue of "systemic chatter" (Vinsky and Prevatt-Hyles, 2021) is also an important facet of critical allyship. We experience systemic chatter ambiently as we go through the world picking up social cues about meaning making, but we may experience it more acutely when we engage in practice within institutional settings or within organizational contexts.

Systemic chatter may be defined as a metaphor that reminds people who are seeking to engage in anti-oppressive practice and allyship about what is wanted by the dominant culture in terms of maintaining the status quo (Vinsky and Prevatt-Hyles, 2021). Healthcare professionals are surrounded by symbols, signs, and other discursive tools that promote particular readings and understandings of organizational processes that generally promote continuation of the status quo.

Systemic Chatter

Systemic chatter can have undue influence on the way healthcare providers (and other helping professionals) assess and eventually frame their work and thus their decision making. For example, if a local hospital system elects to place a poster about *bed-flow and wait times* in a prominent location within a clinical area, healthcare providers and patients are invited to interpret the poster as part of the messaging of the clinical encounter (Rapoport, 1990). Messages about systems issues such as funding, efficiency, resource allocation, institutional liability, deserving and underserving patients and flow targets can have a significant influence on how healthcare professionals see and understand their role; similarly it influences how patients understand their meaning in the healthcare encounter.

Continuing with our example, a poster about "patient flow" placed prominently in a clinical area means that information about patient flow becomes the kind of internal definition of desired practice constituted by hospital administration – perhaps to the exclusion of other things that are not displayed in posters on the wall.

The hospital administration has a point, *but* healthcare providers and patients want to be able to move through the system, *giving* and *receiving the right kind of care* – not just to be pushed through in a manner akin to a conveyor belt. Without enough resources to move people through the system as they access the right kind of care, the messages about patient flow downloads the expectation of patient movement onto singular parts of the system (e.g., the Emergency Department) and to individual care providers who are trying to make decisions about the level of service needed by patients. Reflecting on how "systemic chatter" can shift our understanding of our role in an intervention and using that reflection as a way of reclaiming a broader understanding of care that includes our personal commitment to our profession and our profession's framing of practice goals, is part of engaging as a critical ally.

Understanding the Social Environment

Another aspect of critical allyship is understanding the social environment within which we practice and service users and patients receive care. When we talk about critical allyship, we are concerned about social issues, social problems and the people who are affected and implicated within these social processes. In this section we utilize mental illness to explore the significance of the social construction of illness and healthcare responses as well as considering the importance social context plays in shaping these understanding. While mental illness is the example used, similar vulnerabilities are exposed when the same approach to analysis is used to consider other health conditions. For example, poverty, minority stress (such as racism) and trauma, as well as limited access to fresh food (for example, living in a food desert) can amplify individual risk factors for type 2 diabetes, so understanding how to read social context in to patient experiences is an important part of allyship.

Social issues and social problems are socially constructed; they are named and framed by the communities and societies in which we live and work. Value systems and social norms, or what might also be described as "world views" are fundamental to the creation of social problems. These definitions change over time and so do the social attitudes that surround them. To bring this idea to life, think about previous attitudes towards smoking, a habit endorsed by physicians in the 1950s that is now seen as a dangerous and life limiting activity. Similarly, same sex marriage and cannabis use were both seen as immoral actions in the recent past; but both were legalized in Canada in the recent past.

Defining the terms "social issue" and "social problems" are an important way of identifying how these processes work and how they are related to critical allyship. Social problems are understood as phenomena that are socially constructed, societal in nature, affect a lot of people but can be improved through action (Baines, 2017). Similarly, social issues are phenomena that have not yet become social problems but are beginning to affect a mass of people that is likely to evolve into a social problem if prevention activities are not undertaken to modify the context.

The way that social issues and social problems are constructed often leads to the development of specific interventions designed to respond to these problems most effectively. In some instances, we may describe these as evidence-based practices, or simply as "best practices". The design of the solution follows very closely behind the social construction of these issues. For example, if a society believes that people abuse healthcare services and seek mental health services when they are not really needed, we might solve this problem by trying to prevent or discourage patients from using these services – except in very specific circumstances such as when there is imminent risk to self or others. We might also educate service providers to ration services, or to disqualify or screen out people who they feel might be overusing the system. However, if we frame risk in a more generous way, and suggest that resources will be allocated in response to need, then we would refocus the issues and concerns that healthcare providers emphasize.

To reinforce the idea that generosity (rather than scarcity) is a possibility in healthcare policy, consider the healthcare funding model in some jurisdictions. For example, in Canada, **until 1990** the funding model that supported provincial healthcare systems *provided dollar for dollar matching funds for healthcare expenditures* recognized under the Canada Health Act without any funding caps. Scarcity is enacted as part of healthcare policy; it is part of the social construction of social problems.

Social problems and issues are socially constructed, which makes the idea of processes like mental illness more complicated and complex. If we believe that mental illnesses are biological phenomena produced by physical and biological processes, then we can safely say that mental illnesses are *not* a social problem. However, if we look at the social effects of mental illness which include personal, physical, and emotional suffering, difficulty engaging in normative social activities such as living independently, and as something that may result in unemployment or eviction, we can see how quickly mental illness is wrapped up in other social problems like homelessness. Reexamining the social environment and reframing the issues allows deeper appreciation for the role of critical allyship in responding to experiences of oppression.

Most people do not believe that mental illness is simply a biological process. Rather they believe there are many complex elements that go into the making of mental illness that include some biological factors and a very long list of economic, social, emotional, and political factors that come together to produce mental illness – which affects a lot of people (about 20% of the population), but can be improved with intervention (CMHA, 2021).

Figure 13.1 illustrates how analysis of mental illness can be made more complex when we consider the social influences that affect the presence of mental illness and the way in which it is experienced by individuals and the community. Understanding mental illness as a social problem opens the door to multiple forms of intervention and prevention, and points to some of the ways that allies can work in partnership with people living with the experience of mental illness.

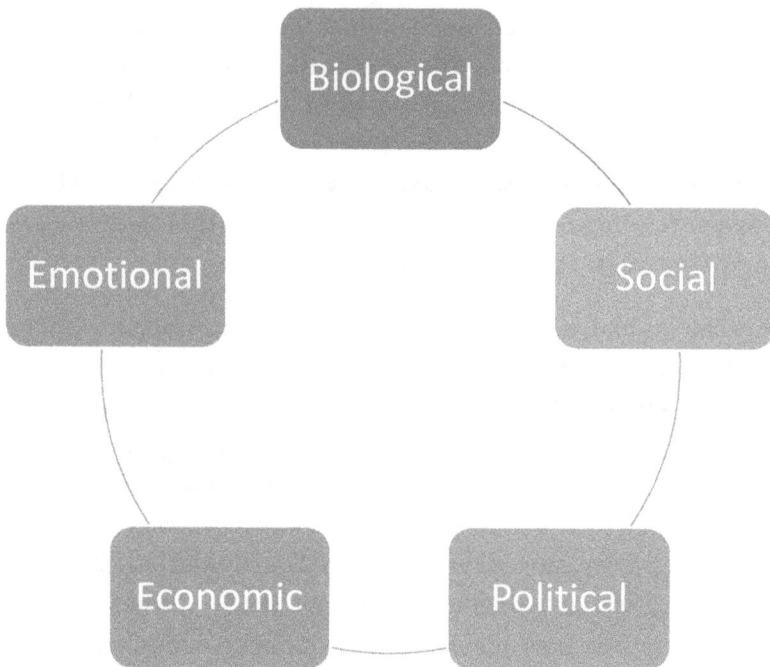

Figure 13.1. *A social problem approach to mental health*

As critical allies, if we think about our role in responding to mental illness, we can see that the most powerful and dominant voices framing mental health as a social problem are not the voices of the people who are most acutely affected by this social phenomenon. In most psychiatry departments there are few if any physicians who identify as having a serious mental illness. Similarly, there are few hospital systems where members of senior leadership have disclosed mental health conditions, just as there are very few universities training healthcare professionals where instructors and professors share stories of their own experiences of mental illness. Yet, if 20% of the population experiences mental illness, it is statistically impossible for *no one* in these contexts to have lived experience of mental illness (CMHA, 2021).

Without lived experiences being shared or brought to light in the personal and professional contexts, it is likely that we are missing important knowledge about lived experiences such as that of living with mental illness. If no one is willing to disclose because of the persisting stigma of mental illness, then it is necessary to find other ways to include these voices in order to understand how critical allyship can inform mental health practices. Developing processes by which people want to share their identities and lived experiences for the purpose of enhanced understanding and service is part of the work of critical allyship. Is it time to take a risk?

Understanding Community and Community Functions

The first step in understanding the communities we wish to serve as allies is unearthing the experiential knowledge, the "lived experience" present in our communities; for many privileged allies, this is in part a matter of "showing up" (Selvanathan et al., 2021). The idea of *showing up* means making the time and engaging the effort to be present at community events, activities, and gatherings to listen and learn more about social issues and problems of concern. Showing up means being present *and* opening yourself up; exposing yourself to knowledge and information that you may not already know and that may challenge some of the assumptions and beliefs that we hear as systemic chatter and that we hold dear as part of our professional identity. For the people with whom you wish to be allies, showing up is a practical action that reflects the allies' willingness to spend their time and energy on an issue that may not affect them directly.

Allies may not receive much attention or even be noticed when they first start showing up, but showing up repeatedly has meaning and will eventually lead to being recognized at the very least, as a familiar face. Being familiar may be the first step to becoming an ally. Doing the "grunt work", folding flyers, setting up chairs, cleaning up after coffee is served or emptying the trash at the end of the event is another way of showing up and it has particular meaning when you are someone who is understood to hold a privileged social standing – if this comes from a sincere place of wanting to be present, it sends a message of humility. For many marginalized groups who have little funding or support, practical help means a lot – proving yourself through a willingness to do this kind of practical work is part of the process of building trust and relationships, and may lead to deeper and richer involvement.

The next most important step, according to many community activists and critical allies is "shutting up" (Baines, 2022; Bishop, 2020; Selvanathan et al., 2020). Because the voices of affected people are rarely the most dominant voices, one of the roles of an ally is to make space for the voices of those affected by the issues, and amplifying or promoting those voices within your own sphere of influence rather than taking up the space yourself. A great example of promoting voices is the work of Brian Goldman (2023), the host of a Canadian radio podcast, "White Coat, Black Art". Goldman's podcast tells the story of healthcare from "the other side of the gurney". Goldman invites care recipients and other professionals who provide allied healthcare (no pun intended) to explore and explain the meaning of care with a particular emphasis on innovations that challenge some of the hierarchical elements present in healthcare systems and in professional identities.

Inclusion Strategies

How Do We Build Spaces for Critical Allyship?

If one of the key roles of an ally is amplifying the voices of the people we wish to support and help, then we might understand allies to bring important resources to the cause when they open up new spaces, places, and audiences to the voices of people affected by social issues and social problems. Allies circulate in communities that may be unique (but overlapping) with those of the people they wish to serve. Therefore, using influence and resources to create spaces for allyship and for those most deeply affected by the social problem is important. In making this space, you may want to think about how to support those with whom you are aligned to engage, educate, and have voice. That being said, it is important to get buy-in, sanction, and support from the community you wish to serve before initiating any work on your own (Baines, 2022; Bishop, 2020; Selvanathan et al., 2020).

To begin this process, the literature suggests you should engage in critical reflexivity to inventory the spaces, places, and organizations to which you have access and to consider how you might use these resources to support allyship goals based on the needs and wants of the community. For example, a psychiatrist concerned with the issues of mental health stigma might begin by considering where they work and what committees, teams, groups, or other spaces and places may exist to support allyship efforts. Dr. Francine Grant might try to get other trans people who are not necessarily physicians to sit on some of the committees at the local health authority, or on some of the national and international committees on which she serves; she might ask trans patients to do the same within the local health authority. This would take the pressure off Francine by helping the institutions she works in to hear the voices of trans people who do not hold the high social position of a doctor and to think about how their lived experience and narrative provides new and different understanding beyond what Francine knows.

Few organizations operate alone; most organizations are linked into networks, affiliate groups, and associations that represent issues and concerns to a range of constituents, often in the context of geographic settings such as local, regional, national, or international levels. Tapping into these networks and considering how the various levels (or layers of the organization) become institutional or organizational allies by providing spaces, resources, and opportunities to educate, organize, or engage in knowledge mobilization is another form of allyship. For example, most regions where individuals must travel long distances to seek medical treatment have organizations or agencies that provides resources and supports to health travelers.

Communities often have cultural groups or services (e.g., Native Friendship Centre, Women's Centre, Cancer Assistance Program) that provide services or supports to individuals based on certain aspects or types of identity (culture/ethnicity, gender, type of illness). These organizations provide services locally but are often also affiliated with national organizations providing certain types of services in a local context, and/or may use a national approach to service. Dr. Vida must refer patients out of the local area, often requiring patients to travel long distances to receive care. By creating relationships with service organizations in the receiving community, Dr. Vida may be able to provide patients with important supports by referring them to both the healthcare provider or facility and community resources that are a part of ensuring wellbeing. Forming these relationships takes time and effort, but the time and effort would likely produce better outcomes for the patients she serves and would enhance their trust in Dr. Vida.

Mentoring

Most successful healthcare professionals have received mentoring from other successful people along their path. The guidance, support, connections, and resources provided by mentors, formal and informal, help to facilitate access to opportunities that are likely to produce desired end results. For example, being able to ask an instructor or professor for a letter of reference, or being briefed on how best to answer potential job interview questions.

For many people who experience marginalization or oppression, access to mentors may be limited or may require a lot of cultivation, which means extra work, extra risk and the potential of rejection for marginalized and oppressed people who already face day to day challenges and stresses. Another potential critical practice of allyship is stepping up as a mentor for someone who comes from an equity-deserving community who may find it challenging to make connections otherwise. Mentorship is discussed in greater detail in Chapter 4.

As a critical ally, there are options for engaging in mentoring and considering mentoring as a long-term investment that follows a spectrum or an evolutionary process as a helpful schema, with the possibility of the relationship evolving into one of sponsorship, collaboration and/or partnership. In instances where a mentorship turns into a sponsorship, allies often engage in a process of challenging systemic processes. Mobilizing resources to support the work of marginalized collaborators is an important way of demonstrating support for equity-deserving persons while creating examples and resources that may be used to support ongoing/future collaboration.

Nixon (2019) suggests that mentoring is really the first phase in the process of supporting marginalized people to succeed in systems that have long blocked their participation. Mentors are described as teachers who support and share knowledge with protégés. Critical allies build relationships or trust and respect with individuals who might eventually be open to engaging with the mentor as a protégé, seeking to understand the knowledge of a mentor, even if they do not blindly accept all they share.

Mentors can transform their relationship with a protégé into one of collaboration when they seek to sponsor this individual by resourcing or mobilizing resources to support their advanced participation and engagement in the system. As collaborators, critical allies can expand this resource to support marginalized and oppressed people within their community to participate more actively and consistently within the system. Modelling collaboration is modelling change in institutions where hierarchy is the norm. In this traditional setting bound by hierarchy, the norm is for a retained power and resource balance on the part of the mentor over the duration of the relationship.

Critical allies also engage in critical considerations of succession planning. If you are in a position that affords you some power and privilege, who are you supporting to take over your role in the future? By mentoring, sponsoring, and collaborating with individuals from marginalized and equity deserving groups, you can ensure they have a seat at the table well into the future. Succession planning is an important part of allyship.

Vignette Wrap-up

As a critical ally in the trans community, Dr. Francine Grant understands that her status as a medical doctor gives her considerable power, credibility, and socioeconomic status to which many other trans people in the community do not have access. Francine's analysis of her self-identity, professional identity, and the role she was being asked to occupy as a guest speaker led her to understand that if change within the medical system was to take place, she needed to find a way to expand the voices reflecting the lived experiences of trans people within the healthcare system. To achieve this goal, Francine worked with a local LGBTQ+ community group to start a "speakers training program" called Trans Toast Masters.

The Trans Toast Masters group has built slowly over the last couple of years. Now when Francine is asked to speak, she either requests that the organization elects to have a "panel" of speakers and attends together with members of the group, or she defers the offer to the speakers' club and can say with confidence that the group is ready, willing, and able to respond to these requests.

Connection with the LGBTQ+ community group has also supported Francine in networking with organizations in other communities to refer out of area speaker requests to these organizations. When Francine does elect to serve as a speaker, she encourages those who make the request to make donations to these organizations so that she can continue to support the community in practical ways.

Dr. Vida began consulting with other practitioners working in rural and remote communities to better understand the context of distance referrals and to understand resources for supporting the resourcing of the clinical spaces in which she practiced. After joining an online community and sharing some of her knowledge and expertise, she began to better understand how rural and remote practitioners work to consult with each other and with experts outside of the local community to best care for patients in place. Included in this, Dr. Vida has attended some local healing events where traditional practices have been discussed as a way of demonstrating that traditional care and medical care can be collaborative and complementary activities.

Dr. Vida also worked with the health authority and local community groups to apply for grants to better equip her clinic to provide health consultations remotely. Dr. Vida has used the close-knit nature of the community to help work with community groups, to try to mobilize resources, apply for grants, and improve the conditions and resourcing of the community so that her clinic is more comfortable and inviting for patients. This included the development of an art gallery in the clinic that showcases the work of local artists on a rotating basis, which brings the community into the clinic and makes patients want to see what is on display in the office! By *showing up* in the community, local people feel more secure that Dr. Vida cares about local people, is committed to the community and is there for the long haul.

Key Takeaways

This chapter on allyship has presented a number of ideas designed to provide practical suggestions as well as a theoretical foundation for thinking about allyship. The following key takeaways are action-oriented steps that healthcare professionals who are seeking to become critical allies can use to begin this process:

- Critical reflection and critical reflexivity are fundamental to becoming an ally.
- Considering the social construction of social issues and social problems broadens the potential for change making.
- Showing up, shutting up, honouring and amplifying the voices of marginalized and oppressed people is important allyship work.
- Unlearning and relearning are a part of the allyship process; this may be a challenge that includes giving up long-held beliefs and approaches to make room for new knowledge and understandings.
- Understanding the networks surrounding the organizations you work within allows you to use these networks to meet your allyship goals and to amplify the resources that exist within this system to benefit marginalized and oppressed populations.
- Understanding the places, spaces and systems you work in will allow you to use your power and influence to mobilize resources and supports and to create systemic change that benefits marginalized and oppressed individuals and groups.
- Allies engage in mentoring to support the success of members of marginalized and oppressed groups.
- Succession planning can be part of allyship.

Conclusion

Allyship is a way of engaging in social change making that centers collaboration with equity-deserving individuals and groups. Allyship in healthcare contexts is an active process of creating social change and enhancing social justice as a process shared with groups and individuals who have life experience of marginalization and oppression. Perspectives of allyship and critical allyship require practitioners to interrogate what they know and how they know it, the standards of their profession and workplaces, as well as the responses of those with whom they wish to become allies.

The questions and reflective activities contained in this chapter are included to support healthcare professionals preparing for engagement in the practice of critical allyship. Remembering that allyship is an ongoing process of becoming that requires practice is an important way of framing the practice of allyship.

On a Parting Note...

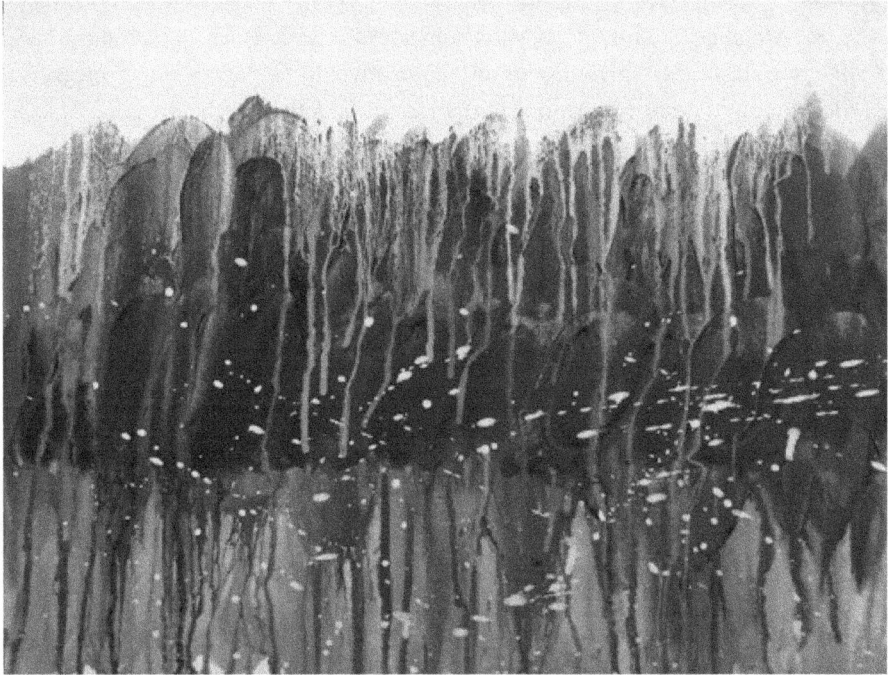

Original artwork by second author, Albina Veltman

References

Arif, S., Afolabi, T., Mitrzyk, B.M., Thomas, T.F., Borja-Hart, N., Wade, L. and Henson, B. (2022) 'Engaging in authentic allyship as part of our professional development', *American Journal of Pharmaceutical Education*, 86(5).

Baines, D. (2017). Resistance in and outside the workplace: Ethical practice and managerialism in the voluntary sector', in *Practical social work ethics*. Oxfordshire: Routledge, pp. 239-256.

Baines, D. (2022). *Doing Anti-Oppressive Social Work, 4ᵗʰ Ed.: Rethinking Theory and Practice*. Halifax: Fernwood Publishing.

Bishop, A. (2020). *Becoming an ally: Breaking the cycle of oppression in people*. Halifax: Fernwood Publishing.

Bishop, A. (1994). *Becoming an ally: Breaking the cycle of oppression*. Halifax: Fernwood Publishing.

Cambridge Dictionary. (2023). *English Dictionary* [online]. Available from: https://dictionary.cambridge.org/dictionary/english/

Canadian Mental Health Association [CMHA]. (2021). *Fast facts about mental health and mental illness; Mental health and mental illness: What's the difference?*[online]. Available from: https://cmha.ca/brochure/fast-facts-about-mental-illness/

Dyck, E. (2013). *Facing eugenics: Reproduction, sterilization, and the politics of choice*. Toronto: University of Toronto Press.

Freire, P. (2020). Pedagogy of the oppressed, in *Toward a Sociology of Education*. Oxfordshire: Routledge, pp. 374-386.

Horton, M. and Freire, P. (1990). *We make the road by walking: Conversations on education and social change*. Philadelphia: Temple University Press.

Kendall, M. (2020). *Hood feminism: notes from the women that a movement forgot*. New York: Viking.

La Rose, T. (2017). Digital media stories through multimodal analysis: A case study of erahoneybee's song about a child welfare agency', in *Methods for Analyzing Social Media*. Oxfordshire: Routledge, pp. 156-168.

May, J. (2021). 'Bias in science: Natural and social'. *Synthese*, 199(1-2), pp. 3345-3366.

Nixon, S.A. (2019). The coin model of privilege and critical allyship: Implications for health', *BMC Public Health*, 19(1), pp.1-13.

Pourbairamian, G., Bigdeli, S., Arabshahi, S.K.S., Yamani, N., Sohrabi, Z., Ahmadi, F. and Sandars, J. (2022). Hidden curriculum in medical residency programs: A scoping review', *Journal of Advances in Medical Education & Professionalism*, 1990(2), p. 69.

Rapoport, A. (1990). The Meaning of the Built Environment: A Nonverbal Communication Approach. Beverley Hills: Sage Publications.

Rose, D. (2016). We are all mentally ill: grassroots efforts to provide LGBTQ affirmative psychotherapy & social services, 1960-1987: Oral History Project, Seattle, Washington. Master's Thesis, Smith College, Northampton.

Sakamoto, I., and Pitner, R. O. (2005). Use of critical consciousness in anti-oppressive social work practice: Disentangling power dynamics at personal and structural levels, *The British Journal of Social Work*, 35(4), pp. 435-452.

Schwartz, R.C. and Blankenship, D.M. (2014). Racial disparities in psychotic disorder diagnosis: A review of empirical literature, *World journal of Psychiatry*, 4(4), p. 133.

Selvanathan, H. P., Lickel, B., and Dasgupta, N. (2020). An integrative framework on the

impact of allies: How identity-based needs influence intergroup solidarity and social movements, *European Journal of Social Psychology*, 50(6), pp. 1344–1361.

Shragge, E. (2007). In and against" the community: Use of self in community organizing, p.p. 159 – 179. In, D. Mandell (ed.) *Revisiting the use of self: Questioning professional identities*. Toronto: Canadian Scholars' Press.

Sumerau, J.E., Forbes, T.D., Grollman, E.A. and Mathers, L.A. (2021). Constructing allyship and the persistence of inequality', *Social Problems*, 68(2), pp. 358-373.

Taylor, C., and White, S. (2001). Knowledge, truth and reflexivity: The problem of judgment in social work', *Journal of Social Work*, 1(1), pp. 37-59.

Vinsky, J. and Prevatt-Hyles, D. (2021). Anti-Black racism education in human service organizations: The Liberation Practice International (LPI) critical reflective practice model–"The LPI Model"', in J. Fook (ed.) *Practicing Critical Reflection in Social Care Organisations*. Oxfordshire: Routledge, pp. 49-80.

Wong, Y.L.R. and Vinsky, J. (2021). Beyond implicit bias: Embodied cognition, mindfulness, and critical reflective practice in social work, *Australian Social Work*, 74(2), pp. 186-197.

Chapter 14
The Moral Imperative to Redress the Equity Balance

Marissa Joseph, MD

❖

"Wrong does not cease to be wrong because the majority share in it."
—Leo Tolstoy, 1882

❖

Abstract: Equity in medicine is a moral imperative that must be addressed in order to ensure that all people receive fair, accessible, equitable, and non-discriminatory care. In order to address these inequities, institutions and leaders must (1) provide safe spaces for dialogue, (2) facilitate a culture shift that embeds equity, diversity and inclusion (EDI) into the institutional climate, (3) shift away from tokenism of the corporate scorecard, and (4) embed the language of microaffirmations into clinical education and leadership. This chapter will explore these four aspects of equity and the moral imperative to redress the equity balance in the field of medicine, with particular attention to the role of intentionality, and the concept of equity as an institutional brand within the spheres of clinical education, leadership, and institutional identity.

Keywords: brand, culture, diversity, equity, inclusion, injustice, intentionality, institution, justice, medicine, microaffirmations

Introduction: Inequity in Medicine

Medicine is a field of paramount responsibility. A great deal of trust is placed onto medical professionals to care for the health and wellbeing of others by deploying limited healthcare resources in a fiscally and ethically responsive manner. Thus, medical stewardship comes with some key accountabilities at all levels, from the frontline up through the ranks to systems administrators. As illustrated in preceding chapters, the ethical conduct of the profession has been variable over time, with some key gaps increasingly being revealed. Specifically, the field of medicine has been one of inequity and disparity for certain populations. Established structures and practices within the field have perpetuated harm and injustice for many. This has been seen in the lack of representation of minority groups in medical education and leadership, the lack of access to high-quality healthcare for marginalized populations, and the lack of consideration of the effects of structural racism on individuals and groups.

Equity is an important concept in medical practice because it ensures that all individuals, regardless of race, gender, religion, or any other differences, are treated fairly and have access to quality healthcare. However, due to the history of racism, medicine has not been a field of equity. It has been steeped in bias and prejudice, leading to a lack of access to quality healthcare for racialized persons. This has led to disparities in health outcomes, including lower life expectancy and higher rates of morbidity and mortality.

The embodiment of racism in medicine dates back to the early 1800s. The medical profession has traditionally been dominated by "white, male, middle-class professionals" who have held a monopoly on the tools and knowledge necessary to provide healthcare (Byrd and Clayton, 2001). This has led to a systemic marginalization of the voices and experiences of racialized populations. Moreover, racialized people were often excluded from medical education and training. This exclusion was further compounded by the fact that medical professionals often held racist views about non-White populations. These racist views, combined with a lack of access to healthcare, led to worse health outcomes for under-represented communities (Byrd and Clayton, 2001). Despite advances in medical technology, medical care, and medical education, disparities in access to medical care remain a pervasive problem. Those at the wrong end of the equity imbalance are still more likely to receive lower quality care, and are also more likely to be diagnosed with and suffer from preventable and treatable illnesses (Mahajan et al., 2021).

Furthermore, there is ongoing lack of diversity among medical professionals, which further contributes to inequity.

Defining Equity

In order to address the moral imperative to redress the equity balance in the field of medicine, it is important to first define what is meant by equity. The World Health Organization (WHO, 2023) defines equity, as "the absence of avoidable, unfair and remediable differences among groups of people, whether those groups are defined socially, economically, demographically, or geographically or by other dimensions of inequality (e.g., sex, gender, ethnicity, disability, or sexual orientation)". Thus, individuals should not be denied access to medical care based on their background and identity. Additionally, this definition implies that any disparities in access to medical care should be identified and addressed.

Health and access to healthcare are fundamental human rights (WHO, 2023), thus addressing health injustice in the field of medicine is an ethical obligation. Inequity in medicine is unacceptable given the implications for health status, health outcomes and self-actualization. Together, these implications drive the moral imperative to redress the equity balance in medicine.

The Issues

The Impact of Social Determinants on Health

❖

"These inequities in health, avoidable health inequalities, arise because of the circumstances in which people grow, live, work, and age, and the systems put in place to deal with illness."
—WHO, 2008

❖

It is important to recognize the role that social determinants of health play in influencing access to healthcare. Social determinants of health are factors such as socioeconomic status, education, employment, housing, and access to healthcare that shape an individual's health and can impact an individual's access to medical care. Individuals from lower socioeconomic backgrounds have lower access to quality healthcare than those from higher socioeconomic backgrounds (Bushnik et al., 2020). Additionally, individuals from certain racial and ethnic minorities have been found to have lower access to quality healthcare than those from majority racial and ethnic groups.

Action on social determinants of health to address health equity has been named a fundamental part of public health practice (Shahi et al., 2019). Furthermore, the Quintuple Aim includes health equity as one of the five components necessary to achieve quality improvement in healthcare (Nundy et al., 2022). As the Quintuple Aim, health equity is only achieved when everyone can attain their full potential for health and wellbeing (WHO, 2023).

Redressing the Equity Balance Requires Intentionality

Intentionality is essential in examining the structures of inequality in the field of medicine, as it allows for a critical analysis of the motivations and consequences of the existing systems. In doing so, it can provide insight into how change can be made, and what new structures and practices can be implemented to promote equity and justice.

Intentionality in anti-racism work is the conscious effort to embed anti-racism into all aspects of work, including decision-making, policy, practice, and culture. This can be seen in the way institutions, organizations, and individuals strive to create more equitable environments while actively dismantling systems of oppression. In order to create meaningful change, anti-racism work must be approached with understanding of the history and power dynamics that have allowed racism to persist. This understanding must be applied to the current context to develop strategies to counter racism. Intentionality in anti-racism work requires ongoing reflection on the impact of decisions and actions, and the commitment to make changes based on that reflection. A key concept in anti-racism work is "intersectional" thinking (Shahi et al., 2019). Intersectionality is defined as a framework for understanding how various aspects of a person's identity, such as race, gender, class, and other social categories, intersect and overlap, resulting in unique and complex experiences of oppression and privilege (Crenshaw, 1989).

The concept of intersectionality recognizes that racism is deeply intertwined with other oppressions such as classism, sexism, and ableism, and that these oppressions must be addressed to create equitable outcomes. Intentionality in anti-racism work is necessary to ensure that all forms of oppression are addressed, rather than just one form. Intentionality in anti-racism work also requires an understanding of the power dynamics that exist and how individuals and organizations can use their power to challenge racism.

Recognizing the role privilege plays in perpetuating racism can be used to impugn systems of oppression. It also includes understanding how systemic racism is perpetuated through institutional policies, practices, and culture, and how this can be challenged. In addition, intentionality in anti-racism work means actively engaging in dialogue with those who may have different perspectives or experiences of racism. This can be done through listening to and learning from the lived experiences of marginalized groups, as well as through engaging in difficult conversations about racism. Finally, intentionality in anti-racism work requires ongoing evaluation of progress. This includes tracking progress and outcomes, reflecting on the impact of decisions and actions, and making changes as needed to ensure that progress is being made towards a more equitable society.

Intentionality in anti-racism work is essential in order to create meaningful and lasting change. Analysis of the history and power dynamics that have allowed racism to persist, an intersectional approach to addressing oppressions, and an understanding of how privilege and power can be used to challenge racism. By engaging in intentional anti-racism work, individuals, organizations, and institutions can create more equitable outcomes and dismantle oppressive systems that are not solely limited to racial oppression.

Examining Long-Standing Structures and Practices

The first step towards addressing equity in the field of medicine is to examine long-standing structures and practices that continue to perpetuate inequities. Structural inequities are often hidden or ignored, as they are embedded in the culture and norms of an organization or society. Structural inequity can be defined as the systematic differences in access to resources and opportunities based on socially constructed categories such as race, gender, class, and sexual orientation (Harris and Pamukcu, 2020).

An intentional approach is essential to identify and challenge existing power structures and systems of oppression. This requires an understanding of how current practices and systems have been shaped by the history and culture of the institution, and how these systems have contributed to the marginalization of certain groups. It also requires an understanding of the impact of these structures and practices on the lives of those who are most affected by them. Additionally, it is important to recognize the role of institutional leaders in perpetuating these inequities and to identify ways in which they can be held accountable for their actions and the institutional history where reparation is necessary.

A Century of Inaction: Institutional Racism in Medical School Admission

- In 1918, a motion to ban Black students from the School of Medicine was adopted by Queen's University Senate in Kingston, Ontario, Canada.
- There were 15 Black medical students enrolled at Queen's when the ban was enacted.
- *Black students were not welcomed back until 1965.*
- *Although this anti-Black practice was no longer enforced after 1965, it remained on the books as policy until 2018,* after its existence was brought to light by Edward Thomas, a Cultural Studies PhD candidate.
- The ban was revoked by Senate 100 years after its adoption and Queen's University offered a public apology.

- One of those students was Ethelbert Bartholomew, a member of the class of 1918. After being expelled, Mr. Bartholomew worked as a porter for Canadian Pacific Railways and died in 1954.
- In a 2019 convocation ceremony, Queen's University conferred a posthumous Doctor of Medicine degree upon Dr. Bartholomew, which was accepted by members of his family (Queens Alumni Review, 2020).

Pause and Reflect

Queen's University Ban of Black Medical Students Repealed in 2018 (Queens Alumni Review, 2020)

1. Does this policy impact your view on the culture at this institution?
2. Although the exclusion of Black medical students was no longer enforced after 1965, the policy remained on the books until 2018 when it was brought to light by a student. Do you think the policy may have exerted any influence after 1965? Does the lack of enforcement alter the impact of discriminatory policies?
3. Are you aware of any discriminatory policies at your institution?

The Opportunity to Bridge the Equity Gap

❖

"Of all the forms of inequality, injustice in health is the most shocking and the most inhuman"
—Martin Luther King, 1966

❖

Redressing inequities in healthcare is an opportunity to level the playing field and create more equitable access to quality healthcare. Moreover, pursuing health justice is "doing the right thing" because it upholds the fundamental principles of fairness, equity, and respect for all individuals, most notably the concept that health and access to healthcare are fundamental human rights (WHO, 2023). In order to correct these inequities, there must be a comprehensive and collaborative effort between providers, payers, and policymakers to implement policies and practices that promote health equity. It is important to examine the underlying structures and practices that lead to disparities in healthcare, in order to develop strategies to address equity and promote inclusion. The opportunity to narrow the health equity gap entails an examination of the role of institutions and leaders (Section 14.5.1) and the role of healthcare providers (Section 14.5.2).

The Role of Institutions and Leaders

In order to effectively redress the equity balance, institutions and leaders must play a critical role. According to Barenboim et al. (2021), creating a safe space for dialogue is essential in fostering an environment of trust and respect that is necessary for meaningful change to occur. Institutional leadership have a responsibility to create safe spaces and promote dialogue around issues of equity, diversity, and inclusion (EDI). This is especially important in the field of medicine, where there is often a power imbalance between those in positions of power and those who are most affected by the existing systems.

It is imperative to create policies and procedures that enable an environment of respect and understanding, and create opportunities for those who have been traditionally marginalized to participate in the decision-making process. Furthermore, it is important for institutions and leaders to take a proactive approach to embedding EDI in the institutional climate. This can include training and resources for faculty and staff, particularly at critical juncture points such as initial appointment or recruitment, onboarding, and annual renewal of institutional appointments or privileges.

Institutions and leaders should utilize the principles of critical allyship to devise and implement EDI-focused policies, and create an environment where all individuals are respected and valued. Creating this type of culture can provide the foundation for further change as it allows for open dialogue and encourages honest discussions about the inequities. However, at all costs, institutions must avoid "diversity regimes" as these do not yield meaningful and sustainable transformation. Thomas (2018) describes diversity regimes as "a set of meanings and practices that *institutionalizes a benign commitment to diversity,* and in doing so obscures, entrenches, and *even intensifies existing racial inequality by failing to make fundamental changes in how power, resources, and opportunities are distributed"*. To this end, intention must be authentic and action carefully considered with a view towards transformation rather than short-term gains. Action on creating anti-oppressive climates can include:

i.   Mandating the implementation of initiatives such as cultural safety training, anti-discrimination policies, and diversity hiring initiatives.

ii. Developing a clear mission statement that outlines the commitment to EDI, providing diversity training and education for staff, and implementing EDI policies and procedures.

iii. Providing support for members of marginalized populations by offering resources such as counseling and mental health services, mentorship, and support groups.

iv. Facilitating open dialogue by creating a culture of inclusion and respect for all individuals. This can include hosting events such as town hall meetings, EDI workshops, and panel discussions to encourage open dialogue on the importance of EDI.

v.   Instituting changes in recruitment and hiring processes to ensure that they are equitable and diverse. The implementation of a *diversity monitor* may be instrumental in fostering critical dialogue within recruitment panels, with consistent use ideally coalescing in a reflexive and intentional institutional approach to recruitment and advancement.

vi. Embedding EDI in the institutional climate by developing a measurable EDI plan that outlines specific goals, objectives, and strategies for EDI. This plan should be evaluated and updated regularly to ensure that it is reflective of the current EDI needs of the institution. The plan should be embedded in the institution's strategic plan.

vii. Shifting institutional culture by engaging in proactive leadership and creating a shared understanding of EDI.

viii. Allocation of resources towards EDI initiatives and ensuring that they are properly staffed and funded.

ix. Institutions should establish a system of accountability to ensure that EDI policies and procedures are being implemented properly.

> To reiterate, at all costs, institutions must avoid "diversity regimes" as these are largely about checkboxes and scorecards and less about meaningful and sustainable action.

The above framework requires clear expectations for action on equity, diversity and inclusion (EDI), creating an environment where diverse perspectives are welcomed and respected, so that staff can actively engage in conversations about EDI. Additionally, medical institutions can ensure that their practices are equitable and inclusive by reviewing policies, procedures, and processes to ensure that they are not biased or discriminatory. The Queens University anti-Black policy that lay dormant from 1965 to repeal in 2018 underscores the necessity for active policy and procedure review to ensure safe spaces for staff, learners and patients.

The Role of Healthcare Providers

One example of a structural inequity in healthcare is the disproportionate representation of certain demographics in medical training and education. Studies have found that racial and ethnic minorities are underrepresented in medical schools (Williams et al., 2016). This lack of diversity in medical education can lead to a lack of cultural understanding and empathy when it comes to treating diverse patients. In order to address this structural inequity, institutions must ensure that their medical education programmes are accessible to all students, regardless of race, gender identity, ability, and socioeconomic status amongst other aspects of social identity. In addition, medical institutions must examine the implicit biases and stereotypes that are perpetuated in their culture and policies.

Implicit biases are unconscious schemas that form a mental shortcut of sorts, based on our past experiences, to quickly categorize people and situations. Implicit bias is defined as the attitudes or stereotypes that affect our understanding, actions, and decisions in an unconscious manner (Sabin, 2022). These beliefs can influence our decisions and behavior, often without us being aware of it. Devine (1989) noted biases based on racial stereotypes occur automatically and without conscious awareness even by persons who do not endorse racist beliefs. Studies have found that implicit bias can lead to disparities in healthcare, as providers may be more likely to provide different levels of care based on a patient's race or gender (Sabin, 2022). In order to address this issue, medical institutions must ensure that their policies and culture do not perpetuate any form of discrimination or bias.

This can be done in a number of ways. First, medical professionals must strive to be more aware of the history of racism in medicine and its effects on marginalized peoples. This awareness can foster analysis and ultimately strategic planning. Second, medical professionals must work to increase diversity among their ranks. Strategies include actively recruiting medical professionals from underrepresented backgrounds, offering scholarships and grants to medical students from underrepresented backgrounds, and ensuring that medical schools are providing an equitable and inclusive learning environment (Barnabe et al., 2023). Healthcare institutions directly affiliated with medical schools can influence and instrumentally support medical schools and residency training programs in these endeavours whilst also applying similar initiatives to their nursing and allied health professional programs and recruitment efforts.

Third, medical professionals must strive to provide equitable access to healthcare. This can be achieved in part through advocacy to reduce barriers to healthcare, such as cost and distance, as well as concrete action on cultural competence so as to provide culturally safe care and approach cultural humility. This requires understanding the unique needs of individuals, and providing care that is tailored to those needs. Cultural humility is an approach which incorporates self-questioning and immersion into patients' point of view, to work with individuals, families, and communities based upon respect of their culture and beliefs by using active listening and flexibility, which all serve to confront and address personal and cultural biases or assumptions (Kibakaya and Oyeku, 2022). It encompasses an attitude of openness and willingness to learn and understand other perspectives and values.

Cultural humility requires a commitment to self-examination, self-reflection, and a willingness to recognize, respect, and learn from the power dynamics that may exist between individuals and groups. It is important to recognize one's own privilege and power, and to actively seek to reduce health disparities. Finally, medical professionals must strive to reduce health disparities in under-represented populations. This can be done by increasing access to preventive care, providing more community-based care, and improving health literacy. Medical professionals must strive to create a more equitable healthcare system that is accessible and tailored to the needs of all individuals. By doing so, they can ensure that all people are able to receive the quality healthcare to which they are entitled as a fundamental right.

Clinical Vignette: The Story of Henrietta Lacks (Nature, 2020)

- Henrietta Lacks, a Black woman, died in 1951 at the age of 31 of cervical cancer.
- Her cervical cancer cells gave rise to the immortal **HeLa** cell line, after her treating physicians distributed samples of her cells **without her consent** to other researchers, who discovered their remarkable capacity to replicate and survive.
- Over time, the cells were shared extensively with other scientists across the globe, resulting in the immortal **HeLa** cells playing an extraordinary role in biologic research and clinical advancements that underpin much of modern medicine today (see Chapter 1).
- Henrietta Lacks' cells enabled multiple Nobel Prize–winning discoveries and medical advances for the treatment of countless medical conditions, including infections and cancer. Most recently, **HeLa** cells have been used in research for vaccines against the COVID-19 virus.

Clinical Vignette Analysis

- The injustice that characterizes Henrietta Lacks' story illustrates the racial inequities that are embedded in research and healthcare systems:

    o She did not have a voice and her body was used without her consent, granted this was not unusual for the prevailing social environment at the time, and Henrietta Lack's experience predated the Nuremberg Code and formalization of research ethics.

o   None of the biotechnology or other companies that profited from her cells passed any of the significant monetary gains or recognition back to her family.

o   Doctors and scientists repeatedly failed to ask her family for consent as they revealed her name publicly, gave her medical records to the media, and even published her genome.

Inclusion Strategies

❖

"Striving for racial equity- a world where race is no longer a factor in the distribution of opportunity- is a matter of social justice."
—Turner, 2016

❖

Equity as an Institutional Brand

Equity is not only smart business, but essential for business survival and success. Companies with a diversity of perspectives, ideas, and backgrounds are better equipped to understand the needs of their customers, develop innovative solutions, and compete in the global economy (Turner, 2016). The concept of equity as an institutional brand has been gaining traction in recent years as businesses look to move away from performative allyship and demonstrate a more meaningful commitment to social responsibility. Institutions must take concrete steps to ensure they are living up to their equity brand.

Equity as a brand embraces the concept of emphasizing fairness and ethical practices across all areas of operations. In a traditional business this includes everything from employee wages and benefits to customer service and product development. The goal is to create an environment of fairness and trust in which all stakeholders are treated equally and with respect. Equity as a brand is a concept that has also become increasingly important in medical institutions. Conceptualizing equity as a brand in healthcare crystallizes a commitment to provide quality care to all its patients, regardless of race, gender, socioeconomic status, or any other factor.

Equity as a brand is different from traditional corporate social responsibility initiatives, which often focus on short-term goals and ineffective tokenistic gestures. For example, mandating compulsory diversity training to encourage employees to examine their biases has short term impact and has been associated with animosity towards equity-seeking groups (Shahi et al., 2019). Instead, equity as a brand is intended to be a long-term commitment to creating an equitable and inclusive culture.

As the cultural and political landscape shifts, so have the ways medical institutions approach issues of equity. Traditionally, medical institutions have adopted tokenistic approaches to equity, such as providing access to care for minority populations or hiring staff from diverse backgrounds. However, this approach has been largely unsuccessful in promoting true equity and has instead perpetuated existing medical disparities. A more comprehensive and effective approach is needed to ensure that equity is no longer a tokenistic concept, but a true shift in vision.

To establish equity as a brand, medical institutions must first focus on identifying and addressing existing disparities in care such as inequities in access to care, in outcomes, and the patient experience. In addition, medical institutions must also focus on creating an inclusive environment for all staff and patients, regardless of background. This can be achieved through initiatives that create a diverse and inclusive workforce that ideally replicates the diversity of the population served, providing ongoing cultural safety training, and developing policies and procedures that promote equity. Once these steps have been taken, medical institutions must then create a comprehensive plan to promote equity as a brand. This includes utilizing marketing and promotional materials to spread awareness of the institution's commitment to equity, as well as implementing initiatives to ensure that equity is a part of all aspects of the institution's operations. Additionally, medical institutions must also focus on creating an environment of accountability and transparency, as this will ensure that any initiatives taken to promote equity are effective and sustainable.

By taking a comprehensive approach to addressing existing disparities and promoting an inclusive environment, medical institutions can ensure that equity is no longer a tokenistic concept, but one that is embedded in the core values of the institution. This means eliminating the corporate scorecard approach, which focuses on checking boxes to demonstrate corporate social responsibility, to one that focuses on daily practice. Shifting away from inauthentic and superficial allyship such as tokenism and towards a focus on EDI as an institutional brand can help to create a culture of equity that is truly embedded in the institutional climate (Zheng, 2023). This approach should focus on creating an equitable environment that is accessible to all individuals, regardless of race, gender, or any other differences.

Leaders should also be aware of the power dynamics in their organization and work to ensure that all individuals are treated with respect and given the same opportunities. Look around the C-suite (i.e., corporate executives) in healthcare organizations- who sits around the table and how did they get there? What characterizes in-group membership at the C-suite level and successive tables below the C-suite? What are the barriers to ascending from the lower-level ranks? Leaders reflecting on these questions will come closer to understanding the actual culture regardless of the intentions espoused. To be able to reflect on these questions is to be able to recognize the intention-action-reality gap and subsequently determine how real the institution's commitment to action on EDI. In the Canadian context, for example, there have been increased calls for organizations to consider action on EDI as an essential factor to success and sustainability in the COVID-19 Pandemic recovery efforts as exemplified in a recent statement by the Chief Commissioner of the Canadian Human Rights Commission (see Box 14.1).

"There have been renewed calls for action on these vital human rights issues as Canada continues to adapt to the new realities created by the pandemic.

...to ensure that Canada comes out of this crisis better than it went into it.

...and to ensure that no one is left behind.

For Canadian businesses, this shift means that to be a leader in your fields, you must also be a leader in anti-racism, diversity, equity and inclusion."
—MC Landry, Chief Commissioner, Canadian Human Rights Commission (Landry, 2021)

Box 14.1 *Leadership on equity, diversity and inclusion is critical to success*

Embedding the Language of Microaffirmations

Focusing on equity as an institutional brand requires a dynamic approach that deploys multiple strategies and tools. Microaffirmations can be used as part of the armament for shifting towards equity and justice. According to Molina et al. (2019), this shift can be facilitated by focusing on microaffirmations such as recognizing and celebrating the unique contributions of individuals which can help to create an institutional culture that is truly inclusive and equitable (see Box 14.2).

The use of microaffirmations can be a powerful tool in medical education, leadership, and institutional identity as well. Microaffirmations are positive and encouraging expressions of recognition, appreciation, and support for individuals, groups, and organizations. They emphasize the value and importance of all perspectives, throughout the power paradigm and can reinforce core values of inclusion. In addition to creating safe spaces and promoting dialogue, it is important for institutions and leaders to embed the language of microaffirmations into the institutional climate. These small, everyday acts of kindness and respect can have a profound impact on individuals and institutions. Examples of microaffirmations include using inclusive language, recognizing and celebrating diverse perspectives and experiences, and creating opportunities for dialogue and collaboration across different identity groups.

- **Appreciative inquiry:** "Can you tell me what you are working on that is going well?"
- Recognition and validation of experiences and feelings: *"That situation must have been difficult."*
- Reinforcing and rewarding positive behaviors: *"Congratulations on your certificate!"*
- **Intentional inclusion**: "I am on the plenary committee for an upcoming conference; I really enjoyed the presentation you gave, and I think you should present at this meeting. I'd like to forward your name to the organizers."
- **Acknowledging all team members by name and role:** "This is Dr. _____, a resident working on your care team."
- Utilizing and encouraging the use of microinterventions:
  - make the invisible visible
  - disarm the microaggression
  - educate the perpetrator, and
  - seek external reinforcement or support.

Box 14.2 *Examples of microaffirmations (adapted from molina et al., 2019, and sue et al., 2019)*

Microaffirmations can be used to foster a sense of collaboration and support. Microaffirmations can also be used to acknowledge the unique strengths, talents, and contributions of medical students and residents; as they absorb this messaging, they are in turn likely to transmit similar attitudes and behaviours to their future learners and to their professional environments, which is necessary to becoming successful as inclusive medical professionals.

Microaffirmations can create an environment of mutual respect and acceptance among medical students and faculty. Their use acknowledges the perspectives and contributions of all members of the medical education community and encourages learners to respect and appreciate the diversity of backgrounds and experiences. This can help to create a more unified and cohesive learning environment and can help to foster a sense of connection between medical learners and faculty. By incorporating microaffirmations into clinical education, leadership, and institutional identity, institutions and leaders can create an environment of inclusion and respect. Embedding the language of microaffirmations into medical education, leadership, and institutional identity can have a positive impact on the learning environment, the leadership team, and the institution as a whole.

Key Takeaways: Four Steps Towards Redressing the Equity Balance in Medicine

Step 1: Examination of the long-standing structures and practices that continue to perpetuate inequities.

Step 2: Institutions and leaders to provide safe spaces for dialogue and facilitate an intentional and explicit culture shift that embeds equity, diversity and inclusion into the institutional climate.

Step 3: Institutions to incorporate equity as an authentic institutional brand.

Step 4 Embed the language of microaffirmations into the clinical education, leadership, and institutional identity.

Conclusion

In conclusion, redressing the equity balance in medicine requires sustained instrumental action at all levels of the clinical setting, healthcare institutions and affiliates, particularly where the affiliate is a medical education and training program. To bridge the equity gap, it is important to be intentional in examining long-standing structures and practices that continue to perpetuate inequities.

Institutions and leaders have a responsibility to create safe spaces, facilitate open dialogue, and embed equity, diversity and inclusion into the institutional climate. Additionally, it is important to incorporate the language of microaffirmations into clinical education, leadership, and institutional identity in order to create an environment of inclusion and respect.

On a Parting Note...

Justice ever changing, will not be rearranged

Though it's hard to keep up, we must stay in the loop

Transformation is coming, it's here and it's loud

The spark of hope granting, it's time to be proud

Justice is rising, for all of us to see

The future is right, a soft touch

Equity.

© Marissa Joseph, 2023

References

American Medical Association and Association of American Medical Colleges Centre for Health Justice. (2021) *Advancing Health Equity: Guide to Language, Narrative and Concepts* [online]. Available from: https://www.ama-assn.org/system/files/ama-aamc-equity-guide.pdf

American Medical Association and Association of American Medical Colleges Centre for Health Equity. (2021) *AMA's Organizational Strategic Plan to Embed Racial Justice and Advance Health Equity 2021–2023* [online]. Available from: https://www.ama-assn.org/system/files/2021-05/ama-equity-strategic-plan.pdf

Barenboim, H. E., Fraser, K., Hood Watson, K., and Ring, J. (2021). Racism and persistent disparities: Difficult conversations on the road to equity. *The International Journal of Psychiatry in Medicine, 56*(5), pp. 302-310.

Barnabe, C., Osei-Tutu, K., Maniate, J. M., Razack, S., Wong, B. M., Thomas, B., and Duchesne, N. (2023). Equity, diversity, inclusion, and social justice in CanMEDS 2025. *Canadian medical education journal, 14*(1), pp. 27–32. https://doi.org/10.36834/cmej.75845.

Braveman P. (2006). Health disparities and health equity: concepts and measurement. *Annual review of public health, 27*, pp.167–194.

Braveman, P., and Gottlieb, L. (2014). The social determinants of health: it's time to consider the causes of the causes. *Public health reports, 129*(1_suppl2), pp.19-31.

Bushnik, T., Tjepkema M., and Martel, L. (2020) *Socioeconomic disparities in life and health expectancy among the household population in Canada* [online]. Available from: https://www.doi.org/10.25318/82-003-x202000100001-eng

Byrd, W. M., and Clayton, L. A. (2001). Race, medicine, and health care in the United States: a historical survey. *Journal of the National Medical Association, 93*(3 Suppl), pp.11S–34S.

Cogburn C. D. (2019). Culture, Race, and Health: Implications for Racial Inequities and Population Health. *The Milbank quarterly, 97*(3), 736–761. https://doi.org/10.1111/1468-0009.12411

Crenshaw, K.W. (1989). Demarginalizing the Intersection of Race and Sex: A Black Feminist Critique of Antidiscrimination Doctrine, Feminist Theory and Antiracist Politics, *University of Chicago Legal Forum*: Vol. 139, Article 8 [online]. Available from: https://scholarship.law.columbia.edu/faculty_scholarship/3007.

D'Angelo, I., Demetriou, C., and Jones, C. (2020). Microaffirmations as a tool to support the process of inclusive education. *Education Sciences and Society*, 11(1), pp. 124-139. https://doi.org/10.3280/ess1-2020oa9429.

Devine PG. (1989). Stereotypes and Prejudice: Their Automatic and Controlled Components. *Journal of Personality and Social Psychology*, 56, pp. 5–18.

Ekpe, L. and Toutant, S., (2022). Moving Beyond Performative Allyship: A Conceptual Framework for Anti-racist Co-conspirators. In *Developing Anti-Racist Practices in the Helping Professions: Inclusive Theory, Pedagogy, and Application* (pp. 67-91). Cham: Springer International Publishing.

Enders, F. T., Golembiewski, E. H., Orellana, M. A., DSouza, K. N., Addani, M. A., Morrison, E. J., Benson, J. T., Silvano, C. J., Pacheco-Spann, L. M., and Balls-Berry, J. E. (2022). Changing the face of academic medicine: an equity action plan for institutions. *Journal of clinical and translational science*, 6(1), e78. https://doi.org/10.1017/cts.2022.408

Estrada, M., Young, G. R., Nagy, J., Goldstein, E. J., Ben-Zeev, A., Márquez-Magaña, L., and Eroy-Reveles, A. (2019). The Influence of Microaffirmations on Undergraduate Persistence in Science Career Pathways. *CBE life sciences education*, 18(3), ar40. https://doi.org/10.1187/cbe.19-01-0012

Galarneau, C. (2018). Getting King's Words Right. *Journal of Health Care for the Poor and Underserved* 29(1), 5-8. https://doi:10.1353/hpu.2018.0001.

Harris, A. P., and Pamukcu, A. (2020). The Civil Rights of Health: A New Approach to Challenging Structural Inequality. *UCLA L. Rev.*, 67, p.758. https://doi.org/10.1146/annurev.publhealth.27.021405.102103

Huber, L. P., Gonzalez, T., Robles, G., and Solórzano, D. G. (2021). Racial microaffirmations as a response to racial microaggressions: Exploring risk and protective factors. *New Ideas in Psychology*, 63, 100880.

Kibakaya, E. C., and Oyeku, S. O. (2022). Cultural Humility: A Critical Step in Achieving Health Equity. *Pediatrics*, 149(2), e2021052883. https://doi.org/10.1542/peds.2021-052883

King G. (1996). Institutional racism and the medical/health complex: a conceptual analysis. *Ethnicity & disease*, 6(1-2), pp. 30–46.

Koehn, S., Neysmith, S., Kobayashi, K., and Khamisa, H. (2013). Revealing the shape of knowledge using an intersectionality lens: Results of a scoping review on the health and health care of ethnocultural minority older adults. *Aging and Society*, 33(3), pp.437-464. https://doi: 10.1017/S0144686X12000013.

Landry. M.C. Canadian Human Rights Commission. (2021). *The Big three" Key inclusion principles for Canadian businesses* [online]. Available from: https://www.chrc-ccdp.gc.ca/en/resources/the-big-three-key-inclusion-principles-canadian-businesses

Mahajan, S., Caraballo, C., Lu, Y., Valero-Elizondo, J., Massey, D., Annapureddy, A. R., Roy, B., Riley, C., Murugiah, K., Onuma, O., Nunez-Smith, M., Forman, H. P., Nasir, K., Herrin, J., and Krumholz, H. M. (2021). Trends in Differences in Health Status and Health Care Access and Affordability by Race and Ethnicity in the United States, 1999-2018. *JAMA*, *326*(7), pp. 637–648. https://doi.org/10.1001/jama.2021.9907.

McMillan Boyles, C., Spoel, P., Montgomery, P., Nonoyama, M., and Montgomery, K. (2023). Representations of clinical practice guidelines and health equity in healthcare literature: An integrative review. *Journal of nursing scholarship: an official publication of Sigma Theta Tau International Honor Society of Nursing, 55*(2), pp. 506–520. https://doi.org/10.1111/jnu.12847.

Molina, R. L., Ricciotti, H., Chie, L., Luckett, R., Wylie, B. J., Woolcock, E., and Scott, J. (2019). Creating a Culture of Micro-Affirmations to Overcome Gender-Based Micro-Inequities in Academic Medicine. *The American journal of medicine, 132*(7), pp. 785–787. https://doi.org/10.1016/j.amjmed.2019.01.028.

Nature. Henrietta Lacks: science must right a historical wrong. (2020). *Nature, 585*(7823), p. 7. https://doi.org/10.1038/d41586-020-02494-z.

Nundy, S., Cooper, L.A. and Mate, K.S. (2022). 'The quintuple aim for Health Care Improvement'. *JAMA*, 327(6), p. 521. https://doi.org/10.1001/jama.2021.25181.

Queens Alumni Review. (2020). Queen's School of Medicine: Confronting exclusion [online]. Available from: https://www.queensu.ca/alumnireview/articles/2020-07-17/queen-s-school-of-medicine-confronting-exclusion

Rowe, M. (2008). Micro-affirmations and micro-inequities. *Journal of the International Ombudsman Association, 1*(1), pp. 45-48.

Sabin, J. A. (2022). Tackling implicit bias in health care. *New England Journal of Medicine, 387*(2), pp.105-107.

Shahi A, Karachiwalla F, and Grewal N. (2019). Walking the walk: The case for internal equity, diversity, and inclusion work within the Canadian public health sector. *Health Equity.* 3(1):183-185. https://doi: 10.1089/heq.2019.0008.

Thomas, J.M. (2018). Diversity regimes and racial inequality: A case study of diversity university. *Social Currents, 5*(2), pp. 140-156. https:// doi: 10.1177/2329496517725335.

Tolstoy, Leo. & Patterson, David. (1983). First Edition, September 1, 1983, *Confession / Leo Tolstoy; translation and introduction by David Patterson,* New York: W.W. Norton & Company.

Turner, A. (2016). The business case for racial equity. *National Civic Review,* 105, pp. 21-29. https://doi.org/10.1002/ncr.21263.

Veenstra G. (2011). Race, gender, class, and sexual orientation: intersecting axes of inequality and self-rated health in Canada. *International journal for equity in health,* 10, p.3. https://doi.org/10.1186/1475-9276-10-3.

Williams, J. S., Walker, R. J., and Egede, L. E. (2016). Achieving equity in an evolving healthcare system: opportunities and challenges. *The American journal of the medical sciences,* 351(1), pp. 33–43. https://doi.org/10.1016/j.amjms.2015.10.012

World Health Organization. (2008). *Closing the gap in a generation: health equity through action on the social determinants of health. Final Report of the Commission on Social Determinants of Health* [online]. Available from: https://www.who.int/publications/i/item/WHO-IER-CSDH-08.1

World Health Organization. (2023). *Health equity* [online]. Available from: https://www.who.int/health-topics/health-equity#tab=tab_1

Yepes-Rios, M., Lad, S., Dore, S., Thapliyal, M., Baffoe-Bonnie, H., and Isaacson, J. H. (2023). Diversity, equity, and inclusion: one model to move from commitment to action in medical education. *SN Social Sciences,* 3(3), p.61. https://doi.org/10.1007/s43545-023-00650-6.

Young, M. E., Thomas, A., Varpio, L., Razack, S. I., Hanson, M. D., Slade, S., Dayem, K. L., and McKnight, D. J. (2017). Facilitating admissions of diverse students: A six-point, evidence-informed framework for pipeline and program development. *Perspectives on medical education,* 6(2), pp. 82–90. https://doi.org/10.1007/s40037-017-0341-5.

Zheng L. (2023). *To Make Lasting Progress on DEI, Measure Outcomes.* Harvard Business Review. Jan 27 2023. Available from: https://hbr.org/2023/01/to-make-lasting-progress-on-dei-measure-outcomes

Chapter 15
Nurturing Equity through More Courageous Conversations

Irina Mihaescu, MD

❖

"We can't afford for the world to be equal to start feeling seen"
—Michelle Obama, 2020

❖

Abstract: This chapter examines inequity as a source of complexity in the healthcare environment. Health equity is now recognized as an essential facet of healthcare improvement, thus nurturing conversations about equity in medicine is essential to centering the issue as a determinant of health and wellbeing for physicians and patients alike. This chapter will discuss strategies for initiating courageous conversations about equity in medicine, explore how physicians can be equitable in their practice, examine ways of leading with equity and consider strategies for promoting equitable clinical environments. Vignettes will be used to examine the spectrum of microaggressions and ways in which microaffirmations can be used as an antidote.

Keywords: *burnout, clinician wellbeing, microaffirmations, microaggressions, microassaults, microinequities, physician bias*

Introduction

Medical environments are characterized by being volatile (V), uncertain (U), complex (C), and, at best, ambiguous (A) (Sinha and Sinha, 2020). This is an occupational hazard of clinical work and one that cannot easily be managed. However, Zhivotovskaya (2019) proposes that clinicians can start to shift this VUCA environment into a MUCA environment, where volatility becomes mastery (M), uncertainty becomes understanding (U), complexity becomes collaboration (C), and ambiguity becomes agility (A). When we focus more on mastery, understanding, collaboration, and agility, we start to transform the healthcare system from the inside out. One aspect that is currently missing and urgently requires a MUCA approach is improving equity within the medical profession.

The Quadruple Aim (Williams et al., 2019) is a four-arm framework to optimize healthcare. The four arms advocate for:

1) A reduction of adverse events;
2) Improving the patient experience and the process of healthcare delivery;
3) Lowering allocation costs by utilizing evidence-based modalities of care and/or increasing the return on investment; and
4) Improving clinician wellbeing and health, which has been shown to affect the other three aims.

Achieving equity in each of the four arms is fundamental to fulfilling the Quadruple Aim, and in fact equity has been proposed as a fifth arm, or Quintuple Aim (Nundy et al., 2022). The impact on clinician wellbeing is perhaps the most important of all as this has direct impact on patient safety. Physicians play a central role in the healthcare team, and are thus in a position to lead change. Individually and as key healthcare team members, physicians can situate equity, diversity and inclusion as a priority by choosing to learn and lead with equity in the interprofessional and clinical spheres.

Inequity in medicine will continue to perpetuate poor health outcomes until it is given due recognition and concerted action is taken to address the adverse impacts on health and wellbeing (Nundy et al., 2022). There is a moral imperative to build equitable healthcare communities and collegial spaces. Physicians have a fiduciary duty to do no harm and to lower the risk for adverse patient outcomes. Marginalized physicians and patients have incredible adaptive skills and valuable experiences that can inform innovation and improvement in medical spaces. Additionally, addressing equity in clinical spaces is pivotal to improved clinician wellbeing and health outcomes.

A decade of research has shown that clinician wellbeing improves patient outcomes and that patients suffer worse outcomes and worse care experiences when cared for by physicians with burnout (National Academies of Science, Engineering, and Medicine, 2019). Swensen and Shanafelt (2020) make a compelling case as to why patient wellbeing needs to start with physician wellbeing, a priority that most healthcare institutions ignore at the risk of adverse patient outcomes, legal risks and physician attrition, including through suicide.

The Issues

A Background on the Context of Systemic Biases

The current climate in Western medicine is predicated on historical biases that continue to permeate current practices. In North America, the 1910 Flexner report (Flexner, 1910) was instrumental in shaping the climate of medicine and subsequently perpetuating biases that have remained ingrained in the field through the last century. The world was relatively isolated at the time and many people did not easily travel between continents and countries. As such, communities were much more myopic, and most people shared the same belief systems, biases, and ancestry as their neighbours. In North America, this was made worse through active marginalization and stereotyping of people as described in *The 1619 Project* (Hannah-Jones, 2019), the "cheap labour" movement (including the building of the Canadian railroad), and the atrocities of the residential school system concurrent with other assimilation initiatives for Indigenous North Americans.

Despite awareness of these issues, as well as ongoing globalization, international migration, and virtual technologies that allow remote communication and greater interconnectedness, not much has changed systemically in terms of institutions and the policies and procedures that guide the way in which healthcare is conceptualized, delivered, and overseen. When we adhere to policies and procedures designed without awareness of, or concern for, inherent biases in the system and interpersonally, we disregard the importance of context within these clinical spaces.

There is a benefit to following standardization, whether in clinical care or in hiring policies and procedures, but there is also a loss, and that loss is the loss of diversity in the clinical workforce. This is especially true if these standardizations, policies, and procedures are not routinely reviewed with an eye towards identifying bias and diversity. Healthcare, military, and government institutions are amongst the most challenging environments within which to enact change (Hogshead, 2010). Innovation and alignment with current cultural norms and societal blueprints cannot occur in environments that are notoriously difficult to change due to their premise and mandate to create stability, order, and standardization. It is critical to note that standardization can have unintended detrimental effects, especially if not revisited routinely.

The medical field is now seen as a place of innovation, although historically, the field has shown resistance to change and often did not value people who "do things differently" (Obenchain, 2021). Some of the greatest physicians of the last century, despite creating penicillin, recognizing the role of handwashing in puerperal fever, and discovering other life-saving interventions, were often seen as threats to the status quo of standardized medicine and effectively treated as outcasts. Thus, the healthcare community can be a formidable resistor to people ("thinkers outside the box"), innovation and system change. Standardization provides a level of comfort and order. Change and innovation require comfort with some degree of discomfort and uncertainty. Innovation and change require curiosity and open-mindedness that may have been lost through years of training and clinical practice indoctrinated with the ethos of standardized practices, policies, and procedures.

The Opportunity to Nurture Equity

Leading with Equity

One of the key reflections for leaders is to ask themselves how to nurture leadership in equity and who should be involved. This burden is often disproportionately placed on persons who are Black, Indigenous, and People of Colour, as well as other groups who are already marginalized. Although their voices are critical at the table, it is important not to assume that every marginalized person has an interest, willingness, or capability to lead with equity. Allies are important, and this is nowhere more important than in reflecting on the spaces that allies, should or should not be in. There are spaces where allies may not fully belong or need to insert themselves. Instead, this may be a moment for the ally to leverage their referral networks instead, in order to find someone who can, and will speak genuinely about their struggles and successes in navigating this marginalized space in medicine and beyond. An ally who finds that they are not of a background concordant to the situation can still be involved peripherally, rather than inserting themselves and relying on marginalized colleagues and patients to teach, educate, or inform of allies of failures and missed reflections.

Leading with equity also necessitates a willingness and ability to build social capital. Social capital is the ability to get to know team members and know their personal and professional values, likes, and dislikes (Cameron and Spreitzer, 2013). It is extending a helping hand when one can, and trusting that the kindness will be reciprocated. The underlying basis of social capital theory rests on building reciprocal personal connections, often guided by a set of shared values, norms, and identities; for example, "we are both mothers", "we are all physicians", or "we are all in this specialty". To build a shared social identity, even amongst all these differences, leaders must look for the commonality in the work they do. For many, this becomes the patient outcomes and professional satisfaction when patients do well.

A common social identity is also built when people feel that they belong at work, or at the very least, when they feel that they are doing meaningful work. This requires transparency, accountability, and shared decision-making with their teams, or at least a rationale for why they chose to do what they did. Many leaders fall short in this regard, believing that they are somehow "protecting" their teams by not sharing the way they arrived at a decision, or perhaps feeling it is not "leader-like" to offer details to the people impacted by these decisions.

One of the key practices for great leadership transparency is the Five "I"s, adapted from Shanafelt et al.'s (2015) Five Leadership Behaviors. They are to include, inform, inquire, invest and indulge team members. This means:

- Including the team members in decision making as much as is possible (including lateral colleagues);
- Informing them of the rationale and decisions ahead of time (including how these decisions may impact them);
- Inquiring as to their suggestions for improvement (you may be surprised at what you hear back);
- Investing them with the capacity to build bridges, lead with equity and develop their ideas;
- Indulging these efforts and initiatives with celebration and recognition of the participants.

The Five "I"s build a culture of innovation and allow clinicians to speak up when they see something amiss or when they may have an idea that would best solve a problem at the local or institutional level.

Aside from healthcare leadership, every physician, whether they recognize it or not, is a leader in their own right. They lead patients through decisions every day, and they lead their teams of allied health clinicians through a myriad of situations and directives. There is currently an epidemic of physicians in mental health crises, who are sometimes, from a psychological standpoint, suffering more than their patients at any given time (Canadian Medical Association, 2021).

It is imperative we work on equity to allow physicians the opportunities and safe spaces to sustain both professional and personal wellbeing. Mental health equity, whether in the local medical communities, societies, or the microcosm of the clinical environment, starts with understanding and building equitable spaces amongst physicians and other clinicians, one where they are able to honor and learn about their mental health, and are not forced or coerced into roles and commitments that are beyond their capacities or abilities.

Motivating teams and individuals alike works better with a focus on strengths and abilities rather than focusing on deficits. Recognizing the diversity of strengths that each physician brings to the table facilitates the building of bridges instead of chasms of shame and embarrassment over difficulties and current struggles. It behooves all physicians to pay attention to the mental health equity of their colleagues, so that this can trickle down into patient care and a bedside manner that is aware, context-driven, and strengths-focused.

An idealized vision of healthcare equity starts by imagining equity, diversity, and inclusion (EDI) metrics as a key prognostic tool of the institution. Much like clinician wellbeing has taken on the fourth pillar of the Quadruple Aim, EDI metrics have since been proposed as the Quintuple Aim (Nundy et al., 2022), joining its previous aims of clinician wellbeing, patient outcomes, improved patient experiences through the system, and return on investments or conscious resource allocation. Given that physicians are themselves healthcare consumers, there should be a collective vested interest in equity-leaning systems transformation.

Inclusion Strategies

Strategies Towards Becoming an Equitable Physician

Becoming a more equitable clinician starts with understanding the basics of social differences and how these differences contribute to a diversity of perspectives, ideas, and solutions. This can cause discomfort given varied outlooks on the world and one's place within that context. The key is to cultivate the capacity to be able to shift this discomfort to discourse and dialogue, allowing for more voices at the table, especially those that have traditionally been silenced.

Equity begins with internal awareness – understanding how differences shape experiences and sense of place, interpretation of events, and understanding. Equity then follows with a systemic awareness whereby intentional policy is at the center of the inclusion and integration process. The caveat here is that intentional policies need to truly *value* the differences that create diversity within the healthcare milieu, and thereby avert performative tokenism for the sake of a standardized checkbox. This same intentional policy applies to clinician wellness initiatives. It requires a willingness to speak up when it is necessary and helpful instead of utilizing silence as an avoidance of discomfort. To become a more equitable clinician, one must be willing to recognize that silence imparts violence, and the impact of this silence is extremely hazardous to colleagues, patient outcomes, fiscal bottom lines, and clinician wellbeing in the long term. What follows are five strategies for cultivating greater equity in your practice as a physician.

Strategy 1: Recognizing Biases in Clinical Care

Did you know?

Among CEOs of Fortune 500 companies, 58% are over 6 feet tall. Whereas only 14.5% of the U.S. population is over 6 feet tall (Meyer, 2009).

Is a 6-foot male candidate for the surgery residency program smarter and more capable of leading than their 5-foot counterparts? Are they inherently more talented? Did they put in greater effort than their peers? Or were they merely endowed with "good" genes, associated with wealth and social class benefits, imbued through good nutrition and environments that allowed them to reach the maximum potential of their genetic blueprint?

Many of the social determinants of health including gender, housing, income, education, food security, access to appropriate health care, and early childhood events can impact one's ability to access privileges. In healthcare, as in other spaces, awareness of those who are not at the table, but should be, is essential to understanding the effects of systemic exclusion on health systems as well as on patients and colleagues from routinely excluded biosocial backgrounds.

Various factors modulate the ability to achieve self-actualization. Raphael (2009) identified 14 specific social determinants of health that are shown to have strong effects upon the health of Canadians. Their effects are proven to be stronger than those associated with behaviours, such as diet, physical activity, and tobacco and alcohol use.

Table 15.1. *The 14 social determinants of health as identified by Raphael (2009)*

Social Determinants of Health	
	o Gender
o Aboriginal status	o Housing
o Disability	o Income and income
o Early life	distribution
o Education	o Race
o Employment and working	o Social exclusion
conditions	o Social safety net
o Food insecurity	o Unemployment and job
o Health services	security

As evident in Table 15.1, the social climate very much shapes health status but, in addition, also shapes the quality of clinical care, based on how these social factors are adapted into clinical metrics. The impact of medicalizing social factors is evident, from the metrics used to assess cognitive function in National Football League (NFL) concussion patients from racialized backgrounds, to the way in which adjustments are made in kidney function and blood pressure management for African Americans (for more information on race correction, see Chapter 11). These race adjustments rest on a bedrock of inherent biases about the innate intelligence, intellectual potential, pain tolerance and normative physiological function in people of color. These racialized metrics were largely status quo and remained unquestioned until very recently (see Chapter 1 and 11).

Equitable spaces allow physicians to evaluate their patients' complaints and current symptomatic profile through the lens of context and an awareness of the power differential between healthcare provider and patient. A physician who is aware of their own implicit and explicit biases (with "noticing" being a key component of equity) is more likely to recognize instances when they are unfairly or prematurely dismissing or not considering real patient and cultural complaints that can affect patients' health and longevity. Equity in medicine emphasizes preventative medicine for earlier detection and intervention by catching biases before they exert an impact on treatment decisions. This is the business case for equity, whereby race correction is eliminated, thus pathology is detected earlier so that higher cost services, such as end-stage surgeries and dialysis, can be prevented, or at least delayed, which inherently costs the system and its participants less.

The *equitable physician* can also be better attuned to the strengths and assets that the patient and the culture bring. This allows the physician to further empower the patient through the use of their own strengths to aid in their health journey, rather than focusing on the patients' deficits. Focusing on the patient's deficits tends to centre the burden of the patient's care on the physician, which is a recipe for physician burnout in the long term. Despite their own discomfort with the subject or disagreement with the context of the topic a physician who is equitably aware can discuss taboo topics that they may otherwise avoid, which could impact the ability of the patient to recover. Topics like religion, culture, sexuality, gender, and race can then be freely discussed and incorporated into the clinical treatment plan.

Much of the work of becoming a more equitable physician lies in the ability to tolerate discomfort and knowing and recognizing the inherent biases and differences between oneself and others. Equity is also about *value*-ing others' differences and trusting that this diversity brings enrichment and progress to conversations, institutions and to the exam room.

Strategy 2: Identifying Microaggressions, Microinequities and Microassaults

Self-evaluation for unconscious biases is important in monitoring for the various ways in which these biases emanate. Physicians who are unaware of their implicit biases may not recognize when they act on their unconscious biases. These expressions of bias can take the form of microinequities and subconscious microaggressions or be more conscious, in the form of microassaults and intentional microaggressions.

Microaggressions –Sue and colleagues (2007) note that "microaggressions are brief, everyday exchanges that send denigrating messages to people of color because they belong to a racial minority group". Microaggressions capture a spectrum of identity microrelations including microassaults, microinsults, and microinvalidations. Simply put, microaggressions are small acts of disrespect, disregard, and invalidation (Rowe, 2008). These are often unconscious negative messages that come from stereotypes. Common examples are statements like, "I want to speak to the doctor", when speaking to a female doctor (assuming she's a nurse), or inappropriate invitations, such as, "bring your wife", or "please join us to celebrate Christmas" when speaking to 2SLGBTQ+ or non-Christian people. A few examples are shown in Table 15.2 and the concepts are discussed in greater detail in Chapters 8 and 10.

Table 15.2. *Examples of microaggressions (adapted from Sue et al., 2007)*

Microaggression	Message
"You're not from around here, are you?" "Where are you from from? Where are your parents from? Where are your people from?"	You don't look like the rest of us. You are not from this country.
"I'm color blind when it comes to race. When I look at you, I don't see color."	Denying a person of color's lived experiences. Implying that racial and ethnic differences bear no meaning on lived experience. Denying the individual as a being with unique ethnoracial experiences and perspectives.
"It's not that hard to be successful in this country if people work hard enough" "If you put in the work, you'll be successful like any other hardworking person...."	People of color shouldn't just expect things to be handed to them because of their race. People of color need to work harder if they want to get ahead like the rest.
Person of color in high status or successful roles mistaken for a service worker e.g., male physician of color mistaken for janitor, female cardiac surgeon mistaken for support staff	How did *you* get there? What did you do to get there? People of color rarely occupy high-status positions.

Microinequities – "[a]pparently small events which are often ephemeral and hard to prove, events which are covert, often unintentional, frequently unrecognized by the perpetrator which occur wherever people are perceived to be different" (Rowe, 2008). Microinequities in essence are practices and experiences that devalue, overlook and marginalize on the basis of minority identity. Microinequities are the principal scaffolding for discrimination and are often unconscious. Common examples include inequitable job assignments, passing minorities over for promotions, or failure to provide schedules/food/space needed by a particular group to do their work or meet basic physiological functions, such as lactation rooms.

Microassaults – Microassaults describe any of the actions in Table 15.2 being done with deliberate intent to cause harm through exclusion or demeaning someone else (Sue, et al., 2007). These are conscious assaults. The key differentiator is intent to cause harm. An example would be saying, "go back to where you came from!" when speaking to a visible minority born in the country.

The SCARF model (Rock, 2008) is a summary of important discoveries from neuroscience about the way people interact socially. Our judgements about others, whether patients or colleagues, are often triggered by social threats against status (S), certainty (C), autonomy (A), relatedness (R), and fairness (F). The SCARF model was designed to encompass triggers that affect everyone in all cultures on a daily basis, and proves a helpful model to monitor which of these common triggers often arise within equity and diversity discussions.

Arnold et al. (1991) introduced the idea of a "Power Flower", which was meant to be used as a tool to "identify who we are (and who we aren't) as individuals and as a group in relation to those who wield power in our society". This concept has had many iterations since then, and today many refer to it as a "Privilege Flower" because it can also be used to identify the privilege of individuals or groups in relation to others.

Identities are multidimensional and complex. The intersection of the multiple aspects of an individual's social identities contributes to unique experiences of concurrent power, oppression and privilege. Thus, a heterosexual cis-male physician who identifies as a racialized minority is one in relational privilege to a non-physician of the same background when one considers the physician's cisgender and heterosexual orientation, education, and income level. Concurrently, the physician occupies a place and space of relational power by virtue of cisgenderism and the sociopolitical influence their occupation confers while also living an experience of racial oppression. These intersectional relations of power, oppression and privilege are here described as an Identity Matrix.

The author's rendition of an Identity Matrix, adapted from the original Power Flower work by Arnold et al. (1991) is illustrated in Figure 15.1. The concept of the Identity Matrix is based on a web of identities, with the most advantageous confluence of identities in the central spoke. In contrast, the outer margins of the web include identities of decreasing privilege and power concurrent with increasing spaces of oppression. The web of identities is much like the spider web: the spun silk concentrically becomes "weaker" in the outermost margins as there is increased social vulnerability in these marginalized spaces. The margins are distal to the seat of power and effectively have the least influence and access to choice opportunities. Within each of the outside strata, the same relational dynamics occur, with like inhabitants of a strata differing in key ways such as educational attainment, ability, age and so forth.

As a reflective exercise, in a safe space, take some time to review Figure 15.1 and utilize it as a self-assessment tool. Circle the layers of the web that apply to you. Identify the areas in which you have privilege/power or find yourself at an intersection of oppression/domination. Although this can result in some personal discomfort, it can allow us to compassionately learn about ourselves and how we can deepen our genuine understanding of ways to advocate for spaces free of judgement, social injustice and structural violence.

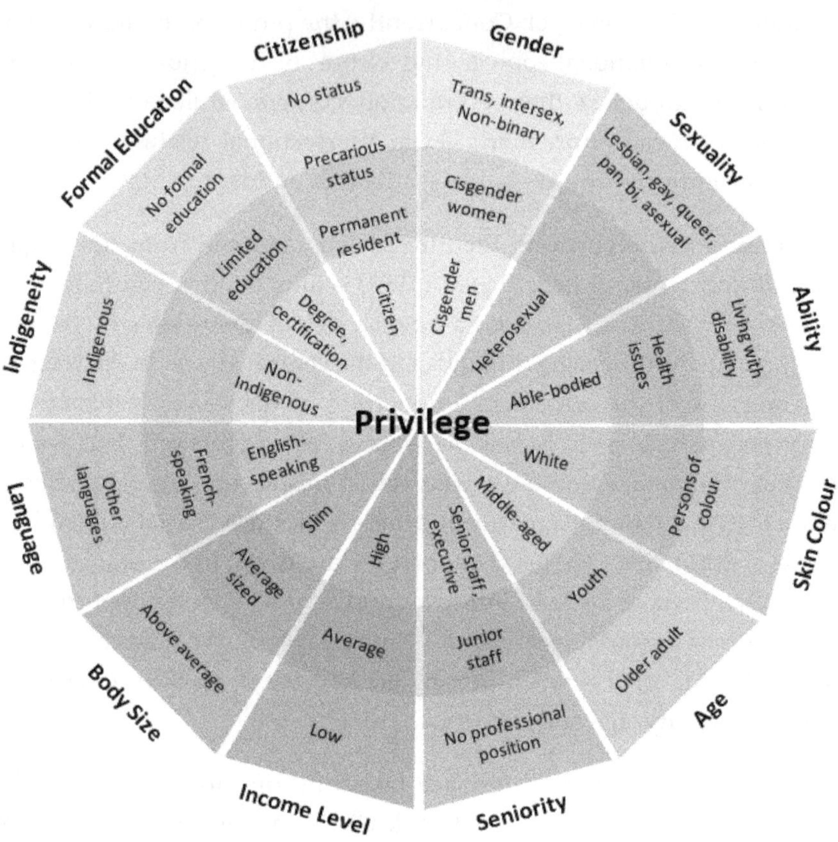

Figure 15.1. *The Identity Matrix: a complex web of identities reflecting the relational confluence of power, privilege and oppression (adapted from Arnold et al., 1991)*

The Project Implicit from Harvard (1998) can help physicians and medical leaders identify their own implicit biases and safeguard against them becoming complicit within their unconscious. The inner work and reflective capacity of the physician and medical leader is pivotal to systems-level equity and equitable practices. It begins with a willingness to sit with the discomfort of personal biases, associate discriminations (making assumptions about others based on whom they spend time with), perceptual discriminations, as well as any direct or indirect discrimination noticed in the medical and learning environment. For non-marginalized medical staff, it starts by understanding and being comfortable with the discomfort of recognizing their own privilege on the Privilege Flower. Allies are needed but can also be misused and harmful if the ally does not recognize the part they play in this "othering" as a result of their own privileges.

The importance of purpose, of being genuine with one's intentionality cannot be underscored. When purpose is inauthentic or mired in "fragility" or "saviour" complexes, it can have more deleterious than beneficial effects. Equity work that is done with intentionality but with inauthentic purpose, perhaps for leveraging the institutional brand, will only serve to further marginalize those already marginalized, perpetuating the social, economic, and health related inequities that are all too prevalent. There is benefit to familiarity with the concept of "White fragility" and the myriad of ways in which the dominant or "standard" culture in Western countries tends to defend the "good White self", as illustrated in Table 15.3.

Table 15.3. *Defending the "good White self" (adapted from Schoen and Johnson, 2021)*

Defense	Examples
Denial or minimization of oppression and White privilege	Minimizing/denying difference, insistence on "color blindness"
	Ascribing the blame to the person/people of colour – "He has such a big chip on his shoulder, he's reading too much into what happened", "She's too sensitive, too defensive, and it's not like I meant any harm."
Enactment on the interpersonal level	Avoidance, withdrawal or refusal to engage in interaction because it's an "attack" when you meant no harm. The withdrawal may be emotional, intellectual, social and/or physical
	Shifting the discussion to own experience of oppression
	Defensiveness – "I'm being attacked but I'm not the problem". "What about the big chip on his/her shoulder?"

Defense	Examples ...*continued*
Enactment on the intrapersonal level	Refusal to explore/accept/acknowledge our racial/racist conditioning
	Desire to be anti-racist without giving up any privileges
	Judging and separating oneself from other White people "I'm not racist like some White people can be, I have Asian friends", "I'm not like other White people"
	Intellectualization – focusing on the intellectual understanding of a situation to minimize the anxiety-provoking/difficult emotions you are feeling
Making Use of Racialized Persons	Expecting overtures to racialized persons to be acknowledged and expecting gratitude, redemption, approval, or acceptance in return - "my friendship with him will help him"
Reinstatement of the White racial equilibrium	Refocusing the encounter on the White person's distress in response to the interaction- the aggressor becomes the victim

Strategy 3: Attunement to Identity Suppression

A pervasive climate of inequity is ripe with necessity for people to "cover" and "code-switch" on a consistent and frequent basis (see Chapter 9). *Covering* demands people to hide or avoid visual clues that would reveal their culture, beliefs, sexual orientation, or anything else that places them in a minority category. *Code-switching* entails adjusting language and gestures to better blend into the dominant culture; these key elements of blending in for acceptability within the dominant culture are explored in detail in Chapter 9.

From 2SLGBTQ2+ identities, to neurodiverse and marginalized populations, the inherent exhaustion of covering up and identity switching in order to avoid drawing negative attention and "fit in" erodes wellbeing within what is already a demanding healthcare profession. The inability to be one's authentic self and the burden of being tolerated when difference cannot be masqueraded accumulate over time in a field that thrives on standardization and stability.

Navigating the biases that exert the pressure to code-switch can begin by observing the immediate practice environment for visible expressions of diversity and the level of meaningful overt celebrations of diversity. If it is a diverse group, how are ethnoracial minority colleagues treated? Are gender and sexual minority identities freely expressed? Is inclusive language expected and used? Are some non-Western holidays and cultural events acknowledged? It may also be instructive to observe colleagues for differences in their interactions with concordant groups relative to majority in-groups. Open inquiry about observed shifts in identity revelation may be informative in spaces where there is healthy dialogue.

Professional Vignette

Tiffany arrives on her first day as a specialist physician at a new cardiology clinic with a little excitement and some trepidation. Her last clinic was quite dysfunctional and insistent on doing things "the way they've always been done". Despite Tiffany's research experience and novel publications on the use of stents in cardiology, she was consistently met with resistance from medical leaders and the management team. The implication was to "not fix what isn't broken". However, Tiffany noticed that many of her patients were doing better on this new stent and wanted to ensure her patients had good outcomes. She would spend hours in the operating room trying to get the surgery "just right" and caring for her patients in post-operative recovery. She was determined and passionate about her field but during the last year she had become more and more disillusioned with her work.

Tiffany grew up in a biracial family, a "third space" where she experienced multiple cultures and family traditions. Her father, a physician, originally from North Africa and a Muslim man, warned her to "just survive" residency. He had experienced his fair share of difficulties and even some violence. In the rural community where she was training, Tiffany, heeding her father's advice, decided to remove her hijab. After residency, she chose to wear a hijab in her urban-setting clinic, replacing it with a surgeon's cap when she operated on patients. This was not an easy decision for her, as she knew it would incite questions from people who were confused about her background. However, she thought it would be safer in the city and now that she had a "real" attending job. She still received multiple questions from the daycare staff at her children's school, and from colleagues and civilians at the corner coffee shop.

Tiffany hopes this new clinic will embrace her innovative spirit and be open to her research, unlike her previous workplace. She wants to feel valued for her abilities and her forward-thinking attitude. At her previous place of work, she was not invited out to dinners and openly disdained in meetings for "novel" suggestions. One colleague went so far as to try and block her from having operating room access, citing that Tiffany was single-handedly "destroying" the cardiology profession. For months she was pressured to be the only one reading electrocardiograms and echocardiographs, a task she would have preferred to do more minimally. Tiffany's mother is of Asian descent, and despite growing up in Canada, people still made assumptions. Medical students would often ask for Tiffany's help with the math components of their rotations. They never outwardly said it, but Tiffany always wondered whether it was her partial Asian heritage that made them siphon her into this role.

As Tiffany walks into this new clinic, she notices that the walls are filled with art by diverse painters and there are "safe space" stickers on most of the chairs in the waiting room. Later that week, Tiffany overheard an old residency colleague at a local restaurant. He worked in the same cardiology clinic, and, although not part of the leadership team, she had overheard him discussing with his family that his workplace is "only hiring colored people to fill a quota now". They retorted with comments about how the most qualified person should get the job.

Tiffany remained hopeful, although partially cautious. After many conversations with the medical directors, she knew they were committed to intentional hiring practices and their purpose for doing this, including revising their policies and procedures, was largely inspired by their own desire for a more holistic clinic that served the populations they saw every day. They hoped Tiffany would become part of the solution. She had thought long and hard about this, as she wasn't sure if she wanted to be part of the diversity efforts her new medical directors were so passionate about. Many people through the years assumed that she would be interested in such a role. She was even asked to fill such a role at her old clinic but refused when she recognized the position would be more performative than personal.

Her new medical directors seemed to value her opinions, her diverse perspectives and innovative operating techniques. During a pre-hiring discussion, one of the medical directors encouraged Tiffany to speak a little louder. This caused her discomfort as she didn't know how to address it directly. She had spoken loudly, unlike her usual demeanour, many times in residency and at her old work so that she would be taken more seriously. She found this exhausting.

Professional Vignette Analysis

Tiffany has to make multiple micro-decisions each day to preserve social civility and protect herself from judgement. This *code-switching* uses up emotional energy, leaving her depleted and exhausted. She must function and perform despite the extra stress and effort, which many in medicine may not notice, and do not recognize signs of in their colleagues and patients.

Reflective Exercise

Reflecting on Tiffany's experiences, which microaggressions are evident? How would you construct Tiffany's relative positions within the Identity Matrix (Figure 15.1) relative to yours?

For colleagues and patients who are constantly on high alert for when they need to "cover up" and code-switch while navigating subtle and overt microaggressions, their ability to succeed and perform requires a resilience that others in the medical space do not need to draw on. It is this very resilience and adaptability that is most needed at the table in order to rework and re-examine standardized policies and procedures on which our systems have been based for millennia. Patients and colleagues whose voices and experiences have not been seen and heard are exactly the adaptable influences and perspectives needed for healthcare systems and communities to grow more socially responsive and minimize the risk of complacency.

❖

"It is not the strongest of the species that survives, nor the most intelligent that survives. It is the one that is the most adaptable to change."
— Charles Darwin, 1859

❖

Strategy 4: Implementing and Encouraging More Courageous Conversations

To be able to shift the medical climate towards equity and diversity, as physicians we must become comfortable with discomfort in a way that perhaps we have not been exposed to before. The inherent silence created by the aversion to "making waves" and disrupting the status quo will only serve to further disparage and create chasms in diversity efforts.

The work starts with inner reflection and recognition of the ways in which physicians have inadvertently and maybe even explicitly contributed to the problem in the past. It starts with looking at our own biases and "fragility", but it also necessitates a commitment to becoming comfortable with discomfort when difficult conversations about race, equity, and diversity arise.

One helpful skill to use in these circumstances is the "pause, relax, open" (PRO) acronym, introduced by Schoen and Johnson (2021). This can be used as an internal reminder to pause, relax our bodies, and open our minds to curiosity about what is causing our own inner discomfort and tension. It also behooves us to take this further and reflect, alone or in affinity groups, on our experiences, and take the necessary steps to correct our distorted perceptions of the situation at hand. Many of the inner and outer discomforts arise from a lack of understanding of the impact that systemic factors have in this narrative of inequity and privilege.

> **Skill box – The PRO method** (Schoen and Johnson, 2021)
>
> A helpful method to use when you are feeling discomfort in conversations:
>   Pause
>   Relax
>   Open

Wilber et al. (2008) remind us that "everything is just information, when your response takes it elsewhere then it's no longer information." That unexamined response becomes the basis of internal judgements and many of our biases. To clarify, judgement as a character trait is not "bad". We need it every day as physicians. However, the danger is in its overuse.

So, how can physicians crusade for more courageous conversations around equity, diversity, and inclusion? The starting point should focus on equity and not just equality. It is essential to tie equity in with the Quadruple Aim, creating an enduring fifth arm of healthcare improvement. As such, the Quintuple Aim should form the basis of closing the equity gap. The business and moral case for the equity imperative could not be clearer given the critical interaction between healthcare improvement and clinician wellbeing.

As physicians become more aware of inequities and learn to tolerate some discomfort (about biases, privilege and, for White people, the myriad of ways we defend the "good White self") instead of avoiding it, a larger space is created for constructive dialogue. Policies and procedures should be reviewed with an awareness and keen eye for context-centered processes rather than context neutrality alone. As previously discussed, it is also important to routinely examine standardization, remain aware of the potential harms of standardization and eliminate these harms where they create or perpetuate equity gaps. Physicians must also have an awareness of microinequities and microaggressions in the cultural milieu in which the medical community operates. When inequities and aggressions arise, it is important to reflect on personal and collective responsibility so as to determine when it is constructive, wise and helpful to speak up and when it is not.

It is our fiduciary duty to implement intentional policies and procedures that tackle blatant discrimination and racism in the workplace. This can be done through just and fair procedures that focus on workplace wellbeing, rather than toxic shame, blame, silence, or cancelling procedures. Seeing these as opportunities to continuously improve workplace culture would be prudent for ongoing healthcare systems that can tolerate the changing tides and culture shifts of the new wave of medical students, physicians, and leaders who are much more attuned and aware of these dynamics than the physicians and medical leaders of past decades.

Strategy 5: Nurturing Differences in Clinical Practice

Leadership principles are often centered on the understanding of people's different preferences, strengths, and choices. Not all team members will have the same skills or ways of approaching a situation no matter how standardized the solution. Leadership on equity, diversity and inclusion requires going beyond naming diversity to *value*-ing diversity for the richness it can bring to the healthcare environment and beyond. One of the main adages of positive organizational psychology is to "Know, Grow, Show" your own strengths, and then learn to "Spot, Savour, and Celebrate" strengths in others (Cameron and Spreitzer, 2013).

Microaffirmations as an Antidote to Microaggressions

When clinicians and medical leaders are able to recognize the strengths, preferences and choices of the diverse staff and patients in a medical ecosystem and the context within which these different skills and opportunities arise, microaffirmations can be used in an intentional way to shape more inclusive environments. Microaffirmations are a concept developed by Rowe (2008) as a way to combat the ill effects of microaggressions.

Rowe defines microaffirmations as "apparently small acts, which are often ephemeral and hard-to-see, events that are public and/or private, often unconscious but very effective, which occur wherever people wish to help others to succeed". They are "tiny acts of opening doors to opportunity". Over time and intentional practice, microaffirmations are, or soon become, unconscious processes. They occur when an abiding goal is to help others succeed. It occurs when value is expected from diverse perspectives and differing skillsets. Embedding microaffirmations into the institutional climate is about intention and purpose.

Microaffirmations are not about wise feedback, which is holding someone to high standards while helping them get the necessary training, help, and support they individually need to achieve those outcomes. Microaffirmations are an intentional practice of recognizing the good and the contribution of another, while also understanding the purpose and the "hidden why" of those statements of recognition (see Table 15.4). It is not performative. It is personal.

As an example, land acknowledgement in Canada constitutes a personal reflection of the ways in which settlers have benefited from the genocide of Indigenous peoples and is also an acknowledgment of the ongoing impacts of this genocide. It is a practice focused on microaffirmations and imparts a responsibility for reflexive thinking in the workplace and elsewhere (Native Governance Center, 2019).

Microaffirmations start with getting to know the team, colleagues, and patients. It starts with knowing not only their strengths but also their values, their personal goals, and their aspirations. Research on workplace health and wellbeing has shown over and over again that when teams and leaders understand what the personal goals and values of their people are, without forcing people to hide these personal goals and preferences at work, productivity goes up (Avey et al., 2011). People no longer feel like they need to hide or leave parts of themselves out of their work life. They do not need to engage in covering, passing, or code-switching. They can bring their whole self to work, allowing more psycho-emotional and physical energy for them to be productive and perform at a higher capacity.

Shifting the healthcare climate towards an asset model of microaffirmations and minimizing over-reliance on deficits (which our brains naturally focus on due to negativity bias) becomes an intentional practice over time. Eventually, with practice, it becomes unconscious, just as psycho-therapeutic support can generalize to outside the therapy room with practice, intention, and purposeful action (Reich and Milner, 2020).

Table 15.4. *Examples of microaffirmations (adapted from Rowe, 2008)*

Microaffirmation	Message
Gestures of inclusion and caring	I care about you and this team, and I want you to feel like you belong.
Practicing generosity (social capital)	I'm invested in you so you can be invested in this team.
Consistently giving credit to others	I want you to do well, so you can enjoy doing well too.
Providing comfort and/or support when others in distress (public attack, idea that did not work, organizational or leadership failure)	We are a team and will support you so you can do your work well.
Affirming emotional reactions through verbal acknowledgement, even if not approving of behavior or outcome	I value you as a person and know that emotions are a normal part of life and important clues.
Identifying and validating constructive behaviour	I value this behaviour, please do more of it.
Active listening, using eye contact, open body posture, summarizing statements, and asking qualifying questions to ensure understanding	I value what you are saying and hope I can hear more of your thoughts.
Paying attention to "small things", especially in senior leadership	I notice that we are making gains even if they are small. I'm focused on the process, not the outcome.
Focusing on strengths and success vs. faults and weakness	I notice what is good, not only what is wrong.
Organizationally, encouraging mentoring and building supportive networks	I recognize we all learn from each other and can help each other.

Over time and intentional use of the previously discussed tools and strategies, one may reach a point where a SCARF trigger (described above in Strategy 2) occurs and it does not cause a big emotional reaction or attachment; instead, one may experience a release from the myopia of the moment. It can be an opportune moment to pause, relax, open (PRO) and become curious about the situation and trigger. The person or situational trigger can be seen from a bird's eye view, a top-level perspective that places the trigger in the larger context of the day's events, cultural upbringings, and the systemic factors at play.

Equity work may sometimes necessitate remaining quiet due to physical safety considerations. Most of the time, this work requires stepping up into a brave space of open dialogue that may be difficult to bear and uncomfortable at best, but vitally necessary. At the core of it, equity work is not about altered states like a brief moment of safety or joy, but about altered traits; where behaviour and character strengths of resilience and understanding are at the center.

Clinical Vignette

Jonah got extremely loud during the meeting. He was triggered when the trainer suggested that this seminar on trauma-informed care would not allow time for any emotion. He felt it was performative and without stories, completely impersonal. Jonah had been through his own share of difficulties in his lifetime. As a young, Indigenous man, he was hospitalized in his early 20s with appendicitis. He spent three weeks in the hospital post-op in agonizing pain. His medical team were worried about giving him opioids; without any personal history of addictions, Jonah knew that this was blatant racism, as well as the inherent assumption that his people could somehow tolerate more pain than White patients. It was that experience that motivated him to enter medical school, and eventually graduate and become a psychiatrist. He was tired of the way the medical establishment ignored the traumas and medical necessities of his people.

In his psychiatric practice, he often burned sage between patients, and made sure to allow room for spiritual connections related to the person's ancestry. Many of his patients were Indigenous, but not all of them. He recognized that his response to this training would make people uncomfortable. He also recognized that people would blame him for bringing up the issue of racism when his colleague repeatedly mentioned the *hysteria* of a colleague blaming her difficulties at work on her being of South Asian ancestry, but he didn't care. He was tired of "good White people" telling him they're not like the others, and then making the same mistakes as everyone else. His White colleagues would not take responsibility for the impact of their statements, and continued to focus on their intent to do no harm. Sometimes, they would stay silent in fear, not knowing what to do next.

At one particular meeting, when he called out a racist comment, he got labelled as "difficult" and got reprimanded when the colleague started crying. The others in the room went to comfort the person, and, although, Jonah, himself, is quite empathetic, he was frustrated with the implication of this person's inability to take responsibility for their impact, and then covering this embarrassment with sadness and doubt, allowing them a free pass to excuse their racist comments.

This time as he looked around the room, he saw that most of the trainees were bewildered and looked confused. No one said a word. They reiterated that we need to focus on people's strengths and provide a safe space for this work. Jonah had a choice to either engage further or decide that he did not want to be part of this initiative. Still, he knew how necessary it was for physicians to be trained in trauma-informed care, and, putting his own triggers aside, he opened up a conversation about the social determinants of health, a key metric he felt was missing from the training.

Jonah had grown up on reserve, and it was only through his mother's persistence and ingenious survival skills that he was able to find some sense of stability in his early years. His mother had recently passed from cardiovascular complications, and Jonah had spent days in the hospital at her bedside, ensuring she received the best care. He often had to be the intermediary between a medical system that saw his mother as an Indigenous woman maybe undeserving of full care, and his closest family member who was gravely ill. Being a physician helped him to speak eye to eye with the doctors and medical staff and he was able to advocate for end-of-life care and pain management during her final days. Still, this experience, alongside all the others through his youth, remained fresh for him now. He had recently lost one of the most significant relationships in his life.

He had joined this training, appreciating its value, and hoping for a trauma-informed medical space in which he would feel more at home. When he heard racist comments diminishing a colleague's experiences and dismissing the importance of the social determinants of health in trauma-informed care, he realized that this was not, perhaps, a place of connection, and his sense of isolation and loneliness as a physician grew. He started to wonder what the purpose of the group was, especially if there was no room to discuss their stories and associated emotions, personalizing the initiative for each one of them in the room. He started to wonder if this was all performative and if he was only being invited as a "token" rather than because his voice and perspective was valued and desired. Much of the discussion on strengths thus far seemed superficial and a lesson in social civility rather than in building social capital.

Feeling uncomfortable, one of the other trainees spoke up and surprised Jonah. She said that she felt ashamed of what had just transpired and that, although she can't quite articulate it yet, she would ensure to educate herself more on the topic of racism. She also apologized for the impact it had had on him and others in the group. What was most surprising is how she talked about her shame and embarrassment as being a potential catalyst for change. She seemed to understand that there were different types of shame, and that in diverse spaces some types of shame propel action and change. She continued to point out all the good things that could come from this interaction and commented on how much courage it likely took for Jonah to start speaking out against these things versus remaining silent.

In reflection after this event, Jonah thought about his old cell biology professor from his university. This professor would always take the time to meet with Jonah and help clarify the parts of the material that were confusing. He even advocated for Jonah to get extra test-taking time during his university courses, recognizing that Jonah could meet high standards with some structural support around his studies. It was this professor who convinced Jonah that he could indeed become a physician. He would always recognize the good in Jonah's in-class contributions and would mention how much he valued hearing his perspective and his ideas.

Emboldened, this led Jonah to recognize that he had a powerful voice and one that he need not shy away from, even when others were uncomfortable, especially if he remained steadfast in his deep need to pave the path for other Indigenous physicians. On a more personal level, Jonah wanted to make sure that the spaces he would be a part of could become a little less divided and a little more inclusive of diverse perspectives and ways of knowing and making sense of the world, including and especially of his Indigenous heritage.

Clinical Vignette Analysis

Jonah's experiences in the vignette highlight the importance of being intentional and sincere in this work. Still, as the adage goes, intent does not equal impact, and so it is essential to remain cognizant of this through the process of renewal and re-structuring. Mistakes present opportunities to pause and learn, recognizing that progress rests on intent, commitment and action. Work on equity, diversity and inclusion is never finished, however the work is more than one person or one department alone can do. It requires a concentrated collaborative effort, both inter- and intra-departmentally, creating a boundary-lessness between equity and diversity work at different levels and niches of the institution.

It is wise to remain humble and curious, and be reminded of Schein's work on humble inquiry (Schein, 2013), "if you don't know if you should act, ask". The same goes for saying or not saying something in moments of witnessing subtle or overt microaggressions or microassaults. Intentionality matters. As does *value*-ing someone else's experiences as their own and valid. This helps prevent the fallacy of performative action, both in its own right and in ascribing others' opportunities, successes, or failures to their cultural and marginalized identities: "they only hired her because she's a woman", "he's pulling the race card", "they only accept people of color into medical school now". Such conclusions may stem from errors of underuse or overuse of judgment.

Judgement, when used appropriately and in the right amounts, leaves one analytical, open minded, and logical (see Table 15.5). When judgment is underused, people appear illogical, naïve, and close-minded. When overused, as often occurs in medicine, people can become narrow-minded, cynical, and rigid in their beliefs. They may forget or be too tired and exhausted to recognize that someone else is struggling and that these struggles are bigger than their own individual effort or history of trauma, reflecting larger societal barriers and microaggressions that build over time.

Table 15.5. *Characteristics of judgement as being overuse/underuse/optimal use (adapted from VIA Institute on Character, 2022)*

Underused	Optimal	Overused
o Illogical o Naïve o Close-minded	o Analytical o Open-minded o Logical	o Narrow-minded o Cynical o Rigid

When one's judgement is called into question, it can bring up feelings of shame. It is wise to remember the "both/and" dialectic in these moments of shame; that two opposing truths can exist at the same time. One's intention may be authentic *and* they may have made a mistake, playing out these very common scenarios of White fragility and White saviourism. It is also wise to remember that there are three types of shame, broadly categorized as:

- "Good" shame that leads to change;
- "Destructive" shame that can lead to negative self-talk, self-injury, or self-criticism; and
- "Externalized shamelessness" that manifests as instantaneous rage and violence towards others

There is a space for "good" shame in this work, one that brings about change and causes inner reflection, ongoing learning, and decolonization.

Key Takeaways

- Nurturing conversations about equity in medicine is essential to centering the issue as a determinant of health and wellbeing for physicians and patients alike.

- Health equity is now proposed as a fifth domain of healthcare improvement, thus constituting a Quintuple Aim framework.
- Addressing equity in clinical spaces is pivotal to improved clinician wellbeing and patient health outcomes.
- Inequitable clinical spaces are perpetuated by designing policies and procedures without awareness of, or concern for, inherent biases in the system and interpersonally.
- Innovation and alignment with progressive cultural norms occur slowly in environments like healthcare due to the mandate to create stability, order, and standardization.
- Standardizations, policies, and procedures should be revisited routinely with an eye towards identifying bias and diversity as order and stability can subvert inclusion and create exclusion.
- The burden of being tolerated, passing and code-switching accumulates over time, contributing to burnout and physician attrition in a field that thrives on standardization and stability.
- Inclusion strategies suggested for cultivating greater equity in clinical practice include:
  o Cultivate internal awareness in order to facilitate the recognition of biases in clinical care
  o Understand and identify microinequities, microaggressions and microassaults
  o Navigate personal and peer biases in order to reduce the pressure on minority peers to masquerade and conform
  o Implement and encourage more courageous conversations about equity
  o Make a commitment to becoming comfortable with discomfort when difficult conversations about race, equity, and diversity arise: Pause, Relax Open
  o Nurture differences amongst peers and patients alike
- Microaffirmations are posited as an antidote to microaggressions and can be skillfully used to validate observed microaggressions.
- Judgements about others are often triggered by social threats against status (S), certainty (C), autonomy (A), relatedness (R), and fairness (F) (SCARF).
- The SCARF model can be useful to monitor and explore common triggers that arise within equity and diversity discussions.

- Leading with equity necessitates a willingness to share social capital.
- Equity-leaning systems transformation requires intention, commitment and action which begin through courageous conversations about equity.

Conclusion

Nurturing equity through more courageous conversations is complex but imperative given the human cost attached to continuing with the status quo. The costs of waiting for the world to be equal and equitable are innumerable, including loss of diversity in the clinical workforce, loss of innovation and adaptability, negative care experiences, and ongoing microaggressions that perpetuate deteriorating mental health and physical health outcomes for patients and clinicians alike.

Physicians have a bird's eye view of the impact of inequitable spaces relative to other industries. Disregarding equity, diversity and inclusion issues in spite of their high valence is akin to "postponing" a deadline: it means overlooking opportunities for prevention and delaying potentially lifesaving interventions. The longer we wait to address the issue, the harder it will be to "right shift" the curve towards a more equitable healthcare environment.

What are the costs of waiting for the world to be equal?

- o   Loss of diversity
- o   Lack of trust (in decision-making, input, feedback given, feedback provided, or lack thereof)
- o   Career development stalled and nonexistent
- o   Turnover (opacity) - why are people really leaving?

Equity work at its core is about relationships and reciprocity. It extends into noticing, naming, navigating, negotiating, and nourishing social capital and conversations about privilege, bias, and microaffirmations. These conversations facilitate an open dialogue and aim to expand the diversity and differences at the local and institutional level. Differences amongst and between patients and physicians alike constitute a rich palette from which we can broaden our scope of equitable practice and care delivery.

There is a famous metaphor of a large circle of people, all watching one person in the center seated on a chair. This centrally seated person has a key hanging out of their left pocket; however, it is not entirely visible to all, and, in fact, only half the circle will notice and be able to appreciate this key. We never know what "key" someone will hold and how this "key" difference will impact the clinical team and the broader institution through initiatives, ideas, or simple skills. As such, a critical asset for fostering courageous conversations about equity is curiosity: to notice and where a voice is needed, to avoid joining a silent majority, and instead align with a vocal minority, knowing that just because it has not been done before, it does not mean it cannot be successful.

On a Parting Note...

Here we are
Standing on shoulders of those who came before.
Mighty and strong,
Supported and upheld.
Grit and grace
Combined to softness and a gentle embrace.
Change in the chaos,
Chaos in the change,
Interruptions and detractions
And a rising in the chest.
We are like lava waiting
To be unboiled and clear revealed,
Lifting up and out
Of our dormant state within.
A moment of openness,
Vulnerability exposed
And here we find our strength
Mired in grit and grace.

©Irina Mihaescu, 2023

References

Arnold, R., Burke, B., James, C., Martin, D. and Thomas, B. (1991). *Educating for a Change*. Toronto: Between the Lines and the Doris Marshall Institute for Education and Action.

Avey, J.B., Reichard, R.J., Luthans, F. and Mhatre, K.H. (2011). Meta-analysis of the impact of positive psychological capital on employee attitudes, behaviors, and performance. *Human Resource Development Quarterly*, 22(2), pp.127–152.

Cameron, K.S. and Spreitzer, G.M. (2013). The Oxford Handbook of Positive Organizational Scholarship. New York: Oxford University Press

Canadian Medical Association. (2021). *A profession under pressure: results from the CMA's 2021 National Physician Health Survey* [online]. Available from: https://www.cma.ca/news/profession-under-pressure-results-cmas-2021-national-physician-health-survey

Flexner, A. (1910). *Medical Education in the United States and Canada: A Report to the Carnegie Foundation for the Advancement of Teaching*. New York: The Carnegie Foundation for the Advancement of Teaching.

Hannah-Jones, N. (2019). *The 1619 Project*. New York: New York Times.

Hogshead, S. (2010). *Fascinate: Your 7 Triggers to Persuasion and Captivation*. New York: HarperCollins Publishers.

Meyer, R. (2009). *The University of Texas at Austin* [online]. Available from: https://news.utexas.edu/2009/12/15/research-shows-height-may-be-predictor-of-financial-success/

National Academies of Sciences, Engineering, and Medicine. (2019). *Taking Action Against Clinician Burnout: A Systems Approach to Professional Well-Being [online]*. Washington, DC: The National Academies Press. Available from: https://doi.org/10.17226/25521

Native Governance Center. (2019). *A Guide to Indigenous Land Acknowledgment* [online]. Available from: https://nativegov.org/news/a-guide-to-indigenous-land-acknowledgment

Nundy, S., Cooper, L.A. and Mate, K.S. (2022). The quintuple aim for health care improvement. *JAMA*, 327(6), p. 521. https://doi.org/10.1001/jama.2021.25181.

Obenchain, T.G. (2021). *Genius Belabored: Childbed Fever and the Tragic Life of Ignaz Semmelweis*. Tuscaloosa: University of Alabama Press.

Project Implicit. (1998) [online]. Available from: https://www.projectimplicit.net/

Raphael, D. (2009). *Social Determinants of Health: Canadian Perspectives*. 2nd ed. Toronto: Canadian Scholars' Press.

Reich, J. and Milner, H.R. (2020). Unit 1: Seeing and Valuing Individuals through an Equity Lens. *Becoming a More Equitable Educator*. University of Alberta Department of Psychiatry, unpublished.

Rock, D. (2008). SCARF: a brain-based model for collaborating with and influencing others. *NeuroLeadership Journal*, 1(1), pp.1-9.

Rowe, M. (2008). Micro-affirmations and micro-inequities. *Journal of the International Ombudsman Association*, 1, pp.45-48.

Schein, E.H. (2013). Humble inquiry: the gentle art of asking instead of telling. San Francisco: Berrett-Koehler Publishers, Inc.

Schoen, K. and Johnson, C.A. (2021). Racial Awareness Training. *Mindfulness Meditation Teacher Certification Program*. Sounds True, unpublished.

Shanafelt, T.D., Gorringe, G., Menaker, R., Storz, K.A., Reeves, D., Buskirk S.J. and Swensen, S.J. (2015). Impact of organizational leadership on physician burnout and satisfaction. *Mayo Clin Proc*, 90(4), pp.432-40.

Sinha, D. and Sinha, S. (2020). Managing in a VUCA World: Possibilities and Pitfalls. *Journal of Technology Management for Growing Economies*, 11(1), pp.17-21.

Sue, D.W., Capodilupo, C.M., Torino, G.C., Bucceri, J.M., Holder, A.M.B., Nadal, K.L. and Esquilin, M. (2007). Racial Microaggressions in Everyday Life: Implications for Clinical Practice. American Psychologist, 62(4), pp.271-286.

Swensen, S.J. and Shanafelt, T. (2020). *Mayo Clinic Strategies to Reduce Burnout: 12 Actions to Create the Ideal Workplace (Mayo Clinic Scientific Press)*. New York: Oxford University Press.

VIA Institute on Character. (2022). *Character Strengths Overuse and Underuse* [online]. Available from: https://www.viacharacter.org/research/findings/character-strengths-overuse-and-underuse

Wilber, K., Patten, T., Leonard, A. and Morelli, M. (2008). *Integral Life Practice: A 21st-Century Blueprint for Physical Health, Emotional Balance, Mental Clarity, and Spiritual Awakening*. Boulder: Integral Books.

Williams, E.S., Rathert, C. and Buttigieg, S.C. (2019). The Personal and Professional Consequences of Physician Burnout: A Systematic Review of the Literature. *Medical Care Research and Review*, 77(5), pp.371-386.

Zhivotovskaya, E. (2019). How Mindfulness Creates a Thriving Positive Organization: The 3 Key Psychological Factors to Success. Presented at the Mindful Leadership Summit 2019.

Chapter 16
Conclusion

Mariam Abdurrahman, MD, Ana Hategan, MD, Caroline Giroux, MD

❖

And once we see, we can never go back and unsee.
—Caroline Giroux, 2023

❖

Beginnings from this Ending....

We thank you for engaging in a courageous exchange with each author through the self-reflective exercises in the chapters and hope you are inspired to continue the dialogue with others, examine your place and build local synergies. To do so, it is necessary to take inventory of our complex web of identities (see Figure 15.1) and our privilege-merit assumptions (see Figure 11.2). Then we must take ownership of our dimensions of privilege and use them as a catalyst to advocate for the groups who, at the moment, are the most oppressed. Engaging in gratitude and celebrating mini victories are important elements in the journey.

The journey towards increased structural competence and integrity in medicine is complex, with no start or finish as time shapes our knowledge and recognition of equity gaps. Recognizing the essential role of time, both past and present, we began this journey by examining the history of medicine for current day relevance (see Chapter 1). Medicine can use history to examine current power structures and inform foundational work on bridging the equity gaps in medicine.

History has been instructive in demonstrating the ways in which culture, institutions, knowledge, society and power intersect to perpetuate primacy and inequity (Amster, 2022). Similarly, medical history is rich with examples of the weaponization of medicine, with evolution to modern day equivalents. For example, the disproportionately observed prevalence of schizophrenia-spectrum disorders in racialized North American persons relative to their White counterparts is postulated as a modern equivalent of utilizing medicine to pathologize race (Faber et al., 2023). Historically, weaponization took the form of pathologizing attempts to fight oppression by naming it a medical diagnosis; e.g., *drapetomania, hysteria and homosexuality*. As Amster (2022) so eloquently captures, "the medical past provides a roadmap for the operational why and how" of the *-isms* and *-phobias* that exist and persist in medical practice today. Thus, time is the most instructive teacher we have in the creation of equity-responsive educational and clinical environments that approach structural competence.

Shifting towards structural competence and integrity requires close examination of the organizing structures of the science and practice of medicine. The role of educational institutions was examined closely (Chapters 2-4, and 10), with note made of the essential role of both the formal and silent curriculum in shaping physician identity and the subsequent attitudes demonstrated towards patients from minority backgrounds. Reframing attitudes and intentionally building capacity for an inclusive environment in medicine begins with the silent curriculum, which is suggested to play the most influential role in the process of enculturation into medicine. Enculturation is intangible, yet its effects pervasive and powerful, thus the need to cast a light on the invisible.

It is critical to align the messaging in the silent curriculum and its explicit (formal) counterpart in order to fill the gap between the explicit vision of a diverse, equitable and inclusive medical profession and the reality of the dissonance within its intricate layers. Similarly, the science and practice of medicine require some courageous conversations at all levels in order for transformative change that better serves patients and providers alike. Such conversations necessitate a dose of courage as they aim to heighten awareness about inequities, address the role of microaggressions, and foster ongoing self-appraisal for implicit biases in the maintenance of inequities. This task is effective only if there is a concerted effort towards a deep culture shift of seeing, acknowledging and addressing the *-isms* and -

phobias. Transformative shifts like these require institution-wide engagement with clear evidence of action within the leadership ranks.

Leaders need to foster a culture of microaffirmations, allow "good" (or constructive, non-paralyzing) shame, and utilize critical self-reflection to propel their programs, teams and institutions forward. In so doing, leaders can lead the charge but co-create the change with physicians, as both can leverage their various levels of privilege to engage in meaningful change making.

Although physicians occupy a space of relative privilege, this exists within a complex web of identities such that the intersectional relations of power, oppression and privilege render a unique identity matrix to each physician (see Chapter 15). These unique identities can be harnessed collectively to enrich local health systems and shape the healthcare environment into one that is more equity responsive. Investment by medical leadership at all levels is essential to reaping these benefits, otherwise academic and clinical institutions stand to replay the minority tax dynamic again and again with no meaningful advancement while burning out their local "diversity champions" (see Chapter 11). Organization-wide engagement and co-creation are essential to forward momentum. Esparza et al. (2022) note that "the placement of responsibility on a select few—rather than the entirety of institutional, departmental, and programmatic leadership—is neither sustainable nor equitable". To this end critical allyship is a necessary journey at both the organizational, programmatic and individual physician level for social change making.

As discussed in Chapter 13, allyship in healthcare contexts is viewed as an active process of creating social change and enhancing social justice as a process shared with individuals and groups who have lived experience of marginalization and oppression. Critical allyship is a more intentional process of engaging in social change making that centers collaboration with equity-deserving populations, communities and individuals concurrent with the praxis of critical reflection on the ally's part. Perhaps the most important takeaway message about allyship is that it is a journey without a destination, in that the multiple route changes and stopovers are more important than getting there lest we fall into the trap of a race without learning and growing along the way.

Critical allyship, individually, programmatically and organizationally, is essential to understanding the prevailing culture and the ways in which it can both sustain and hinder action on equity, diversity and inclusion (EDI). Devising effective and sustainable EDI strategies rests on continued cultural appraisal particularly given the strong influence of the history of medicine and the cultural elements buried in daily practice. Not attending to the culture of medicine would constitute a serious gap, potentially allowing culture to continue to eat strategy (Drucker as cited in Melnyk, 2016).

On the Culture of Medicine

As programs, organizations and individual physicians engage in critical allyship, they become more comfortable with critical reflection, a necessity for understanding the silent aspects of the organizational culture and unearthing what lies hidden in the invisible space between policies and practices. The ability to make the invisible more visible and therefore capable of either being reinforced or diminished is essential to reframing the culture of medicine and the culture of its constitutive structures. Take for example the largely ableist culture of medicine which tends to view disabilities as "an 'anomaly to normalcy', rather than an inherent and expected variation in the human condition" (Rioux and Valentine, 2008). This outlook has hindered a shift towards a more inclusive field for patients and healthcare providers with disabilities (see Chapter 12).

Although all academic and clinical institutions espouse non-discrimination and a zero-tolerance policy to ability-related discrimination, physicians and learners rarely disclose disabilities if they can keep them silent, thus shame and expectations of unfair treatment persist, likely because of the disconnect between the formal messaging and the reality of the medical culture. Similarly, although the formal curriculum addresses the clinical needs associated with various disabilities and espouses care delivery in a non-discriminatory manner, learners are often confronted with a different message during clinical rotations where they observe but cannot necessarily name discriminatory attitudes to patients with disabilities.

Incorporating the spectrum of persons with disabilities in the medical workforce is necessary in order to better serve patients. Thus, ableism is one area of medicine that could be made more visible for cultural reframing and intentional adoption of a more inclusive outlook. In drawing ableism out of the silent curriculum and making it more visible, intentional work can be done on de-adopting the disability tragedy model.

The outlook of temporary able bodiedness continues to be deliberated. The recognition that "ability" can be a temporal and relative state is important in the approach to ableism in medicine. Making this shift requires professional associations and regulatory bodies to move beyond non-discriminatory statements to practical demonstration that it is safe for physicians and learners to disclose that they have disabilities. Similarly, the culture shift requires academic and clinical institutions to remain abreast of innovations in the area concurrent with meaningful engagement and allyship with patients and providers who have disabilities. Creating an equity-responsive academic and clinical environment requires psychologically and physically safe spaces, as both shape the experiences of persons with disabilities.

Medicine and science have long been promulgated as being apolitical, impartial to the -isms and -phobias of the broader society. However, the reality is that the clinical climate is not neutral, and the culture of science has never been blind. Various minoritized groups experience the paradoxical experiences of concurrent hyperfocus and invisibility to the point of erasure. In the North American context, it is noted that Indigenous health professionals must perpetually advocate for visibility in healthcare, with medical trainees learning little about Indigenous health and cultural practices (Jensen and Lopez-Carmen, 2022). Similarly, the presence of epistemic racism in medicine and the sciences is well recognized.

Medical trainees have inadequate exposure to the scope of material and experiences required to serve a diverse patient population. As such, the task of shifting to structural competence is a key responsibility at the medical education and training level. Nurturing the courageous conversations and actions required to make the shift begins with incorporating the language of microaffirmations into clinical education, leadership, and institutional identity.

Of recent, the statement *I trusted my education* is increasingly heard and questions raised about the provenance of medical information and knowledge. This is perhaps most stark when one considers the earlier discussions (Chapters 1, 2, 10, and 11) on the role of curricular materials, clinical practice algorithms and journal publication content in the inaccurate conflation of race and biology. The race correction discussions in Chapters 10 and 11 reveal the insidious presence of racism in medicine, the result being a demarcation of healthcare along racial lines.

This presence of racism in the most fundamental aspects of science and medicine necessitate a concerted systemic shift for any meaningful progress. Health equity must remain the goal, for a true commitment to achieving this Quintuple Aim requires structural action. In addition to attending to the metacommunication around curricular materials, structural action at the education level should also address minority underrepresentation in medicine.

Minority underrepresentation in medicine is prevalent across all stages of the pipeline, from medical school entry to independent practice, from academia to non-academic clinical settings (Boynton-Jarrett et al., 2021; Xierali et al., 2021). Medical learners and physicians recognize this, however, the extent of the role of racism may be underappreciated. While today's medical learners and physicians in practice may agree that racial bias has no place in healthcare, they may not know the relevant history of seminal events that shape the diverse population they serve and shape the trajectory of their minoritized colleagues. This has implications for the appreciation of diversity as a necessity in a representative health workforce. It also has implications for patient care and health equity as discussed so far.

On the –Isms and –Phobias

Identities are complex and multidimensional. The intersection of the multiple aspects of an individual's social identities contributes to unique experiences of concurrent oppression and privilege, with some living the experience of oppression more so than they inhabit their places of privilege. However, it is only when we engage in critical reflection that our various facets of privilege become more conscious and can help identify actions to end the form of oppression that gives us each privilege (Bishop, 1994, pg. 3).

Throughout the book, experiential content has been melded with the literature to facilitate accessibility as equity topics can be charged and uncomfortable, such as occurs with topics like non-conforming identities, gender diversity and racism. In exploring gender diversity, it is quickly apparent that the space for physicians and patients who identify as 2SLGBTQ+ remains small and perilous, while the struggle to dispel erasure is ever present as curricular materials are nearly devoid of 2SLGBTQ+ content and healthcare infrastructure is largely binary.

The pecking order of genders is also apparent in the gendered pay gap. For hospital-based women physicians, the gender pay gap remains notable at 24-34%, exceeding the global 20% gender pay gap across the healthcare sector (Cohen and Kiran, 2020; Dacre et al., 2020; WHO, 2022). Women physicians spend more time with patients and have better patient outcomes, yet their contributions are not valued on par with that of men physicians (Baumkhael et al., 2009; Berthold et al., 2008). Women physicians continue to be impeded by the "sticky floor", the forces that tend to keep women at the lowest levels in an organizational pyramid, despite being at or near parity with men in numbers (WHO, 2022).

Addressing gender equity issues is just and necessary if we are to foster a greater sense of solidarity and inclusion among physicians. This contributes to the sustainability of the healthcare system in terms of physician retention, particularly in academic settings. Although some organizations adopt a blind equality or "see no evil" approach (i.e., color blind, gender blind), this does not translate to the level of recognition and responsiveness required to thrive and reach a fulsome professional potential for many female and gender diverse clinicians. The traditional ways of recognizing and validating professional contributions remain inequitable along gender lines.

The profession stands to lose if meritocracy continues to be a gendered process or one shaped by other -*isms* and -*phobias*. This issue also underlies the diversity-innovation paradox, which is the disconnect between the fundamental goal of scientific progress and uptake of innovation. The disconnect stems from differential uptake of innovations based on the source of innovation. Novel contributions by underrepresented genders and other minorities receive less uptake and increased scrutiny than innovations by the dominant majority. Although diversity breeds innovation, underrepresented groups that diversify organizations have less successful careers within the organizations (Hofstra et al., 2020).

Studies have shown that age, linguistic presentation, personal style preferences, racial features, habitus and other aspects of appearance moderate the way in which the world regards individuals, with significant impacts on both opportunities and barriers, as described in Chapters 7 to 9. Physicians are subject to appearance-related appraisals and may experience a greater level of scrutiny as they are held to a higher critical standard. Therefore, physicians may experience bias, stereotypes, and discrimination from both their colleagues and patients, with the latter affecting patient satisfaction and confidence in their physician.

Harmful stereotypes emanating from a physician's presentation may lead to pressure for conformity within the academic and/or clinical setting in ways that are detrimental to both physician and patient wellbeing. Preceding chapters have tied minority physician wellbeing and burnout risk to the attendant burden of justifying and legitimizing the space they occupy. In combination with the minority tax, the daily experiences of oppression and discrimination that minoritized physicians face creates a burden that drives further inequity and inevitably results in health systems impacts (Esparza et al., 2022; Johnson, 2017; Rodriguez et al., 2015ab; Xierali et al., 2021). Thus, diversity imparts a burden on physicians who occupy the minority space. Yet, diversity is a necessity as a physician workforce with a diverse presentation creates a workforce that can best support the wide and varied patient population of today. Patients are better served when their care better resembles them, and this is only achievable when medicine is as diverse as the population it serves.

In terms of racial diversity, the literature clearly demonstrates that patient care outcomes and experiences of care improve with increased physician-patient concordance. Physicians from minority groups are also more likely to deliver care in underserved settings, care for complex patients and enter primary care (Rodriguez et al., 2015a). Although diversity in medicine is growing, it has not kept apace with population changes, and medicine is yet to resemble the population it serves. The scope of medical racism is deep and broad, and it may be deceptive when racism exists in a sanitized and thus, sanctified form like race correction and tolerance. The smokescreen of tolerance deters the recognition of racism for what it is. It is so effective as to confer on racialized minorities the dubious and intolerable privilege of being tolerated, while also propagating the dynamic of toleration.

In terms of linguistic diversity, the hegemonies embedded in language are apparent when one reflects on the issue of accentism. The history of colonialism and the subsequent expansion of the English language, spoken with a preferred accent, have positioned English as the lingua franca of many Western academic and clinical settings. Perceived competence based on accents and appearances may result in physicians code-switching (i.e., modifying their accent and/or appearance) to better navigate their professional spheres. Thus, in addition to managing their work responsibilities, part of their cognitive load includes managing their dualities of identity. Given that code-switching occurs when there is pressure to modify one's presentation due to discrimination or a fear of retribution, or in exchange for fair treatment (Blanchard, 2021; McCluney et al., 2019), the issue of linguistic bias merits further attention as a distinct avenue of racism.

On Possibilities and Progress

The book utilized questions and reflective activities to support engagement in the practice of seeing, hearing, reflecting, and "doing" in an equity-responsive manner. Throughout the course of the book, the processes and qualities of recognition, reflexivity and critical allyship are encouraged, whether with patients, peers or learners as the physician's role is not confined to a single context in which they encounter individuals and groups who live in the experience of marginalization and oppression.

At the individual level, physicians who engage in allyship with a patient community may very well extend a modified facet of this allyship work to improve the experience of colleagues and medical trainees who have a background of oppression, albeit their allyship in this context may be modulated by the professional relationship. Physicians can also initiate change in their immediate practice by utilizing microinterventions, small everyday actions that convey recognition, support and validation of minoritized patients and colleagues who are targets of microaggressions. Sue et al. (2019) recommend 4 major strategic goals of microinterventions:

i.   make the invisible visible
ii.   disarm the microaggression
iii. educate the perpetrator, and
iv.   seek external reinforcement or support

At the programmatic level, it is essential to incorporate the language of microaffirmations into clinical education, leadership, and institutional identity in order to create an environment of inclusion and respect. The experience of medical education should be in line with accountability to society and future patients by addressing the diversity, accuracy and representativeness of curricular materials as well as examining the dissonance between the formal and silent curriculum when less salubrious messages are embedded in the silence. The content of the null curriculum should also be addressed, for this is where the erasure of some minoritized groups lurks.

Capers and colleagues (2020) propose *bias and racism rounds*, a novel educational forum that is akin to departmental morbidity and mortality rounds. In this forum, departments or sections engage in facilitated rounds to critically review deidentified cases for the role implicit or explicit bias may have played in the course of care. The goal is for the multidisciplinary team to identify opportunities to reduce the impact of bias on care. The rounds enhance the ability to identify, safely discuss and propose local responses that ultimately decrease structural violence.

Physician burnout is linked with increased display of implicit and explicit biases. Thus, the academic environment is also a key venue for action given the rising rates of resident burnout and the observation that resident physicians who experience burnout are more likely to display implicit and explicit biases (Alkozei et al., 2019; Capers et al., 2020; Dyrbye et al., 2019).

At the systems level, it is essential to take concerted action on equity across all levels, from the clinical medical infrastructure to education, research and practice. The clinical infrastructure changes may include examination for and discontinuation of unjustified race correction in laboratory investigations, reference values and treatment algorithms. In terms of research, source data should be more closely examined for inherent biases, the rationale for inclusion and reporting on race must be clear and where race is a proxy for marginalization, this must also be made evident. Data, algorithms and technology should be carefully examined for bias and users made aware of the provenance, assumptions and representativeness of the associated information.

In terms of practice, it is essential to rethink when and how to use race in care delivery, so that race is not conflated with biology and race is no longer posed as the source of pathology (Deyrup and Graves, 2022). The educational setting stands to make shifts in the context of entry into medical education and experience within medical education. Specifically, the entry point must be more equitable and inclusive as the "gatekeeper" function shapes the diversity of the educational body. The experience of medical education should also be addressed in terms of the culture of medicine, curriculum content as noted above, and the experience of minoritized learners. Medical leadership should drive a commitment to equity, diversity and inclusion within the various structures that together constitute medicine and can collectively move medicine towards the Quintuple Aim of health improvement.

On a Parting Note...

Equity, diversity and inclusion generate enrichment, growth and progress, all of which enhance patient outcomes and shift us closer to achieving structural competence. Thus, shifting towards an equity-responsive environment should be viewed as a component of accountability to patients and society. Many strides have been taken in this direction, with many organizations and professional associations examining their spaces, checking their progress and seeking to do better.

As the medical field continues to gain comfort with naming the elephant in the room and acknowledging the field's contribution to the problem, a reflective pause is needed to reaffirm our commitment to truly do no harm, see where harm is being done and speak up, while learning from the past and the present.

Don't just do something, stand there and listen. Then take a deep breath, for the journey is a long one. It is one without a finish, as context, the intersection of identities and the complexity of the human condition are ever changing.

We are at T = zero. Where do we go next and what will your role be? Surely, not to see no evil, hear no evil and speak no evil.

References

Alkozei, A., Killgore, W. D. S., Smith, R., Dailey, N. S., Bajaj, S., & Haack, M. (2017). Chronic Sleep Restriction Increases Negative Implicit Attitudes Toward Arab Muslims. *Scientific reports*, 7(1), 4285. https://doi.org/10.1038/s41598-017-04585-w.

Amster E. J. (2022). The past, present and future of race and colonialism in medicine. *Canadian Medical Association Journal*, 194(20): E708–E710. https://doi.org/10.1503/cmaj.212103.

Amutah, C., Greenidge, K., Mante, A., Munyikwa, M., Surya, S.L., Higginbotham, E., Jones, D.S., Lavizzo-Mourey, R., Roberts, D., Tsai, J., Aysola, J. (2021). Misrepresenting race - the role of medical schools in propagating physician bias. *N Engl J Med.*, 384(9), pp.872-878. https://doi: 10.1056/NEJMms2025768. Epub 2021 Jan 6.

Baumhäkel, M., Müller, U., and Böhm, M. (2009). Influence of gender of physicians and patients on guideline-recommended treatment of chronic heart failure in a cross-sectional study. *Eur J Heart Fail*, 11(3), pp. 299–303. https://doi.org/10.1093/eurjhf/hfn041.

Berthold, H.K., Gouni-Berthold, I., Bestehorn, K.P. et al. (2008). Physician gender is associated with the quality of type 2 diabetes care. *J Intern Med*, 264(4), pp. 340-50. https://doi.org/10.1111/j.1365-2796.2008.01967.x.

Bishop, A. (1994). *Becoming an ally: Breaking the cycle of oppression.* Halifax: Fernwood Publishing.

Blanchard A. K. (2021). Code Switch. *The New England journal of medicine*, 384(23), e87. https://doi.org/10.1056/NEJMpv2107029.

Boynton-Jarrett, R., Raj, A., & Inwards-Breland, D. J. (2021). Structural integrity: Recognizing, measuring, and addressing systemic racism and its health impacts. *EClinicalMedicine*, 36, 100921. https://doi.org/10.1016/j.eclinm.2021.100921.

Capers, Q., 4th, Bond, D. A., & Nori, U. S. (2020). Bias and Racism Teaching Rounds at an Academic Medical Center. *Chest*, 158(6), pp. 2688–2694. https://doi.org/10.1016/j.chest.2020.08.2073.

Cohen, M., & Kiran, T. (2020). Closing the gender pay gap in Canadian medicine. *CMAJ: Canadian Medical Association journal = journal de l'Association medicale canadienne*, 192(35), pp. E1011–E1017. https://doi.org/10.1503/cmaj.200375.

Dacre, J., Woodhams, C., Atkinson C., Laliotis, I., Williams, M., Blanden, J., et al. (2020). Mend the gap: the independent review into gender pay gaps in medicine in England [online]. Available from: https://e-space.mmu.ac.uk/627043/1/ Gender_pay_gap_in_medicine_review.pdf

Deyrup, A., & Graves, J. L., Jr (2022). Racial Biology and Medical Misconceptions. *The New England journal of medicine, 386*(6), 501–503. https://doi.org/ 10.1056/NEJMp2116224.

Dyrbye, L., Herrin, J., West, C. P., Wittlin, N. M., Dovidio, J. F., Hardeman, R., Burke, S. E., Phelan, S., Onyeador, I. N., Cunningham, B., & van Ryn, M. (2019). Association of racial bias with burnout among resident physicians. *JAMA network open, 2*(7), e197457. https://doi.org/10.1001/jamanetworkopen.2019.7457.

Esparza, C. J., Simon, M., Bath, E., & Ko, M. (2022). Doing the Work-or Not: The Promise and Limitations of Diversity, Equity, and Inclusion in US Medical Schools and Academic Medical Centers. *Frontiers in public health, 10*, 900283. https://doi.org/10.3389/fpubh.2022.900283.

Faber, S. C., Khanna Roy, A., Michaels, T. I., & Williams, M. T. (2023). The weaponization of medicine: Early psychosis in the Black community and the need for racially informed mental healthcare. *Frontiers in psychiatry, 14*, 1098292. https://doi.org/10.3389/fpsyt.2023.1098292.

Hofstra, B., Kulkarni, V. V., Munoz-Najar Galvez, S., He, B., Jurafsky, D., & McFarland, D. A. (2020). The diversity-innovation paradox in science. *Proceedings of the National Academy of Sciences of the United States of America, 117*(17), pp. 9284–9291. https://doi.org/10.1073/pnas.1915378117.

Jensen, A., & Lopez-Carmen, V. A. (2022). The "elephants in the room" in U.S. global health: Indigenous nations and white settler colonialism. *PLOS global public health, 2*(7), e0000719. https://doi.org/10.1371/journal.pgph.0000719.

Johnson, T. (2017). The minority tax: an unseen plight of diversity in medical education. *IM Diversity* [online]. Available from: https://imdiversity.com/ diversity-news/the-minority-tax-an-unseen-plight-of-diversity-in-medical-education/

McCluney CL, Robotham K, Lee S, Smith R, Durkee M. (2019). The costs of code-switching. Harvard Business Review [online] November 15, 2019. Available from: https://hbr .org/2019/11/the-costs-of-codeswitching

Melnyk B. M. (2016). Culture Eats Strategy Every Time: What Works in Building and Sustaining an Evidence-Based Practice Culture in Healthcare Systems. *Worldviews on evidence-based nursing, 13*(2), 99–101. https://doi.org/ 10.1111/wvn.12161.

Nundy, S., Cooper, L.A. and Mate, K.S. (2022). The quintuple aim for Health Care Improvement. *JAMA*, 327(6), p.521. doi.org/10.1001/jama.2021.25181.

Rioux, M. H. Valentine F. (2008). Does theory matter? Exploring the nexus between disability, human rights, and public policy. In *Critical Disability Theory: Essays in Philosophy, Politics, Policy, and Law*. Vancouver: UBC Press, pp. 52-53.

Rodriguez, J. E., Campbell, K. M., & Adelson, W. J. (2015). Poor representation of Blacks, Latinos, and Native Americans in medicine. *Family medicine, 47*(4), 259–263.

Rodríguez, J.E., Campbell, K.M. & Pololi, L.H. (2015). Addressing disparities in academic medicine: what of the minority tax?. *BMC Med Educ,* 15(6). https://doi.org/10.1186/s12909-015-0290-9.

Sue, D. W., Alsaidi, S., Awad, M. N., Glaeser, E., Calle, C. Z., & Mendez, N. (2019). Disarming racial microaggressions: Microintervention strategies for targets, White allies, and bystanders. *The American psychologist, 74*(1), pp. 128–142. https://doi.org/10.1037/amp0000296.

Tricco, A.C., Bourgeault, I., Moore, A. et al. (2021). Advancing gender equity in medicine. *CMAJ*, 193(7), pp. E244-50. https://doi.org/10.1503/cmaj.200951.

World Health Organization (WHO). (2022). The gender pay gap in the health and care sector a global analysis in the time of COVID-19 [online]. Available from: https://www.who.int/publications/i/item/9789240052895

Xierali, I. M., Nivet, M. A., Syed, Z. A., Shakil, A., & Schneider, F. D. (2021). Recent trends in faculty promotion in U.S. medical schools: implications for recruitment, retention, and diversity and inclusion. *Academic medicine : journal of the Association of American Medical Colleges, 96*(10), pp.1441–1448. https://doi.org/10.1097/ACM.0000000000004188.

An Equity, Diversity and Inclusion Lexicon

❖

For time and space are ever fluid
As are those who occupy and define that space in time
—Mariam Abdurrahman, 2023

❖

This lexicon is provided as an ***incomplete*** guide to equity, diversity, and inclusion (EDI), in recognition of the shifting sands in which we dwell. This is an ever-changing discourse, sensitive to the awakening and recognition of exclusion, oppression and inequity. As such this lexicon is an evergreen collection that will grow and shift with time and attitudinal changes. The fluidity of the EDI discourse also speaks to the notion that depending on the term there is in fact no one best or 'correct' definition. As noted in Chapter 5, meanings may differ according to those that coined them, institutionalized them, reclaimed them, and/or individually or communally relate to them.

The lexicon is proffered with a view towards increasing the accessibility of the language frequently encountered in the parlance of social justice. While language should unify understanding, it can also itself be a source of confusion. Language can also be divisive - a source of inequity, a barrier to access and discussion, and at the extreme, language recurrently serves as a trigger point for conflict and politicization. Through language, inequitable actions and attitudes are codified into systematic exclusion and oppression, thus language is a powerful counterpoint in the dialogue and actions that seek to redress the balance. Being literate in this language is essential in navigating the complex settings in which medicine unfolds today.

The lexicon is compiled from several sources which are included in the bibliography list for those seeking added reference materials.

Ableism: Bias and discrimination against persons with disabilities that is rooted in a value system where "standard" abilities are seen as normative and superior to disabilities. Ableism perpetuates the view that to have a disability is to be in a diminished state of health. Biases in clinical practice range from viewing persons with disabilities as being "more work", to equating physical differences with cognitive impairment, and providing incomplete clinical assessments based on biased views (e.g., excluding sexual health screening due to an assumption of sexual inactivity). Ableism may be hostile (exclusion, derogatory language, bullying, abuse) or benevolent (patronizing attitudes, decision-making for a competent individual with a disability).

Academic redlining: "The systematic exclusion of students from underrepresented backgrounds from entry into medicine using standardized test hard cut-offs, such as the Medical College Admissions Test (MCAT)", thereby contributing to the lack of diversity in medicine (Rodriguez et al., 2022).

Accentism is when non-native accents are stigmatized or discriminated against. Non-native accents are often judged, marginalised and may be penalised for the way their English sounds.

Agender: a person who does not identify as any gender.

Algorithm bias: Algorithm bias occurs when a clinical care algorithm, such as a screening tool, diagnostic equipment, risk calculator or treatment algorithm utilizes a minority correction factor, thus expanding upon already existing inequities. The bias may occur at any stage, from upstream at the source data level to further downstream at point of use.

Ally: Someone who advocates for and supports members of a community other than their own, reaching across differences to achieve mutual goals.

AFAB/AMAB: Acronyms meaning "assigned female at birth/assigned male at birth".

Asexual: Sometimes called "ace" for short, asexual refers to a complete or partial lack of sexual attraction or lack of interest in sexual activity with others. Asexuality exists on a spectrum where asexual people may experience no, little or conditional sexual attraction.

Anti-racist curriculum: An anti-racist curriculum addresses power dynamics and equity within delivery and content of the curriculum. An antiracist curriculum should facilitate a learner's development of critical reflection skills and social awareness of inequities in such a way that encourages social action.

Bias: "Biases are preconceived notions about individuals or groups that could be based on stereotypes, racism, sexism, or other forms of oppression. Biases allow their users to take "cognitive shortcuts" instead of learning about the individuals or groups" (Rodriguez et al., 2022).

Biphobia: Irrational fear and dislike of bisexual people. Bisexuals may be stigmatized by heterosexual people as well as by lesbians, gay men and transgender people.

Bisexual: A person who is attracted to and may form emotional, romantic and/or sexual relationships with people with the same and people with a different gender and/or gender identity to themselves. People who identify as bisexual need not have had equal experience- or equal levels of attraction- with people across genders, nor any experience at all: it is merely attraction and self-identification that determine orientation.

Cisgender: A person who conforms to gender and/or sex-based societal expectations and is thus "gender normative" or gender conforming. A cisgender person is one whose assigned sex at birth matches their gender identity.

Cisgenderism: Assuming every person to be cisgender, including the expectation that every person must conform to sex- and/ or gender-based societal expectations. Cisgenderism can manifest in distinct forms, such as pathologizing (constructing or treating people's genders, bodies, and experiences associated with their genders and bodies as disordered; e.g., gender dysphoria, gender identity disorder, and disorders of sex development) and misgendering (misclassifying people's genders and bodies; e.g., referring to a man who was assigned female at birth as "she" or "female"). Cisgenderism holds people to traditional expectations based on gender and excludes or subjugates those who do not conform to traditional gender expectations.

Code-switching: Shifting from the linguistic system of one language or dialect to that of another. Beyond the strictly linguistic definition, code switching "involves adjusting one's style of speech, appearance, behavior, and expression in ways that will optimize the comfort of others, in exchange for fair treatment, high-quality service, and employment opportunities" (McCluney et al., 2019).

Coming out: Recognizing one's own sexual orientation or gender identity and being open about it with oneself and/or with others. This often occurs in a significant moment as well as throughout one's life, with each person to whom one chooses to come out.

Critical allyship: An ongoing, active, collaborative and participatory process of alliance that requires critical reflection, social attunement, and action to end the oppression that provides privilege to the ally. Critical allyship emphasizes the action aspect of allyship, rather than simply seeing allyship as an identity based solely on awareness of issues and an openness to listening. The process is always incomplete because of the changing nature and complexity of context and because of the multiple, over-lapping and intersecting realities of marginalization and oppression.

Cultural competence: A combination of attitudes, behaviours, knowledge, protocols and policies that are intentionally deployed by individuals, agencies and organizations to facilitate culturally-informed service delivery within a cross cultural context. Cultural competency exists along a fluid continuum ranging from cultural awareness to cultural sensitivity to cultural competence to cultural humility and then cultural safety.

Cultural safety: In the context of healthcare, cultural safety describes the ability of a healthcare system to deliver care that is culturally appropriate, equitable and critically responsive to power structures. "Cultural safety requires healthcare professionals and their associated healthcare organisations to influence healthcare to reduce bias and achieve equity within the workforce and working environment" (Curtis et al., 2019).

Data inequity: Absence or misrepresentation of data on the health and social determinants of health for racial, ethnic and other minority groups because data is not collected or is reported in aggregate with broader group categories. Essentially, minority data gets lost in majority data, or minority status is not accounted for, or minority groups are not counted. "As a form of structural racism, data omissions contribute to systemic problems such as inability to advocate, lack of resources, and limitations on political power" (Morey et al., 2022).

Decolonization: "The process of deconstructing colonial ideologies of the superiority and privilege of Western thought and approaches" (Antoine et al., 2018: pp. 6-8). In the context of Indigenous populations, Antoine et al. further note that "decolonization involves valuing and revitalizing Indigenous knowledge and approaches and weeding out settler biases or assumptions that have impacted Indigenous ways of being".

Discrimination: Negative behaviour or actions toward a person or group of people based on prejudicial attitudes and beliefs about the person's or group's characteristics, such as sexual orientation, gender, ability, race or other social identity.

Diversity: Differences in appearance, capacity, presentation and social group membership. Refers not only to superficial groupings based on gender, ethnicities and race, it also applies to heterogeneity in age, experience, cultures, religions, socioeconomic status, sexual orientation, mental/physical abilities, and education levels, amongst other variation in the population.

Diversity-Innovation Paradox: The disconnect between the fundamental goal of scientific progress and uptake of innovation; the disconnect stems from differential uptake of innovations based on the source of innovation. Novel contributions by underrepresented minorities receive less uptake and increased scrutiny than those by the dominant majority. Although diversity breeds innovation, underrepresented groups that diversify organizations have less successful careers within the organizations (Hofstra et al., 2020). For example, this is seen with innovations by women and racial minorities in academia.

Enculturation: The socialization process through which people come to learn the dynamics and sociocultural norms, values and worldviews of their microcosm or surrounding society.

Epistemic injustice: Devaluation of knowledge and its sources based on the social identity of the "knower". Epistemic injustice and epistemic racism relate to social hierarchies of knowledge.

Epistemic racism: A facet of systemic racism that discredits or invalidates "the knowledge claims, ways of knowing and 'knowers' themselves" (Beagan et al., 2022). Various groups contend with epistemic racism. In the Indigenous North American context, it is defined as "a colonial mechanism that marginalizes and diminishes the power of Indigenous peoples' voices and knowledge bases" (Sinclaire et al., 2023).

Equality: The state of being equal, thus everyone is given the same amount of resources regardless of differences in their levels of need and ability to access opportunities to utilize the resources meaningfully. In contrast, an equitable approach allocates resources in such a manner as to "level the playing field" by allocating resources differentially based on level of need concurrent with providing the tools and/or accommodations necessary to utilize the resources meaningfully.

Equity: The absence of avoidable, unfair and remediable differences among groups of people. Equity addresses fair allocation of opportunities and resources so that no groups are at a particular disadvantage relative to other groups.

Equity gap: In the context of health, an equity gap refers to disparities in health outcomes and health status metrics that operate along ethnoracial lines, gender, socioeconomic status, other demographic factors and intersectionalities.

Erasure: The process by which the existence of a minority group or perceived non-conforming group is precluded from *conventional* spaces such as healthcare. It may take various forms; e.g., informational erasure of transgender persons in curriculum materials that only contain cisgender patients, infrastructure erasure in which the only washroom facilities available are labeled by binary gender.

Gay: A person whose primary sexual orientation is to members of the same sex or gender. A person of any gender identity can identify as gay, although many female-identified people who are attracted to other female-identified people prefer the term lesbian.

Gender: A system of classifying persons according to socially expected attributes, e.g., constructed roles, behaviours, expressions, and identities; often constructed as a binary framework. People are not born with gender; it is a performative role based on socialization.

Gender-affirming surgeries: Surgical procedures by which a person's physical appearance and function of their existing sexual characteristics are altered to resemble that of the sex or gender to which they are transitioning.

Gender bias: Refers to a person or group receiving different treatment based on their real or perceived gender identity.

Gender creative: Sometimes also known as "gender non-conforming" or "gender expansive"; someone who is gender creative is someone who rejects expected gender roles and stereotypes, expresses a gender identity that is different from the one they were assigned at birth or one that cannot be (or refuses to be) defined within the male/female binary.

Gender discrimination: Refers to a person or group receiving disadvantaged treatment based on their real or perceived gender identity.

Gender dysphoria: The experience of intense, persistent gender incongruence. The Diagnostic and Statistical Manual of Mental Disorders lists gender dysphoria as a diagnosis. However, some argue that this inappropriately pathologizes gender incongruence, while others contend that a diagnosis facilitates access to necessary medical treatment.

Gender expression: The way in which a person expresses their gender identity through clothing, behaviour, posture, mannerisms, speech patterns, activities and more.

Gender identity: One's internal and psychological sense of oneself as male, female, both or neither.

Genderism: Sometimes referred to as cisgenderism. The assumption that all people must conform to society's gender norms, and specifically, the binary construct of only two genders, corresponding to the two sexes (female and male). This belief in the binary construct as the most normal and natural and a preferred gender identity does not include or allow for people to be intersex, transgender, or genderqueer.

Gender nonconforming: A person who does not conform to society's expectations of gender expression based on the gender binary or expectations of masculinity and femininity.

Gender norms: Within the gender binary, these refer to ideas of how boys/men and girls/women should appear, communicate, and behave in society.

Genderqueer: A person who experiences a very fluid sense of their gender identity and who does not want to be constrained by absolute concepts. Instead, they prefer to be open to relocating themselves on the gender continuum.

Gender roles: Within the gender binary, these refer to the roles and responsibilities that are assigned to boys/men and girls/women at home, work, and in society.

Gender relations: Within the gender binary, these refer to relationship dynamics between boys/men and girls/women which can lead to inequities in power.

Gender variant: A synonym for gender nonconforming, which is preferred to gender variant because variance implies a standard normativity of gender.

Gratitude tax: The feeling of obligation that minority faculty have to the academic institution and to future generations of minority physicians for being given the opportunity to be a physician (Rodriguez et al., 2022). The gratitude tax may be enacted by remaining at one's institution out of feeling indebted for the opportunity and not pursuing external opportunities for career advancement.

Health disparity: Health status differences among distinct populations based on demographic variables such as income, education, gender, race and residential neighbourhood.

Health equity tourism: This term was coined in response to the observation of researchers who are experts in other fields but novices in health equity research entering the field of equity research. Lett and colleagues (2022) note that "this phenomenon is the process of previously unengaged investigators pivoting into health equity research without developing the necessary scientific expertise for high-quality work". The concern is that inexpert equity research does not sufficiently attend to the contextual factors that shape inequity and may thus, yield incomplete or inaccurate findings whilst also exacerbating preexisting academic inequity.

Health inequity: Systematic health status differences that occur as a result of avoidable and unjust sociopolitical conditions which create barriers to opportunity.

Heterophily: A tendency for individuals to associate with people dissimilar to themselves. However, homophily is more common than heterophily.

Heterosexual: A person whose primary sexual orientation is to people of a different sex or gender than their own. Heterosexual people are often referred to as "straight".

Heterosexism: The assumption that everyone is, or should be, heterosexual, and that heterosexuality is inherently superior to and preferable to all other sexual orientations.

Heterosexual privilege: Benefits derived automatically by being (or being perceived as) heterosexual that are denied to all other non-heterosexual sexual orientations.

Homophily: A tendency for individuals to associate with people similar to themselves. This presents an inherent source of bias when considerations for positions automatically favour the similar and familiar over the dissimilar within an applicant pool or other group of individuals eligible for the said role.

Homophobia: The irrational fear or hatred of, aversion to, and discrimination against homosexuals or homosexual behaviour.

Homosexual: A person who has emotional, romantic and/or sexual attraction predominately to a person of the same gender. As this term is historically associated with a medical model of homosexuality, most people would prefer to self-identify as gay, lesbian or queer.

Implicit bias: Also known as unconscious bias. Describes the unconscious attitudes, schemas and stereotypes that affect our understanding, actions, and decisions. Because we are unaware of these internalised schemas, we can engage in discriminatory behaviours without conscious intent. Implicit bias training can make individuals aware of their unintentional involvement in the perpetuation of discrimination and inequity as well as the unrecognised advantages and unearned privileges they enjoy based on group membership (Pritlove et al., 2019). Physicians who experience burnout are more likely to display implicit and explicit biases (Alkozei et al., 2019; Capers et al., 2020; Dyrbye et al., 2019).

Indigenization: The process of naturalizing Indigenous knowledge systems and integrating Indigenous ways of knowing and learning with current Western knowledge systems (Antoine et al., 2018: pp. 6-8).

Institutional homophobia or heterosexism: Refers to the many ways that governments, businesses, religious institutions, educational institutions and other organizations set policies and allocate resources such that it discriminates against people who are not heterosexual.

Institutional racism (synonymous with structural racism): Institutionally-based differential access to goods, services, and power based on race. Also described as "racism without racists" as it stems from customs, practices and policies that are codified into the societal infrastructure and thereby "normalized". This form of racism is perpetuated by infrastructure arrangements, differential access to power and resources, and the impact of policies orchestrated by *institutional governance systems that favor White men and women over all others* (Jones, 2000; Rodriguez et al., 2022). "Within academic medicine, institutional racism includes differential access to information, advanced educational opportunities, resources, and having the power to influence decisions, leaders, and policies" (Fritz et al., 2023).

Internalized homophobia: The experience of guilt, shame or self-hatred in reaction to one's own feelings of attraction for a person of the same sex or gender as a result of homophobia and heterosexism. Internalized homophobia is driven by societal norms that stigmatize homosexuality. Internalized homophobia can also motivate prejudice towards others who are homosexual (i.e. external homophobia).

Interpersonal or external homophobia: Overt expressions of internal biases, such as social avoidance, verbal abuse, derogatory humour and physical violence.

Intersectionality: The confluence of multiple social identities such that they create overlapping systems of oppression and privilege in an individual. The interaction of these mutually constitutive elements of oppression and privilege variably shape the lived experience and opportunities of each individual. The term evolved out of Black Feminism and Critical Race Theory, addressing the marginalization of women of color. It was introduced by Kimberlé Crenshaw in 1991, with subsequent expansion of the theory by Patricia Hill Collins.

Intersex: A person who has some mixture of female and male genetic and/or physical sex characteristics. Intersex people may have external genitalia that do not closely resemble typical male or female genitalia, the appearance of both female and male genitalia, the genitalia of one gender and the secondary sex characteristics of a different gender or have a chromosomal make-up that is neither XX nor XY. An outdated term formerly used was hermaphrodite. An intersex person may or may not identify as part of the transgender community.

Internalized racism: "Acceptance by members of the stigmatized races of negative messages about their own abilities and intrinsic worth" (Jones, 2000).

Islamophobia: An irrational fear, aversion, or discrimination against the Islamic religion and those who practice the religion.

Lesbian: A female-identifying individual whose primary sexual orientation is to other female-identifying individuals or who identifies as a member of the lesbian community.

Macroaggressions: Overt and purposefully directed verbal and/or physical racist assaults that typically occur in a public forum. This is the most explicit form of interpersonal racism and may take the form of racial epithets, denigrating gestures or symbols, and physical aggression that leave no doubt about the intention of the perpetrator. In contrast, microaggressions are less tangible but equally distressing as the recipient questions their experience or are questioned about their perception of the experience.

Marginalization: Exclusion from meaningful participation in society, for example the elevated rates of incarceration of Black and Indigenous males in North America.

Microaffirmations: Acts that convey a message of affirmation, validation, inclusion, and/or opportunity. Microaffirmations may be conveyed through body language, tone and word choices that convey inclusion, support, recognition and validation. Microaffirmations are also referred to as micro-moves, micro-gestures, and micro-advantages.

Microaggressions: Brief, commonplace or everyday exchanges that convey disparaging messages to marginalized persons. Microaggressions are often unconsciously delivered. In the context of racism, Sue et al. (2007) describe racial microaggressions as "brief, everyday exchanges that send denigrating messages to people of color because they belong to a racial minority group". The impact of repeated microaggressions culminates over time and can negatively impact the cognitive capacity, mental and physical health, and the productivity of marginalized persons; further information about the impact is captured in Ilan Meyer's Minority Stress Model.

The taxonomy of microaggressions is considered to include three categories: microassaults, microinsults and microinequities. The subtext or metacommunication of these micro messages cut down, put down, deny, overlook or invalidate the reality of marginalized groups (Espaillat et al., 2019; Sue et al, 2007).

Microassault: Explicit aggression that is usually conscious, and may be verbal or nonverbal, towards a marginalized person in relation to aspects of their marginalized identity.

Microinequities: The pattern of being overlooked, under-credited, under-respected, and devalued because of one's minority identity.

Microinterventions: "Everyday words or deeds, whether intentional or unintentional, that communicate to targets of microaggressions (a) validation of their experiential reality, (b) value as a person, (c) affirmation of their racial or group identity, (d) support and encouragement, and (e) reassurance that they are not alone" (Sue et al., 2019: p. 134). By employing microinterventions, they suggest that those witnessing or experiencing microaggressions can regain a sense of self-efficacy and control, which will enhance psychological well-being.

Sue et al. (2019) recommend 4 major strategic goals of microinterventions:

    i.   make the invisible visible
    ii.   disarm the microaggression
    iii.   educate the perpetrator, and
    iv.   seek external reinforcement or support.

Microinvalidation: Comments that dismiss, exclude, or negate the experience or feelings associated with marginalization. For example, comments to the effect that a marginalized person is *reading too much into the situation* or is *being overly sensitive* about responses to their expressed experience of sexism, racism, transphobia, ableism, or other source of marginalization.

By questioning the accuracy of a marginalized persons experience, one superimposes their own perceptions and/or their own experiences as being the more accurate or relevant perspective.

Microinsult: Insensitive comments that demean a marginalized person's heritage or identity.

Minority tax: A spectrum of additional duties and expectations encountered by minorities in institutional environments, often taking the form of expectations to support and promote institutional diversity and inclusion initiatives. These extra duties are time consuming, are not typically considered to be scholarly productivity, and are thus unlikely to contribute to faculty and professional advancement.

Minoritized: In reference to minoritized individuals or minoritized groups to distinguish from the view of minority status being defined by relative numbers and identity differences. Minoritization and marginalization share some similarities but are not synonymous.

A minoritized group is a "social group that is devalued in society and given less access to its resources. This devaluing encompasses how the group is represented, what degree of access to resources it is granted, and how the unequal access is rationalized. Traditionally, a group in this position has been referred to as the minority group. However, this language has been replaced with the term minoritized in order to capture the active dynamics that create the lower status in society, and also to signal that a group's status is not necessarily related to how many or few of them there are in the population at large" (New Discourses, 2020).

Myth of meritocracy: Attribution of success to unearned or unrecognized privileges. Achievements often draw from underlying privilege although the privilege is not recognized and is espoused as merit.

Necropolitics: The relationship between sovereignty and power over life and death. Philosopher Achille Mbembe (2003) coined the term and notes that "the capacity to define who matters and who does not, who is disposable and who is not" is the ultimate purview of a sovereign power on its citizenry. His seminal question is "'under what practical conditions is the right to kill, to allow to live, or to expose to death exercised?" This discourse has sparked much debate in the context of the necropolitical underpinnings of the current COVID-19 Pandemic in which racialized groups bear a disproportionate burden of morbidity and mortality.

Non-binary: An umbrella term for gender identities that fall outside of the man-woman binary, anywhere along the gender spectrum; can include identities such as being agender, genderqueer, gender fluid, or gender nonconforming, amongst others.

Oppression: The systematic subjugation of one group by another through asymmetric power relations due to the dominant group's control of legal and social institutions, customs, and established norms. Social oppression operates at multiple levels (i.e., individual to systems level) and is reinforced by the social norms that enshrine privileges. Iris Young (1990) describes five types of oppression, including exploitation, marginalization, powerlessness, cultural imperialism, and violence.

Othering: "A set of dynamics, processes, and structures that engender marginality and persistent inequality across any of the full range of human differences based on group identities" (powell and Menendian, 2016).

Pansexual: A person who is attracted to other people regardless of gender identity.

Praxis: The process by which theory is put into practice. In the social justice context, praxis involves the use of reflection *in* one's action concurrent with reflection *on* one's action as a means of practicing, exercising, and honing the practical application of social justice ideas, lessons and theories.

Prejudice: An unjustified or biased attitude toward an individual or group of people based solely on their membership in a social group, such as heterosexist attitudes towards the 2SLGBTQ+ community, ableist prejudices towards persons with disabilities.

Privilege: Unearned advantages, benefits, opportunities and access bestowed by social identity such as race, ethnicity, socioeconomic status, gender, sexuality and ability status. Privilege is often conflated with merit in privileged groups, particularly because the social group membership assigns the background advantages required for success while also limiting barriers to success.

Queer: In contemporary usage, queer is an inclusive, unifying, sociopolitical and self-affirming umbrella term encompassing a broad range of sexual and gender expression, including people who identify as gay, lesbian, bisexual, transgender, intersex, genderqueer or any other non-heterosexual sexuality or nonconforming gender identity. Queer is a reclaimed term, which was previously seen as a derogatory term, but many people within the 2SLGBTQ+ community are comfortable using this term.

Questioning: A self-identification sometimes used by those exploring personal issues of sexual orientation and/or gender identity.

Race correction: Also called race norming, or race adjustment. The practice of adjusting medical calculations and parameters (e.g., risk scores, instrumentation settings, treatment algorithms) to account for race. Race correction is in prevalent use, including cardiac risk scores, pulmonary function tests, estimates of glomerular filtration rate, and obstetrics (assessment for vaginal birth after cesarean delivery).

Racial gaslighting: A psychological process in which a racialized individual or group questions their perception of reality with respect to a racialized dynamic, event or interaction. In the professional context, racial gaslighting gradually erodes confidence in one's contributions and experiences, thus interfering with engagement. It can also exacerbate imposter syndrome, isolation, and emotional destabilization (Rodriguez et al., 2022).

Racial trauma: "The individual and/or collective psychological distress and fear of danger that results from experiencing or witnessing discrimination, threats of harm, violence, and intimidation directed at ethno-racial minority groups" (Chavez-Dueñas et al., 2019).

Racism: "A system of structures, policies, practices, and norms that construct opportunities and assigns values based on one's phenotype" (Jones, 2002). Racism is an important modifiable social determinant of health that contributes significantly to health inequities.

Reflexivity: The capacity to understand how one's perspective, assumptions, and identity are socially constructed through the process of reflecting critically on oneself. Through ongoing self-scrutiny, one gains insight into one's biases, preferences, way of being in the world, and ways of seeing the world. Critical reflexivity is a key element in change making and begins with an inventory of the self, the spaces one occupies as well as the places, spaces and organizations to which one has access as a result of one's privilege, which can be leveraged for allyship.

Eric Shragge (2007), a longstanding community organizer in Quebec, Canada, suggests that this deeper concept of critical reflexivity begins with 3 important questions which have been adapted to the healthcare context:

1) Who am I?
2) Who am I as a [medical/healthcare professional]?
3) Who am I in this interaction/intervention?

Reparative or conversion therapy: A range of pseudo-scientific treatments that aim to change a person's sexual orientation from non-heterosexual to heterosexual or a person's gender identity from non-cisgender to cisgender.

Sexual behaviour: Refers specifically to sexual actions or what a person does sexually. Sexual behaviour is not necessarily congruent with sexual orientation and/or sexual identity.

Sexual identity: Refers to a person's identification to self (and others) of one's sexuality. It is not necessarily congruent with sexual orientation and/or sexual behaviour.

Sexual orientation: Refers to how one thinks of oneself in terms of one's emotional, romantic or sexual attraction, desire or affection for another person.

Silent curriculum: Also called the hidden curriculum. The unwritten and unspoken rules that exist outside the formal medical education and training curriculum. The silent curriculum guides assumptions, attitudes, behaviours, expectations, and professional values among physicians, and is transmitted to learners through the process of enculturation into the profession. In contrast, the formal curriculum is explicit, tangible and can be decisively altered.

Social determinants of health: "The environmental conditions in which people are born, live, learn, work, play, worship, and age that affect a wide range of health, functioning, and quality-of-life outcomes and risks" (USDHSS, 2023).

Sociopolitical structures and political power are implicated as key drivers of the social determinants according to the WHO Report, Closing the Gap in a Generation (2008). This is perhaps most evident in the stark life expectancy differences reported by Geruso (2012) for Black versus White Americans, noting that "for males, 80% of the black-white gap in life expectancy at age 1 can be accounted for by differences in socioeconomic and demographic characteristics. For females, 70% percent of the gap is accounted for".

Sponsorship: A professional relationship that provides instrumental support for career advancement. The sponsorship dyad includes a career aspirant or "sponsoree" and a sponsor. The sponsor is in a position of higher professional influence with access to resources and networks. Sponsorship, mentorship and coaching play important roles in professional growth and success, particularly for underrepresented minorities who have not traditionally had access to such resources. Sponsorship is generally essential for significant career advancement, while mentorship alone is not adequate unless the mentor is in an influential role that can open doors for the mentee.

Stereotype threat: The fear or worry on the part of a minority individual about confirming a negative stereotype of a minority group to which they belong when performing a task on which they aspire to do well. Steele and Aronson (1995) theorized that racialized individuals may underperform on aptitude tests as a result of fear that their performance may confirm a negative societal stereotype about their race. Stereotype threat is thought to be a contributing factor in the gender and minority gaps in academic presence, academic performance and pursuit of academic opportunities.

Structural competence: Recognition and action on the ways in which institutions, neighborhood conditions, market forces, public policies, and healthcare delivery systems collectively shape symptoms and diseases, resulting in health inequities (Hansen and Metzl, 2017). Structural competence expands the elements of cultural competence and cultural safety through a rigorous framework that accounts for the role of the social determinants of health.

Structural racism: A form of racism that is embedded in the organizing structures of society, including laws, policies, institutions, and practices such that it provides advantages to certain racial groups while disadvantaging others. In the context of health, structural racism divides the health of individuals, communities and populations along racial lines. Structural racism was coined by American sociologist, Joe Feagin (2000) in his book, Racist America: Roots, Current Realities, and Future Reparations.

Feagin described structural racism as *"the complex array of antiblack practices, the unjustly gained political-economic power of whites, the continuing economic and other resource inequalities along racial lines, and the white racist ideologies and attitudes created to maintain and rationalize white privilege and power. Systemic here means that the core racist realities are manifested in each of society's major parts."*

Structural violence: The social arrangements that put individuals and populations in harm's way due to disparate access to resources, social capital, political power, education, and healthcare. These social arrangements inhibit individuals, groups, and societies from reaching their full potential due to differential access to resources. Because these arrangements are so deeply entrenched in the societal fabric and inform our ways of understanding the world, they can be imperceptible.

Syndemic: The disproportionate occurrence of two or more health conditions clustered within a given population, with the health conditions occurring in excess as a result of synergistic interaction between noxious social forces and biological disease processes in a vulnerable populace.

Syndemic orientation: A biosocial framework that postulates upstream social, political, and structural determinants can contribute more to health inequities than biological factors or personal choices.

Temporarily able bodied (TAB): The concept that everyone is temporarily able-bodied, because as life events and the effects of aging accrue, disability is bestowed in varying degrees. This is in contrast to the ableist view of disabilities as "an 'anomaly to normalcy', rather than an inherent and expected variation in the human condition" (Rioux and Valentine, 2008). The TAB outlook has met with variable reception as there is concern that it represents a euphemism about disability and may inadvertently also perpetuate ageism. Similarly, the use of "differently able" instead of disability is not favoured as it is also euphemistic and chiefly serves to eliminate the discomfort of the group doing the naming.

Tolerance-based racism: Unintended consequence of the underlying power dynamic between a dominant majority group that exercises non-interference towards minority group differences. The negative attributes of the toleration dynamic stems from the construction and amplification of the minority group's "otherness" which facilitates the propagation of racism.

Transgender or trans: Someone whose gender identity or expression differs from their assigned gender or assigned sex at birth. The person's gender identity differs from societal expectations of masculinity or femininity. Transgender is often used as an umbrella term that includes people who identify as Two Spirit, intersex, genderqueer and non-binary.

Transition: A complicated, multi-step process that can take years as transgender people align their anatomy and (or) their gender expression with their gender identity.

Transphobia: Irrational fear or dislike of persons who are, or are perceived to be, transgender.

Two Spirit: A term used by some North American Indigenous people to describe those people in their cultures whose nature is comprised of both male and female spirits. People who identify as Two Spirit may also identify as gay, lesbian, bisexual, transgender, intersex, or have multiple gender identities.

Upstander: The concept of transforming from a passive bystander observing micro-/macroaggressions silently to assuming an active stance of critical allyship. Upstanders may collaborate with marginalized colleagues to address micro-/macroaggressions, utilize their privilege to provide equitable access to professional opportunities, and speak up when innovative ideas arising from marginalized colleagues are silenced or credited to others.

White fragility: Coined by Robin DiAngelo (2019) to describe a spectrum of emotional and behavioural responses exhibited by White persons in response to being confronted by their participation and/or benefit from racial inequality, injustice and/or oppression. The spectrum of response may include avoidance, denial, or defensiveness which reduces the discomfort and other negative emotions arising from the encounter. DiAngello theorizes that these responses are subconsciously designed to silence conversations around race and maintain the comfortable, White status quo.

White saviourism: The belief that White persons have a benefactory and/or fiduciary duty to uplift, save, educate and protect their non-White counterparts; the concept originated from rhetoric about global health work, peacekeeping and missionary work conducted by persons and agencies from wealthy White nations in developing countries. More recently, the concept was reactivated by author, Teju Cole's (2020) views about the White Savior Industrial Complex (WSIC) which he argued was more about the saviour's own emotional validation of privilege than helping others. Marginalized groups are denied agency in this context as they are seen as passive targets for the saviours' performative benevolence.

Conclusion

The lexicon included here is not exhaustive, nor is it static as the equity, diversity and inclusion conversation is rich with dynamic ideas, new insights and nuances. This lexicon is provided as a guide to further understanding as we collectively strive to engage in uncomfortable conversations about the elephant in the exam room.

The lexicon is an evergreen collection that is anticipated to grow and shift with time. As healthcare providers, it is essential to understand the terminology as the terminology conveys a reality. To understand and speak a mutual language that is respectful and knowledgeable about the realities that surround us is powerful in building bridges, whether in relation to the patient in front of us, the communities we serve, or the colleagues and learners we act in concert with to deliver care.

Bibliography

Ackerman-Barger, K., Boatright, D., Gonzalez-Colaso, R., Orozco, R., & Latimore, D. (2020). Seeking inclusion excellence: understanding racial microaggressions as experienced by underrepresented medical and nursing students. *Academic medicine: journal of the Association of American Medical Colleges*, 95(5), pp. 758–763. https://doi.org/10.1097/ACM.0000000000003077.

Alkozei, A., Killgore, W. D. S., Smith, R., Dailey, N. S., Bajaj, S., & Haack, M. (2017). Chronic Sleep Restriction Increases Negative Implicit Attitudes Toward Arab Muslims. Scientific reports, 7(1), 4285. https://doi.org/10.1038/s41598-017-04585-w.

Antoine A., Mason R., Mason R., Palahicky S., Rodriguez de France C. (2018). Pulling together: A guide for Indigenization of post-secondary institutions. Pressbooks Ed. A professional learning series. BCcampus. Indigenization, Decolonization, and Reconciliation pp. 6–8 [online]. Available from: https://opentextbc.ca/indigenizationcurriculumdevelopers

Asare, J.G., What Is White saviorism and how does it show up in your workplace? Forbes September 30, 2022 [online]. Available from: https://www.forbes.com/sites/janicegassam/2022/09/30/what-is-white-saviorism-and-how-does-it-show-up-in-your-workplace/.

Beagan, B. L., Bizzeth, S. R., Sibbald, K. R., & Etowa, J. B. (2022). Epistemic racism in the health professions: A qualitative study with Black women in Canada. *Health (London, England : 1997)*, 13634593221141605. Advance online publication. https://doi.org/10.1177/13634593221141605.

Bishop, A. (1994). *Becoming an ally: Breaking the cycle of oppression.* Halifax: Fernwood Publishing.

Butler, K., Yak, A., and Veltman, A. (2019). "Progress in medicine is slower to happen": qualitative insights into how trans and gender nonconforming medical students navigate cisnormative medical cultures at Canadian training programs. *Academic medicine*, 94(11), pp. 1757-1765.

Canadian Institutes of Health Research (CIHR). (2020). *What is gender? What is sex?* [online]. https://cihr-irsc.gc.ca/e/48642.html

Capers, Q., 4th, Bond, D. A., & Nori, U. S. (2020). Bias and Racism Teaching Rounds at an Academic Medical Center. Chest, 158(6), pp. 2688–2694. https://doi.org/10.1016/j.chest.2020.08.2073.

Carbado, D. W., Crenshaw, K. W., Mays, V. M., & Tomlinson, B. (2013). Intersectionality: Mapping the movements of a theory. *Du Bois review: social science research on race*, 10(2), pp. 303–312. https://doi.org/10.1017/S1742058X13000349

Chavez-Dueñas, N. Y., Adames, H. Y., Perez-Chavez, J. G., & Salas, S. P. (2019). Healing ethno-racial trauma in Latinx immigrant communities: Cultivating hope, resistance, and action. *The American psychologist*, 74(1), pp. 49–62. https://doi.org/10.1037/amp0000289.

Cambridge Dictionary. (2023). *English Dictionary* [online]. Available from: https://dictionary.cambridge.org/dictionary/english/.

Cole, T. *In* BMJ GH Blogs. The White Savior Industrial Complex in Global Health [online]. Posted on March 11, 2020. Available from: https://blogs.bmj.com/bmjgh/2020/03/11/the-white-savior-industrial-complex-in-global-health/

Cornell Law School Legal Information Institute. (2020). *Gender bias* [online]. Available from: https://www.law.cornell.edu/wex/gender_bias

Crenshaw, K.W. (1989). Demarginalizing the intersection of race and sex: A Black feminist critique of antidiscrimination doctrine, Feminist Theory and antiracist politics, *University of Chicago Legal Forum*: Vol. 139, Article 8 [online]. Available from: https://scholarship.law.columbia.edu/faculty_scholarship/3007.

Crenshaw. K. (1991). Mapping the margins: intersectionality, identity, and violence against women of color. *Stanford Law Review,* 43(6), pp. 1241–1300.

Curtis, E., Jones, R., Tipene-Leach, D., Walker, C., Loring, B., Paine, S. J., & Reid, P. (2019). Why cultural safety rather than cultural competency is required to achieve health equity: a literature review and recommended definition. *International journal for equity in health, 18*(1), 174. https://doi.org/10.1186/s12939-019-1082-3.

D'Angelo, I., Demetriou, C., and Jones, C. (2020). Microaffirmations as a tool to support the process of inclusive education. *Education Sciences and Society,* (2020/1).

Diangelo, R.J. (2019). White Fragility: Why It's So Hard for White People to Talk About Racism. London: Allen Lane, An Imprint of Penguin Books.

Dyrbye, L., Herrin, J., West, C. P., Wittlin, N. M., Dovidio, J. F., Hardeman, R., Burke, S. E., Phelan, S., Onyeador, I. N., Cunningham, B., & van Ryn, M. (2019). Association of racial bias with burnout among resident physicians. JAMA network open, 2(7), e197457. https://doi.org/10.1001/jamanetworkopen.2019.7457.

Emmerich N. Bourdieu's collective enterprise of inculcation: The moral socialisation and ethical enculturation of medical students. *British Journal of Sociology of Education.* 2015 Oct 3;36(7):1054-72.

European Institute for Gender Equality (EIGE). (2016). *Gender norms* [online]. Available from: https://eige.europa.eu/thesaurus/terms/1194

European Institute for Gender Equality (EIGE). (2016). *Gender roles* [online]. Available from: https://eige.europa.eu/thesaurus/terms/1209

Farmer, P. E., Nizeye, B., Stulac, S., and Keshavjee, S. (2006). Structural violence and clinical medicine. *PLoS medicine*, 3(10), e449. https://doi.org/10.1371/journal.pmed.0030449.

Feagin, J. R. (2000). *Racist America: roots, current realities, and future reparations.* New York, NY: Routledge.

The 519 Church Street Community Centre. (2020). The 519 Glossary 2020 [online]. Available from: https://www.the519.org/educationtraining/glossary

Flentje, A., Heck, N. C., Brennan, J. M., & Meyer, I. H. (2020). The relationship between minority stress and biological outcomes: A systematic review. *Journal of behavioral medicine*, 43(5), 673–694. https://doi.org/10.1007/s10865-019-00120-6.

Fraser, S. L., Gaulin, D., & Fraser, W. D. (2021). Dissecting systemic racism: policies, practices and epistemologies creating racialized systems of care for Indigenous peoples. *International journal for equity in health*, 20(1), 164. https://doi.org/10.1186/s12939-021-01500-8

Fritz, C. D. L., Obuobi, S., Peek, M. E., & Vela, M. B. (2023). Cultivating anti-racism allies in academic medicine. *Health equity*, 7(1), pp. 218–222. https://doi.org/10.1089/heq.2022.0024.

Galtung J. (1969). Violence, peace and peace research. *J Peace Res* 6, pp. 167–191.

Geruso M. (2012). Black-white disparities in life expectancy: how much can the standard SES variables explain?. *Demography*, 49(2), pp. 553–574. https://doi.org/10.1007/s13524-011-0089-1.

Hansen, H. and Metzl, J.M. (2017). 'New medicine for the US health care system: training physicians for structural interventions', *Academic Medicine: Journal of the Association of American Medical Colleges*, 92(3), p.279.

Harrison, C., & Tanner, K. D. (2018). Language Matters: Considering Microaggressions in Science. *CBE life sciences education*, 17(1), fe4. https://doi.org/10.1187/cbe.18-01-0011.

Hartland, J., and Larkai, E. (2020). Decolonising medical education and exploring White fragility. *BJGP open*, *4*(5), BJGPO.2020.0147. https://doi.org/10.3399/BJGPO.2020.0147.

Hofstra, B., Kulkarni, V. V., Munoz-Najar Galvez, S., He, B., Jurafsky, D., & McFarland, D. A. (2020). The diversity-innovation paradox in science. *Proceedings of the National Academy of Sciences of the United States of America*, *117*(17), pp. 9284–9291. https://doi.org/10.1073/pnas.1915378117.

Howard, S., Saewyc, E.M., Cameron, C., et al. (2021). *Promoting 2SLGBTQI+ health equity: Best practice guidelines* Jan 12 2022 [online]. Available from: https://rnao.ca/sites/rnao-ca/files/bpg/2SLGBTQI_BPG_June_2021.pdf

Jones C. P. (2000). Levels of racism: a theoretic framework and a gardener's tale. *American journal of public health*, *90*(8), 1212–1215. https://doi.org/10.2105/ajph.90.8.1212.

Jones, C.P. (2002). Confronting institutionalized racism. *Phylon*, 50 (1), pp. 7-22. https://doi:10.2307/4149999.

Langston University. (2020). *Gender discrimination defined* [online]. Available from: https://www.langston.edu/title-ix/gender-discrimination-defined

Lett, E., Adekunle, D., McMurray, P., Asabor, E. N., Irie, W., Simon, M. A., Hardeman, R., & McLemore, M. R. (2022). Health Equity Tourism: Ravaging the Justice Landscape. *Journal of medical systems*, *46*(3), 17. https://doi.org/10.1007/s10916-022-01803-5.

Levine, R. B., Ayyala, M. S., Skarupski, K. A., Bodurtha, J. N., Fernández, M. G., Ishii, L. E., & Fivush, B. (2021). "It's a Little Different for Men"-Sponsorship and Gender in Academic Medicine: A Qualitative Study. *Journal of general internal medicine*, *36*(1), pp. 1–8. https://doi.org/10.1007/s11606-020-05956-2.

Liu, W. M., Liu, R. Z., Garrison, Y. L., Kim, J. Y. C., Chan, L., Ho, Y. C. S., & Yeung, C. W. (2019). Racial trauma, microaggressions, and becoming racially innocuous: The role of acculturation and White supremacist ideology. *The American psychologist*, *74*(1), pp. 143–155. https://doi.org/10.1037/amp0000368.

Mbembe, A. (2003). Necropolitics. *Public Culture*, *15*(1), 11-40. https://doi.org/10.1215/08992363-15-1-11

McCluney, C.L., Robotham, K., Lee, S., Smith, R., and Durkee, M. (2019). The costs of code-switching [online]. *Harvard Business Review*. Available from: https://hbr.org/2019/11/the-costs-of-codeswitching

McMaster University Michael G. DeGroote School of Medicine. (2015). *Glossary of diversity-related terms* [online]. https://mdprogram.mcmaster.ca/students/diversity-affairs/diversity-affairs-resources/glossary-of-diversity-related-terms

Merriam Webster (2022). Available from: https://www.merriam-webster.com/dictionary/racism.

Metzl, J.M., Hansen, H. (2014). 'Structural competency: theorizing a new medical engagement with stigma and inequality', *Social Science and Medicine*, 103, pp. 126–133.

Meyer I. H. (2003). Prejudice, social stress, and mental health in lesbian, gay, and bisexual populations: conceptual issues and research evidence. *Psychological bulletin, 129*(5), 674–697. https://doi.org/10.1037/0033-2909.129.5.674.

Morey, B. N., Chang, R. C., Thomas, K. B., Tulua, , Penaia, C., Tran, et al. (2022). No equity without data equity: Data reporting gaps for Native Hawaiians and Pacific Islanders as structural racism. *Journal of health politics, policy and law, 47*(2), pp. 159–200. https://doi.org/10.1215/03616878-9517177.

New Discourses. (2020). Minoritize [online]. Available from https://newdiscourses.com/tftw-minoritize/

Page S. (2017). Diversity bonuses and the business case. *The Diversity Bonus.* Princeton, NJ: Princeton University Press.

powell, j.a. Menendian, S. (2016). The Problem of Othering: Towards Inclusiveness and Belonging. In *Othering and Belonging: Expanding the circle of human concern* [online]. Berkley, CA: Haas Institute. Available from https://www.othering andbelonging.org/the-problem-of-othering/

Pritlove, C., Juando-Prats, C., Ala-Leppilampi, K., and Parsons, J. A. (2019). The good, the bad, and the ugly of implicit bias. *Lancet (London, England), 393*(10171), 502–504. https://doi.org/10.1016/S0140-6736(18)32267-0.

Rioux, M. H., and Valentine, F. (2008). Does theory matter? Exploring the nexus between disability, human rights, and public policy. In *Critical Disability Theory: Essays in Philosophy, Politics, Policy, and Law.* Vancouver: UBC Press, pp. 52-53.

Rodríguez, J. E., Figueroa, E., Campbell, K. M., Washington, J. C., Amaechi, O., Anim, T., et al. (2022). Towards a common lexicon for equity, diversity, and inclusion work in academic medicine. *BMC medical education, 22*(1), 703. https://doi.org/10.1186/s12909-022-03736-6.

Rukadikar, C., Mali, S., Bajpai, R., Rukadikar, A., & Singh, A. K. (2022). A review on cultural competency in medical education. *Journal of family medicine and primary care, 11*(8), pp. 4319–4329. https://doi.org/10.4103/jfmpc.jfmpc_2503_21.

Sandset T. (2021). The necropolitics of COVID-19: Race, class and slow death in an ongoing pandemic. Global public health, 16(8-9), pp. 1411–1423. https://doi.org/10.1080/17441692.2021.1906927.

Shragge, E. (2007). In and against" the community: Use of self in community organizing, p.p. 159 – 179. In, D. Mandell (ed.) *Revisiting the use of self: Questioning professional identities*. Toronto: Canadian Scholars' Press.

Sinclaire, M., Lavallee, B., Cyr, M., & Schultz, A. (2023). Indigenous Peoples and Type 2 Diabetes: A Discussion of Colonial Wounds and Epistemic Racism. *Canadian journal of diabetes*, S1499-2671(23)00031-X. Advance online publication. https://doi.org/10.1016/j.jcjd.2023.01.008.

Singer, M., Bulled, N., Ostrach, B. and Mendenhall, E. (2017). 'Syndemics and the biosocial conception of health', *The Lancet*, 389 (10072), pp. 941-950.

Steele, C. M., & Aronson, J. (1995). Stereotype threat and the intellectual test performance of African Americans. *Journal of personality and social psychology*, 69(5), pp. 797–811. https://doi.org/10.1037//0022-3514.69.5.797.

Sue, D.W., Capodilupo, C., Torino, G., Bucceri, J., Holder, A.B., Nadal, K.L., et al. (2007). Racial microaggressions in everyday life: implications for clinical practice. *American psychologist*, 62, pp. 271–286.

Sue, D. W., Alsaidi, S., Awad, M. N., Glaeser, E., Calle, C. Z., & Mendez, N. (2019). Disarming racial microaggressions: Microintervention strategies for targets, White allies, and bystanders. *The American psychologist*, 74(1), pp. 128–142. https://doi.org/10.1037/amp0000296.

The Centre. (2006). *LGTB health matters: an education & training resource for health and social service sectors* [online]. Available from: http://www.sexualhealth centresaskatoon.ca/pdfs/p_lgbt.pdf

The 519 Church Street Community Centre. (2020). The 519 Glossary 2020 [online]. Available from: https://www.the519.org/educationtraining/glossary

Tricco, A.C., Bourgeault, I., Moore, A. et al. (2021). Advancing gender equity in medicine. *CMAJ*, 193(7), pp. E244-50. https://doi.org/10.1503/cmaj.200951.

United States Department of Health and Human Services (USDHSS). (2023). Healthy People 2030. Social determinants of health [online]. Available from: https://health.gov/healthypeople/priority-areas/social-determinants-health

University of Michigan School of Social Work. (2023). What is privilege, oppression, diversity and social justice? [online]. https://ssw.umich.edu/privilege-oppression-diversity-and-social-justice

Veltman, A., and La Rose, T. (2019). LGBTQ mental health: What every clinician needs to know, *Psychiatric times*, 36(12), pp. 21-23.

Williams DR, Lawrence JA, Davis BA. (2019). Racism and health: evidence and needed research. *Annu Rev Public Health*, 40, pp. 105-125.

World Health Organization (2019). *HA60 Gender incongruence of adolescence or adulthood*. International classification of diseases,11th revision [IDC-11]. Available from: https://icd.who.int/browse11/l-m/en#/http://id.who.int/icd/entity/90875286

World Health Organization (2018). *Health inequities and their causes* [online] 20 Feb 2018. Available from: https://www.who.int/news-room/facts-in-pictures/detail/health-inequities-and-their-causes

World Health Organization. (2023). *Health equity* [online]. Available from: https://www.who.int/health-topics/health-equity#tab=tab_1

World Health Organization. (2008). *Closing the Gap in a Generation* [online]. Available from: https://www.who.int/publications/i/item/WHO-IER-CSDH-08.1

Young, Iris Marion. (1990). Five Faces of Oppression (Chapter 2). In *Justice and the politics of difference*. Princeton, NJ: Princeton University Press. pp. 39–65